Podiatry
SOURCEBOOK

Health Reference Series

First Edition

Podiatry
SOURCEBOOK

Basic Consumer Health Information about Foot Conditions, Diseases, and Injuries, Including Bunions, Corns, Calluses, Athlete's Foot, Plantar Warts, Hammertoes and Clawtoes, Clubfoot, Heel Pain, Gout, and More

Along with Facts about Foot Care, Disease Prevention, Foot Safety, Choosing a Foot Care Specialist, a Glossary of Terms, and Resource Listings for Additional Information

Edited by
M. Lisa Weatherford

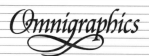

Omnigraphics

615 Griswold Street • Detroit, MI 48226

Podiatry sourcebook

Bibliographic Note

Because this page cannot legibly accommodate all the copyright notices, the Bibliographic Note portion of the Preface constitutes an extension of the copyright notice.

Each new volume of the *Health Reference Series* is individually titled and called a "First Edition." Subsequent updates will carry sequential edition numbers. To help avoid confusion and to provide maximum flexibility in our ability to respond to informational needs, the practice of consecutively numbering each volume has been discontinued.

Edited by M. Lisa Weatherford

Health Reference Series

Karen Bellenir, *Series Editor*
Peter D. Dresser, *Managing Editor*
Joan Margeson, *Research Associate*
Dawn Matthews, *Verification Assistant*
Jenifer Swanson, *Research Associate*

EdIndex, Services for Publishers, *Indexers*

Omnigraphics, Inc.

Matthew P. Barbour, *Vice President, Operations*
Laurie Lanzen Harris, *Vice President, Editorial Director*
Kevin Hayes, *Production Coordinator*
Thomas J. Murphy, *Vice President, Finance and Controller*
Peter E. Ruffner, *Senior Vice President*
Jane J. Steele, *Marketing Coordinator*

Frederick G. Ruffner, Jr., *Publisher*

© 2001, Omnigraphics, Inc.

Library of Congress Cataloging-in-Publication Data

Podiatry sourcebook : basic consumer health information about foot conditions, diseases, and injuries, including bunions, corns, calluses, athlete's foot, plantar warts, hammertoes and clawtoes, clubfoot, heel pain, gout, and more; along with facts about foot care, disease prevention, foot safety, choosing a foot care specialist, a glossary of terms, and resource listings for additional information / edited by M. Lisa Weatherford.-- 1st ed.
    p. cm. -- (Health reference series)
    Includes bibliographical references and index.
    ISBN 0-7808-0215-2
    1. Podiatry. 2. Foot--Diseases. I. Weatherford, M. Lisa. II. Series.

RD563 .P593 2001
617.5'85--dc21

                                                                2001036477

∞

This book is printed on acid-free paper meeting the ANSI Z37.48 Standard. The infinity symbol that appears above indicates that the paper in this book meets that standard.

Printed in the United States

Table of Contents

Part III: Diseases that Affect the Foot

Part IV: Foot Injuries

Part V: Additional Help and Information

Preface

About This Book

Podiatry is the field of medicine that specializes in foot care and diagnosis and treatment of related problems. Formerly known as "chiropody," modern podiatry covers the entire range of foot problems from a simple case of Athlete's foot to long-term conditions caused by accidents and diseases. Using the most up-to-date practices and equipment, podiatrists, like other medical specialists, care for their patients both in an office setting and in hospitals. The diagnosis of foot problems can include visual inspections, x-rays, and other sophisticated testing tools. Podiatric treatment options may include prescription medicines, orthotics, physical therapy, and surgery.

This *Sourcebook* offers general information about the practice of podiatry and a range of foot-related diseases, conditions, and injuries. Also included is specific information about a variety of treatment options, everyday things you can do to care for your feet, foot safety at work and at play, and where to find additional information.

How to Use This Book

This book is divided into parts and chapters. Parts focus on broad areas of interest. Chapters are devoted to single topics within a part.

Part I: Your Feet provides general information about foot care, including tips on choosing a podiatrist, facts about problems associated with shoe fit, and an overview of common treatment options. Also included is special information for specific populations such as children, pregnant women, people with diabetes, athletes, and the elderly.

Part II: Foot Conditions addresses common conditions of the foot including bone, nerve, and skin problems, infections, and congenital abnormalities.

Part III: Diseases that Affect the Foot offers information about foot-related problems caused by a variety of diseases, including diabetes, Parkinson's disease, gout, and AIDS.

Part IV: Foot Injuries provides facts about sprains and fractures and disorders associated with overuse. Information on the diagnosis and treatment of foot-related sports injuries is also included, along with tips for injury prevention.

Part V: Additional Help and Information provides a glossary of terms used in podiatry, a list of medical resources including associations, organizations, and government agencies, and a directory of resources specific to foot safety.

Bibliographic Note

This volume contains documents and excerpts from publications issued by the following U.S. government agencies: National Institute on Aging (NIA), National Institute of Arthritis and Musculoskeletal and Skin Diseases, and National Institute of Diabetes and Digestive and Kidney Diseases, and the U.S. Food and Drug Administration (FDA).

In addition, this volume contains copyrighted documents from the following organizations, publications, and individuals: *Advances in Wound Care: The Journal for Prevention and Healing; Consultant;* American Diabetes Association; American Orthopedic Foot and Ankle Society; Barry H. Block, DPM, JD; Center for Sports Medicine; Foot Health Network; Foot Talk; Gaynor Minden, Inc.; Drew A. Harris, DPM, MPH; Mark A. Jenkins, MD; Katy Keller, PT; Mayo Foundation for Medical Education and Research; Medical Multi Media Group; *Medical Sciences Bulletin;* Nidus Information Services; *Occupational Hazards;* OnHealth Network; *Orthopaedic Nursing; Patient Ca;,* Podiatry Online; *Podiatry Today;* Rice University; Douglas H. Richie, Jr., DPM; Seaford Foot Care; *The London Free Press; The Physician and Sportsmedicine;* The Prescription Foot Orthotic Laboratory Association; and Dennis White, DPM.

Full citation information is provided on the first page of each chapter. Every effort has been made to secure all necessary rights to reprint the copyrighted material. If any omissions have been made, please contact Omnigraphics to make corrections for future editions.

Acknowledgements

In addition to the organizations listed above, special thanks are due to document engineer Bruce Bellenir, researchers Jenifer Swanson and Joan Margeson, verification assistant Dawn Matthews, and permissions specialists Maria Franklin and Carol Munson.

Note from the Editor

This book is part of Omnigraphics' *Health Reference Series.* The series provides basic information about a broad range of medical concerns. It is not intended to serve as a tool for diagnosing illness, in prescribing treatments, or as a substitute for the physician/patient relationship. All persons concerned about medical symptoms or the possibility of disease are encouraged to seek professional care from an appropriate health care provider.

Our Advisory Board

The *Health Reference Series* is reviewed by an Advisory Board comprised of librarians from public, academic, and medical libraries. We would like to thank the following board members for providing guidance to the development of this series:

Dr. Lynda Baker, Associate Professor of Library and Information Science, Wayne State University, Detroit, MI

Nancy Bulgarelli, William Beaumont Hospital Library, Royal Oak, MI

Karen Imarasio, Bloomfield Township Public Library, Bloomfield Hills, MI

Karen Morgan, Mardigian Library, University of Michigan-Dearborn, Dearborn, MI

Rosemary Orlando, St. Clair Shores Public Library, St. Clair Shores, MI

Health Reference Series *Update Policy*

The inaugural book in the *Health Reference Series* was the first edition of *Cancer Sourcebook* published in 1990. Since then, the *Series* has been enthusiastically received by librarians and in the medical community. In order to maintain the standard of providing high-quality health information for the lay person, the editorial staff at Omnigraphics felt it was necessary to implement a policy of updating volumes when warranted.

Medical researchers have been making tremendous strides, and it is the purpose of the *Health Reference Series* to stay current with the most recent advances. Each decision to update a volume will be made on an individual basis. Some of the considerations will include how much new information is available and the feedback we receive from people who use the books. If there is a topic you would like to see added to the update list, or an area of medical concern you feel has not been adequately addressed, please write to:

Editor
Health Reference Series
Omnigraphics, Inc.
615 Griswold Street
Detroit, MI 48226

The commitment to providing on-going coverage of important medical developments has also led to some format changes in the *Health Reference Series*. Each new volume on a topic is individually titled and called a "First Edition." Subsequent updates will carry sequential edition numbers. To help avoid confusion and to provide maximum flexibility in our ability to respond to informational needs, the practice of consecutively numbering each volume has been discontinued.

Part One

Your Feet

Chapter 1

How to Choose a Podiatrist

The typical podiatrist is very competent and of high integrity. There are, however, podiatrists on both ends of the practice spectrum. Some are at the top of the profession with extraordinary expertise in such subspecialties as podiatric surgery, sports medicine, pediatrics, dermatology, rheumatology, and peripheral vascular disease. By taking into consideration the following criteria, you will increase your chances of being treated by the most competent podiatrist available.

1.   American Podiatric Medical Association membership. APMA membership is the first and most important standard in choosing a podiatrist. While membership does not insure skill, it does signify that the practitioner is bound to the ethical standards of the podiatry profession. Competency can be taught, ethics cannot. Members are affiliated through state podiatry societies. You may contact the APMA directly at http://www.apma.org/ or calling them at (800) ASK-APMA.

2.   Referral from a friend or relative. This is a valid way of helping you make a choice. If your friend or relative is satisfied with his or her current foot doctor the probability is that you will be too. Do quiz your friend, however, on the specifics of the quality of the care. How complete was the examination?

"Chapter 12: How to Choose a Podiatrist," by Barry H. Block, D.P.M. J.D., excerpted from *FOOT TALK* at www.foothealth.com/11.htm. © 1996, Barry H. Block, D.P.M. J.D.; reprinted with permission.

Did the doctor inquire about visits to other specialists? Did he or she seem concerned about your friend's health, or did the podiatrist seem rushed and disorganized?

Was your friend given alternatives for treatment or was he or she coerced into surgery that same day? Too often patients are influenced more by the doctor's personality than by the quality of care. So do question your friend thoroughly before following up with a visit.

3. Physician referral. Your family practitioner, internist, or pediatrician is a good source of referral. Establishment of a liaison between your podiatrist and physician benefits you by assuring ready consultation. Sending you to an incompetent doctor would reflect poorly on your physician, so he is putting himself on the line when he refers you to another specialist and you can feel reasonably secure with his choice.

4. Hospital referral. Your local hospital can refer you to a podiatrist who holds staff privileges. Hospitals tend to be very selective in their choice of staff. Hospital affiliation adds to a podiatrist's credentials, even if he does most of his surgery in the office.

5. Board certifications. This can be confusing. Some certifications are meaningful and some are not. All Doctors of Podiatric Medicine (D.P.M.) are "Diplomates" of the National Board of Podiatric Examiners. This designation only means that your podiatrist (as well as every other podiatrist) passed his or her board examinations while in school. The credentials of any podiatrist who lists this title are suspect. The only two valid certifying boards at this time are the American Board of Podiatric Surgery and the American Board of Podiatric Orthopedics and Primary Podiatric Medicine.

6. Specialty organizations. It may be useful for you to find a podiatrist through a specialty organization. If you have a sports medicine problem you may contact the American Academy of Podiatric Sports Medicine. A list of foot surgeons operating through "conventional" incisions (open surgery) can be obtained by writing to the American College of Foot and Ankle Surgeons. For a list of surgeons operating through "minimal incisions" write to the American Academy of Ambulatory Foot Surgeons at Box 1976, Lynnwood, Washington 98036.

7. Telephone directory. This is a poor method of selecting any doctor. You are basically leaving your decision to chance. In general, if you have to choose a podiatrist by this method, do not be influenced by a large size listing. The quality of a podiatrist cannot be measured by the size of a listing. Nor can his skill be measured by the size of his practice. A poor practitioner with a good business sense can do quite well, at least for himself.

8. Advertisements. Solicitations for podiatry services either in newspapers or on radio and television are the poorest ways of selecting a podiatrist. Competent and ethical podiatrists do not need to advertise, and seldom do. Beware of advertisements which promise "free consultation" or "no out-of-pocket expenses." It is possible that you may wind up in a crowded, fast-paced office where you and your feet may be valued below the insurance payment the doctor will ask you to assign to him. You cannot expect quality foot care to be cheap. Choose a quality doctor and expect to assume at least part of the cost. Most ethical podiatrists will be willing to work out an acceptable payment plan with you.

The Profession of Podiatric Medicine

Podiatry is the medical specialty devoted to the diagnosis and treatment of foot disorders. Podiatrists are physicians of the foot trained in the medical and surgical alleviation and correction of foot problems.

Podiatry originated along with dermatology and dentistry as part of cosmetology, the external care of the body. Chiriatry (care of the hands) and podiatry (care of the feet) eventually became combined to form chiropody. This designation held until the twentieth century. The term chiropody has not been used in America for over thirty years, although it is still used in the United Kingdom.

The education and training of podiatrists has improved tremendously in the past thirty years. Today's podiatry student must meet the same entrance requirements as do traditional medical students, including taking the new MCATs [Medical College Admission Tests]. The first two years of podiatry schools are similar to traditional medical school and include such courses as anatomy, biochemistry, histology, microbiology, pathology, pharmacology, and radiology.

The last two years consist of courses that specialize in the feet including foot surgery, biomechanics, podo-pediatrics, peripheral vascular disease, and dermatology. These last two clinical years include externships in hospitals and clinics where the student receives hands-on training. The graduating podiatrist receives the degree of Doctor of Podiatric Medicine (D.P.M.) and then may choose a one, two, or three year podiatric residency.

A Visit to Your Podiatrist—What to Expect

A visit to your foot doctor should be a pleasurable experience. In most cases, a podiatrist can provide you with immediate relief of pain. You should walk out of his or her office feeling better than when you came in.

Entering the office you will probably be met by a receptionist who will ask you to fill out an introductory form and may ask you some questions about your previous health history. Try to be as thorough as possible in answering these questions. The more information you provide the doctor, the easier it will be for him or her to make a proper diagnosis. You'll probably be asked about any medicines you may take, allergies you may have, and about previous surgery. Some patients ask, "What do these questions have to do with my feet? I only have a case of athlete's foot!" Your answers are important. The foot is not autonomous from the rest of the body. Your "athlete's foot" may in fact be a allergic reaction.

The more information you provide the doctor about your feet and the rest of your body, the better he or she will be able to diagnose and treat your condition. The pain in your big toe may be a manifestation of the metabolic disease known as gout. Often a podiatrist is the first to diagnose systemic diseases such as diabetes and congestive heart failure.

The Foot Exam

Once in the treatment room, expect a thorough examination of your feet. The doctor will do several tests to measure the circulation and neurological status of your foot. He will also take measurements for range of motion of your joints. If your problem is orthopedically related, he may ask you to walk, so that he can perform a gait analysis.

Do not be intimidated by the equipment in the office. Even the tub for a relaxing whirlpool can seem ominous. The drills a podiatrist uses to smooth down rough callus tissue might remind you of the dentist's, but will surprise you—they tickle rather than hurt. You may notice ultrasound machines and other physical therapy devices. These are used to help rehabilitate an injured foot or to help speed the healing of a foot which has recently been operated on. Ultrasound machines produce sound waves that are perceived as a warm comfortable feeling. In most cases, you'll walk out of your podiatrist's office a lot more comfortable than when you came in.

X-Rays

X-rays can provide your doctor with important diagnostic information about your feet. They are however never routine. If your doctor orders X-rays of your feet before he has even looked at them, find another doctor. If you have a structural foot problem such as a corn due to a hammertoe or underlying bone spur, your podiatrist may need to take an X-ray of your foot. X-rays may also be necessary to locate a foreign body such as a pin or a piece of leaded glass. Nobody likes X-rays. Fortunately, the X-ray machines used by most podiatrists are similar to the low dose machines used by dentists. The exposure you receive will be a small fraction of that from a large X-ray machine. It is still strongly recommended, though, that you insist on having a lead apron placed over your body. A new type of X-ray machine known as a photon image intensifier requires no lead apron and may soon make conventional X-rays obsolete. These portable machines allow a doctor to instantly scan your bones in the same way that a fluoroscope is used. This allows the doctor to immediately determine if a bone is broken, for instance. There are no films to process. The photon image intensifier gives off approximately the same amount of radiation as your color television set.

Treatment

If your foot problem is minor, you may expect immediate treatment. This may consist of a prescription of a medicine, removal of corns or calluses, or removal of an ingrown nail. If more extensive treatment such as surgery is necessary, you will be told. Most foot surgery is elective and it is in your best interest to go home and "sleep on it." Foot surgery should be performed because you want it—knowing both the risks and benefits. Same day surgery is not recommended, except for ingrown nail correction or the removal of a wart. In all other cases, you should arrange to have the procedure performed at your convenience.

If you have any doubts as to the necessity of the procedure, seek out a second opinion. Many health insurance companies will arrange for this, often at no cost to you.

Fees

Your treatment plan should also include a frank discussion of fees. A podiatrist's fees are generally in line with other medical specialists. Most insurance plans include podiatry in their coverage.

In some cases, such as with foot surgery, the doctor may accept part or all of your insurance as payment. You should come to an understanding with your doctor as to what the fees are before you begin treatment. Do not hesitate to query the doctor, assistant, or receptionist about your financial responsibilities.

Chapter 2

The Adult Foot

This text was prepared by the American Orthopaedic Foot and Ankle Society, a group of doctors who have special interests and training in the problems of the foot and ankle. Its members are medical doctors who, after completing medical school, have taken at least five additional years of training in orthopaedic surgery with additional special training in the care of the foot and ankle.

The Normal Foot

The height of arches and the shape of the toes vary from person to person. It is the deviation from normal arches and toe position that lead to foot problems. (There are 26 bones plus 33 joints in the human foot.)

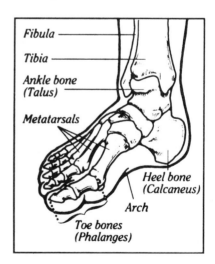

Figure 2.1. *The normal foot.*

"The Adult Foot," excerpted from the American Orthopaedic Foot and Ankle Society (AOFAS) website at http://www.aofas.org. © 1999 AOFAS. Reprinted with permission of the American Orthopedic Foot and Ankle Society.

Skin Problems

Sweaty feet can cause rashes and eczema. Wearing nylon socks in plastic shoes or tightly fitting shoes may not allow the feet to dry properly and can aggravate the problem. Changing socks every day and letting shoes dry out between wearings can help eliminate smelly feet. Wearing thick, soft cotton socks helps draw moisture away from the feet. True athlete's foot is a rash, often between the toes, caused by a fungus infection. Athlete's foot will usually respond to treatment with anti-fungal powders and lotions along with good foot hygiene. Poorly fitting shoes causes most calluses, corns, and blisters. Poor shoe fit can aggravate other foot problems and result in irritation, which may require medical attention.

Toenails

Ingrown toenails often result from trimming the nails too short, particularly at the sides. You should trim your toenails straight across, allowing adequate length to project beyond the skin at the toenail margins. Cuticles should be pushed back with an orange stick or hindu stone and rarely cut.

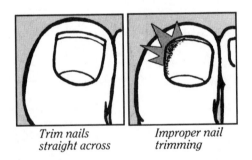

Trim nails   *Improper nail*
straight across   *trimming*

Figure 2.2. Toenail trimming.

First Aid

Pay attention to cuts and bruises of the foot. Like any other injury they should be cleansed and dressed. Generally, minor wounds need little attention. If a wound starts to spread, particularly in lacerations of the sole of the foot, you should consider an emergency visit for stitches.

Puncture wounds are a serious matter and can be dangerous. Nails and the like do not have to be rusty to cause lockjaw (tetanus), or to cause an infection in the foot. You should wear foot protection when walking out-of-doors. Even at the beach, you may encounter hidden obstacles, like glass.

Lockjaw is best treated by immunization protection before you injure your foot. You should have a tetanus booster shot every three to seven years.

Fractures and Sprains

Stubbed toes can be more than just a minor nuisance. If you experience swelling, discoloration, or a persistence of some pain beyond two to three days, you may have a fracture. Neglected fractures, particularly of the large or great toe, can result in painful foot problems and need early evaluation.

Ankle sprains are common, foot sprains less so. If you experience persistent pain and swelling about the foot that interferes with walking, you may need X-rays to determine if you have a fracture.

Bunions

"Bunions," the common name for hallux valgus, is a prominent bump of the great toe at the outer edge of where it joins the foot. This bump is sensitive to pressure caused from wearing shoes that fit too tight. Shoes that are pointed and too narrow squeeze the great toe causing it to drift toward the little toes.

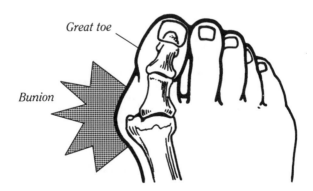

Figure 2.3. Bunions

Treatment: Wearing sandals and bunion shoes can help. Often wearing a pad, available from a drugstore foot counter, will relieve symptoms. If pain persists or shoe fitting is difficult, and the bump is quite noticeable, you should discuss this problem with your physician. Some bunions need surgical correction. Never consider bunion surgery for cosmetic reasons.

There are many operations for bunions, often named for the orthopaedic surgeon who developed the procedure: McBride, Keller, Mitchell, Lapidus to name a few. Most not only remove the bump, but correct what causes the bunion so that it does not grow back. Your orthopaedic surgeon will discuss with you what procedure, if any, is appropriate.

Corns and Hammertoes

Most corns result from pressure when the skin is squeezed between the bones and shoes. Corns can appear over almost any bone of the foot, but most commonly over misshapen, hammertoes. Here the hammertoe causes continued pressure which results in skin irritation and corn formation. Sometimes you will need surgery to relieve the underlying pressure, but a toe pad from a drugstore can treat a mild problem. If the problem persists, your physician can decide if you need surgery. Again, as with bunions, changes in shoe wear will often be all you need.

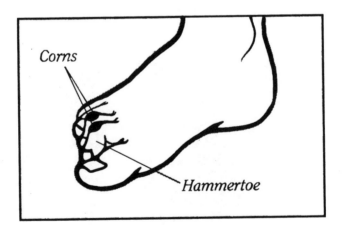

Figure 2.4. *Corns and Hammertoe*

Caution: All swellings of the great toe are not bunions. For example, gout strikes thousands of Americans. This special type of arthritis can be diagnosed only by medical examination and laboratory testing. Diet and special medications can treat gout.

Warts

Warts can look like corns, but tend to occur without pressure from shoes. Warts are the skin's reaction to chronic virus infection. These raised and painful sores, often on the sole of the foot, will sometimes respond to pads and over-the-counter ointment, but often need medical attention.

Caution: Not all painful sores are warts. Reaction to injury, hidden slivers, and old puncture wounds can also result in painful sores. Dark brown or black warts can indicate a type of cancer and should be immediately examined by your physician.

Heel Pain

Pain both below and behind the heel often results from an irritation of the tissues, nerves, or bone of the heel. Called heel spurs, this condition usually indicates a strain and only rarely, a serious bone or nerve problem. Runners and other athletes who subject the arch to strain, may develop heel pain. A direct blow to the heel can also result in this problem (never crush tin cans with your foot).

Treatment: Rest, heat and change of shoe wear will often suffice. If the pain persists, your physician will probably prescribe medication, and shoe modification and specific stretching exercises. In a more serious case of heel pain, your physician will prescribe injections. Rarely is surgery necessary.

Neuromas

Irritation to a nerve can cause it to swell. This condition, known as a neuroma, can occur anywhere in the body. In the foot, walking and shoe pressure can lead to painful neuromas. The most common neuroma, called Morton's neuroma, occurs on the bottom of the foot between the toes. Here, a small nerve to the toe becomes pinched between the toe joints, toe knuckles and the shoe. Neuromas can occur in other places on the foot, often from injury to skin nerves. Pressure from shoes may cause neuromas to become painful.

Treatment: A change in shoe wear, use of pads, and avoidance of irritating activity can help treat a neuroma. Your physician may also recommend medication and injections. If symptoms persist, you may need surgery to release or remove the nerve.

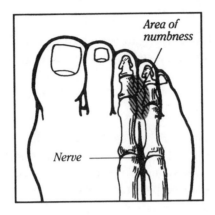

Figure 2.5. Neuromas—pinched nerve

Diabetes

Diabetes and certain other medical conditions which similarly affect the nerves, cause special foot care problems. In some people, diabetes will result in nerve damage. When this happens, the nerves no longer perceive pain and therefore do not warn us of injury. This is particularly true in the foot.

With diabetes, the body's poor defense against infection, and diabetes' damage to blood circulation complicates the problem. Poorly protected from infection by weakened body defenses, and loss of circulation, the foot and toes become more vulnerable to injury.

Patients with diabetes must exercise extreme caution. Properly fitting shoes can help protect your feet and avoid injury. Any injury, no matter how minor, deserves careful attention. You also must always exercise great caution in trimming toenails. Avoid trimming corns and calluses.

Do

- inspect feet daily for pressure spots
- inspect shoes for folds and nails

- bathe feet daily
- tell shoe salesperson you are diabetic
- change shoes at least once a day
- ask your physician to check your feet
- make sure toenails are trimmed

Don't

- go barefoot
- use corn removers
- cut calluses or corns

Shoes

Orthopaedic surgeons do not make shoes. Occasionally they advise you to wear special shoes, or have minor shoe modifications made with pads or wedges.

Shoes should be comfortable, practical and fit well. It is very important that the shoe fits the shape of your foot. Narrow and tight shoes result in foot problems. Make sure your shoes fit comfortably at the time you buy them.

If new shoes need to be "broken in," it means either they were not properly designed or not properly fitted to your feet.

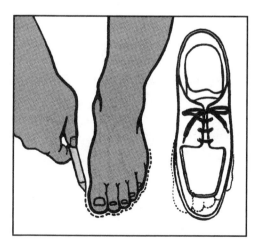

Figure 2.6. Shoe Fit

Cruel Shoes

High-fashion shoes with pointed toes, shoes with thin soles, and shoes with high spike heels, cause crowding of the toes and increased pressure. These can lead to corns, calluses, and neuroma problems in the foot.

Checklist for Shoes

- Good fit; comfortably loose when worn with soft, absorbent socks
- Shaped like the foot; broad and spacious in the toe area
- Shock-absorbent sole; a low wedge type is best; avoid high heels
- Breathable material; canvas or leather, not plastic
- Comfortable the moment you put them on.

Running Shoes

A good running or tennis shoe should have a wide, cushioned heel and sole. The toe box should be deep enough so the toes do not press against the top and long enough to allow free motion and gripping during running. There should be about a thumbnail-length between

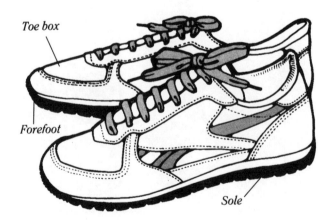

Figure 2.7. *Running Shoes*

the longest toe and the toe of the shoe. If you don't allow enough space for the toes, you can injure the toenails.

Running shoes should have spring in the forefoot; that is, the forefoot of the shoe should tilt up off the ground when the shoe rests flat on the ground.

The running shoe should be flexible but not limp; the heel counter firm and padded to support the heel.

The sole of the shoe should be cushioned enough to absorb much of the shock of running. A soft neoprene sole is a great help in absorbing shock.

Most running shoes have a built in arch support; this is desirable to avoid excessive pronation.

Confused about Foot Doctors?

If you are concerned about your feet and you don't know who to ask, talk to your family physician. Most county medical societies are happy to help you identify medical doctors who specialize in the treatment of specific problems, such as the foot. In larger cities, the telephone book Yellow Pages under "Physicians (M.D.s)" often includes a listing of Orthopaedic Surgeons, members of that specialty of medicine which deals with foot problems. We, too, can help. Write: American Orthopaedic Foot and Ankle Society, 2517 East Lake Avenue, East, Suite 200, Seattle, WA 98102.

Chapter 3

Pregnancy and Your Feet

Definition

Pregnancy triggers many different changes in a woman's body. Many women have common complaints throughout their pregnancy. One of these complaints, often overlooked, is foot pain. Due to the natural weight gain during pregnancy, a woman's center of gravity is completely altered. This causes a new weight-bearing stance and added pressure to the knees and feet.

Two of the most common foot problems experienced by pregnant woman are over-pronation and edema. These problems can lead to pain at the heel, arch, or ball-of-foot pain. Many women may also experience leg cramping and varicose veins due to weight gain. Because of this, it is important for all pregnant women to learn more about foot health during their pregnancy to help make this nine month period more comfortable for them.

Cause

Over-pronation and edema are very common foot problems experienced during pregnancy.

Over-pronation, also referred to as flat feet, is caused when a person's arch flattens out upon weight bearing and their feet roll inward when walking. This can create extreme stress or inflammation

"Pregnancy and Your Feet," from the Foot Health Network website at http://www.foot.com. ©1999-2000 Foot.com, Inc.; reprinted with permission.

on the plantar fascia, the fibrous band of tissue that runs from the heel to the forefoot.

Over-pronation can make walking very painful and can increase strain on the feet, calves and/or back. The reason many pregnant women suffer from over-pronation is due to the added pressure on the body as a result of weight gain. Over-pronation is also very prominent in people who have flexible, flat feet or in people who are obese.

Edema, also referred to as swelling in the feet, normally occurs in the latter part of pregnancy. Edema results from the extra blood accumulated during pregnancy. The enlarging uterus puts pressure on the blood vessels in the pelvis and legs causing circulation to slow down and blood to pool in the lower extremities. The total water fluid in the body remains the same as before pregnancy, however it only becomes displaced. When feet are swollen, they can become purplish in color. Sometimes extra water can be retained during pregnancy, which can add to the swelling. If there is swelling in the face or hands, a doctor should be contacted immediately.

Treatment and Prevention

There are effective ways to treat both over-pronation and edema during pregnancy.

Over-pronation can be treated conservatively with "ready-made" orthotics. These orthotics should be designed with appropriate arch support and medial rearfoot posting to correct the over-pronation. Proper fitting footwear is also very important in treating over-pronation. Choose comfortable footwear that provides extra support and shock absorption. It is important to treat over-pronation for pain relief but also to prevent other foot conditions from developing such as plantar fasciitis, heel spurs, metatarsalgia, post-tib tendinitis and/ or bunions.

Edema in the feet can be minimized and comforted by the following methods:

- Elevate your feet as often as possible. If you have to sit for long periods of time, place a small stool by your feet to elevate them.

- Wear proper fitting footwear. Footwear that is too narrow or short will constrict circulation.

- Have your feet measured several times throughout your pregnancy. They will probably change sizes.

- Wear seamless socks that do not constrict circulation.

- If you are driving for a long period of time, take regular breaks to stretch your legs to promote circulation.

- Exercise regularly to promote overall health; walking is the best exercise.

- Drink plenty of water to keep the body hydrated. This helps the body retain less fluid.

- Eat a well-balanced diet and avoid foods high in salt that can cause water retention.

Swelling is normally similar in both feet. If there is swelling in both feet that are not symmetrical, this may be a sign of a vascular problem and a doctor should be contacted immediately. If any problems persist, consult your doctor.

Chapter 4

Elderly Feet

Disease, years of wear and tear, ill-fitting or poorly designed shoes, poor circulation to the feet, or improperly trimmed toenails cause many common foot problems.

To prevent foot problems, check your feet regularly—or, have them checked by a member of the family—and practice good foot hygiene. Podiatrists and primary care physicians (internists and family practitioners) are qualified to treat most feet problems; sometimes the special skills of an orthopedic surgeon or dermatologist are needed.

Preventing Foot Trouble

Improving the circulation of blood to the feet can help prevent problems. Exposure to cold temperatures or water, pressure from shoes, long periods of sitting, or smoking can reduce blood flow to the feet. Even sitting with your legs crossed or wearing tight, elastic garters or socks can affect circulation. On the other hand, raising the feet, standing up and stretching, walking, and other forms of exercise promote good circulation. Gentle massage and warm foot baths can also help increase circulation to the feet.

Wearing comfortable shoes that fit well can prevent many foot ailments. Foot width may increase with age. Always have your feet measured before buying shoes. The upper part of the shoes should be made of a soft, flexible material to match the shape of your foot. Shoes made

"National Institute on Aging Age Page: Foot Care," from the Administration on Aging website at http://www.aoa.dhhs.gov.

of leather can reduce the possibility of skin irritations. Soles should provide solid footing and not be slippery. Thick soles lessen pressure when walking on hard surfaces. Low-heeled shoes are more comfortable, safer, and less damaging than high-heeled shoes.

Common Foot Problems

Fungal and bacterial conditions—including athlete's foot—occur because the feet are usually enclosed in a dark, damp, warm environment. These infections cause redness, blisters, peeling, and itching. If not treated promptly, an infection may become chronic and difficult to cure. To prevent these conditions, keep the feet—especially the area between the toes—clean and dry and expose the feet to air whenever possible. If you are prone to fungal infections, you may want to dust your feet daily with a fungicidal powder.

Dry skin can cause itching and burning feet. Use mild soap sparingly and a body lotion on your legs and feet every day. The best moisturizers contain petroleum jelly or lanolin. Be cautious about adding oils to bath water since they can make the feet and bathtub very slippery.

Corns and calluses are caused by the friction and pressure of bony areas rubbing against shoes. A podiatrist or a physician can determine the cause of this condition and can suggest treatment, which may include getting better-fitting shoes or special pads. Over-the-counter medicines contain acids that destroy the tissue but do not treat the cause. These medicines can sometimes reduce the need for surgery. Treating corns or calluses yourself may be harmful, especially if you have diabetes or poor circulation.

Warts are skin growths caused by viruses. They are sometimes painful and if untreated, may spread. Since over-the-counter preparations rarely cure warts, get professional care. A doctor can apply medicines, burn or freeze the wart off, or remove the wart surgically.

Bunions develop when big toe joints are out of line and become swollen and tender. Bunions may be caused by poor-fitting shoes that press on a deformity or an inherited weakness in the foot. If a bunion is not severe, wearing shoes cut wide at the instep and toes may provide relief. Protective pads can also cushion the painful area. Bunions can be treated by applying or injecting certain drugs, using whirlpool baths, or sometimes having surgery.

Ingrown toenails occur when a piece of the nail breaks the skin. This is usually caused by improperly trimmed nails. Ingrown toenails are especially common in the large toes. A podiatrist or doctor can remove the part of the nail that is cutting into the skin. This will allow the area to heal. Ingrown toenails can usually be avoided by cutting the toenail straight across and level with the top of the toe.

Hammertoe is caused by shortening the tendons that control toe movements. The toe knuckle is usually enlarged, drawing the toe back. Over time, the joint enlarges and stiffens as it rubs against shoes. Your balance may be affected. Hammertoe is treated by wearing shoes and stockings with plenty of toe room. In advanced cases, surgery may be recommended.

Spurs are calcium growths that develop on bones of the feet. They are caused by muscle strain in the feet and are irritated by standing for long periods of time, wearing badly fitting shoes, or being overweight. Sometimes they are completely painless, but at other times the pain can be severe. Treatments for spurs include using proper foot support, heel pads, heel cups, or other recommendations by a podiatrist or surgeon.

Resources

For more information on foot care, write to either of the following:

American Podiatric Medical Association
9312 Old Georgetown Road
Bethesda, MD 20814-1698
Telephone: 301-571-9200
Toll Free: 1-800-FOOTCARE
Fax: 301-530-2752
Website: http://www.apma.org
E-Mail: askapma@apma.org

The American Orthopaedic Foot and Ankle Society
2517 East Lake Avenue, East, Suite 200
Seattle, WA 98102
Tel: 206-223-1120
Fax: 206-223-1178
Website: http://www.aofas.org
E-Mail: aofas@aofas.org

The National Institute on Aging offers a variety of information about health and aging, For a list of publications, contact:

NIA Information Center
P.O. Box 8057
Gaithersburg, MD 20898-8057
800-222-2225; 800-222-4225 (TTY)

Chapter 5

Diabetic Feet:
Special Care Required

You Can Take Care of Your Feet!

Do you want to avoid serious foot problems that can lead to a toe, foot, or leg amputation? "Take Care of Your Feet for a Lifetime" tells you how. It's all about taking good care of your feet.

Foot care is very important for people with diabetes who have:

• Loss of feeling in their feet.

• Changes in the shape of their feet.

• Foot ulcers or sores that do not heal.

Nerve damage can cause you to lose feeling in your feet. You may not feel a pebble inside your sock that is causing a sore. You may not feel a blister caused by poorly fitting shoes. Foot injuries such as these can cause ulcers which may lead to amputation.

Keeping your blood sugar (glucose) in good control and taking care of your feet every day can help you avoid serious foot problems.

Use this guide to make your own plan for taking care of your feet. Helpful tips make it easy! Share your plan with your doctor and health care team and get their help when you need it.

"Take Care of Your Feet for a Lifetime: A Guide for People with Diabetes," from the National Institute of Diabetes and Digestive and Kidney Diseases (NIDDK), NIH Publication No. 98-4285, November 1997. Visit the NIDDK website at www.niddk.nih.gov.

There is a lot you can do to prevent serious problems with your feet. Here's how.

Take Care of Your Diabetes

Make healthy lifestyle choices to help keep your blood sugar close to normal. Keeping your blood sugar under good control may help prevent or delay diabetes-related foot problems as well as eye and kidney disease.

Work with your health care team to make a diabetes plan that fits your lifestyle. The team may include: your doctor, a diabetes educator, a nurse, a dietitian, a foot care doctor called a podiatrist (pah-di'ah-trist), and other specialists. This team will help you to:

• Know how and when to test your blood sugar.

• Take prescribed medicines.

• Eat regular meals that contain a variety of healthy, low-fat, high-fiber foods including fruits and vegetables each day.

• Increase your physical activity each day.

• Follow your foot care plan.

• Keep your doctors appointments and have your feet, eyes, and kidneys checked at least once a year.

Check Your Feet Every Day

• You may have serious foot problems, but feel no pain. Check your feet for cuts, sores, red spots, swelling, and infected toenails. Find a time (evening is best) to check your feet each day. Make checking your feet part of your every day routine.

• If you have trouble bending over to see your feet, use a plastic mirror to help. You also can ask a family member or care giver to help you.

• Make sure to call your doctor right away if a cut, sore, blister, or bruise on your foot does not begin to heal after one day.

Wash Your Feet Every Day

• Wash your feet in warm, not hot, water. Do not soak your feet, because your skin will get dry.

- Before bathing or showering, test the water to make sure it is not too hot. You can use a thermometer (90° to 95° F is safe) or your elbow.

- Dry your feet well. Be sure to dry between your toes. Use talcum powder to keep the skin between your toes dry.

Keep the Skin Soft and Smooth

- Rub a thin coat of skin lotion, cream, or petroleum jelly on the tops and bottoms of your feet.

- Do not put lotion or cream between your toes, because this might cause an infection.

Smooth Corns and Calluses Gently

- After bathing or showering, use a pumice stone to smooth corns and calluses. A pumice stone is a type of rock used to smooth the skin. Rub gently, only in one direction, to avoid tearing the skin.

- Do not cut corns and calluses. Don't use razor blades, corn plasters, or liquid corn and callus removers—they can damage your skin.

- If you have corns and calluses, check with your doctor or foot care specialist.

Trim Your Toenails Each Week or When Needed

- Trim your toenails with clippers after you wash and dry your feet.

- Trim toenails straight across and smooth them with an emery board or nail file.

- Don't cut into the corners of the toenail.

- If you can't see well, or if your toenails are thick or yellowed, have a foot care doctor trim them.

Wear Shoes and Socks at All Times

- Wear shoes and socks at all times. Do not walk barefoot—not even indoors—because it is easy to step on something and hurt your feet.

- Always wear socks, stockings, or nylons with your shoes to help avoid blisters and sores.
- Choose socks made of cotton or wool. They help keep your feet dry.
- Check the insides of your shoes before you put them on to be sure the lining is smooth and that there are no objects in them.
- Wear shoes that fit well and protect your feet.

Protect Your Feet from Hot and Cold

- Wear shoes at the beach or on hot pavement.
- Put sun screen on the top of your feet to prevent sunburn.
- Keep your feet away from radiators and open fires.
- Do not put hot water bottles or heating pads on your feet.
- Wear socks at night if your feet get cold. Lined boots are good in winter to keep your feet warm.
- Check your feet often in cold weather to avoid frostbite.

Keep the Blood Flowing to Your Feet

- Put your feet up when you are sitting.
- Wiggle your toes for five minutes, two or three times a day. Move your ankles up and down and in and out to improve blood flow in your feet and legs.
- Don't cross your legs for long periods of time.
- Don't wear tight socks, elastic or rubber bands, or garters around your legs.
- Don't smoke. Smoking reduces blood flow to your feet. Ask your doctor or nurse to help you stop smoking.
- If you have high blood pressure or high cholesterol, work with your health care team to lower it.

Be More Active

- Ask your doctor to help you plan an activity program that is right for you.
- Walking, dancing, swimming, and bicycling are good forms of exercise that are easy on the feet.

- Avoid activities that are hard on the feet, such as running and jumping.
- Always include a short warm-up and cool-down period.
- Wear athletic shoes that fit well and that provide good support.

Be Sure to Ask Your Doctor to

- Check the sense of feeling and pulses in your feet at least once a year.
- Tell you if you are likely to have serious foot problems. If you have serious foot problems, your feet should be checked at every visit to your doctor.
- Show you how to care for your feet.
- Refer you to a foot care doctor if needed.
- Decide if special shoes would help your feet stay healthy.

Get Started Now

- Begin taking good care of your feet today.
- Set a time every day to check your feet.
- Note the date of your next visit to the doctor.
- Cut out the foot care tip sheet in this booklet and put it on your bathroom or bedroom wall or night stand as a reminder.
- Complete the "To Do" list at the back of this booklet. Get started now.
- Set a date for buying the things you need to take care of your feet: nail clippers, pumice stone, emery board, skin lotion, talcum powder, mirror, socks, athletic shoes, and slippers.
- Most important, stick with your foot care program—and give yourself a special treat such as a new pair of soft cotton socks. You deserve it!

Tips for Proper Footwear

- Proper footwear is very important for preventing serious foot problems. Athletic or walking shoes made of canvas or leather are good for daily wear. They support your feet and allow them to "breathe."

31

- Never wear vinyl or plastic shoes, because they don't stretch or "breathe."

- When buying shoes, make sure they are comfortable from the start and have enough room for your toes.

- Don't buy shoes with pointed toes or high heels. They put too much pressure on your toes.

Ask Your Doctor about Medicare Coverage for Special Footwear

You may need special shoes or shoe inserts to prevent serious foot problems. If you have Medicare Part B insurance, you may be able to get some of the cost of special shoes or inserts paid for. Ask your doctor whether you qualify for:

- one pair of depth shoes and three pairs of inserts or,

- one pair of custom molded shoes (including inserts) and two additional pairs of inserts.

If you qualify, your doctor or podiatrist will tell you how to get your special shoes.

For More Information

American Association of Diabetes Educators
100 West Monroe Street
Suite 400
Chicago, IL 60603
Toll Free: 800-338-3633
Telephone: 312-424-2426
Fax: 312-424-2427
Website: http:// www.aadenet.org

American Diabetes Association
1701 N. Beauregard St.
Alexandria, VA 22311
Toll Free: 800-DIABETES (800-342-2383)
Toll Free: 800-232-3472 Professional Services
Website: http://www.diabetes.org
E-Mail: customerservice@diabetes.org

American Podiatric Medical Association
9312 Old Georgetown Road
Bethesda, MD 20814-1698
Telephone: 301-571-9200
Toll Free: 1-800-FOOTCARE
Fax: 301-530-2752
Website: http://www.apma.org
E-Mail: askapma@apma.org

Centers for Disease Control and Prevention
Division of Diabetes Translation
Program Development Branch
4770 Buford Highway, NE,
Mailstop K-10
Atlanta, GA 30341-3724
Toll Free: 877-CDC-DIAB (877-232-3422)
Telephone: 770-488-5000
Fax: 770-488-5966
Website: http://www.cdc.gov/diabetes
E-Mail: diabetes@cdc.gov

Juvenile Diabetes Foundation International
120 Wall Street, 19th Floor
New York, NY 10005
Toll Free: 800-JDF-CURE (800-533-2873)
Website: http://www.jdfcure.org
E-Mail: info@jdrf.org

National Institute of Diabetes and Digestive and Kidney Diseases
National Diabetes Information Clearinghouse (NDIC)
1 Information Way
Bethesda, MD 20892-3560
Toll Free: 800-GET-LEVEL (800-438-5383)
Telephone: 301-654-3327
Fax: 301-907-8906
Website: http://www.niddk.nih.gov

Chapter 6

Ten Points of Children's Shoe Fit

Fitting Children's Shoes

1. Always measure both feet. Most children have one foot larger than the other.

2. Children's shoes should feel comfortable immediately. Don't let your child wear hand-me-downs or expect him or her to break in the shoe.

3. Most children don't fully develop an arch until preadolescence and a shoe is not needed to help the arch develop.

4. Children should wear shoes shaped like their foot and that allow plenty of room to wiggle all their toes.

5. Allow a thumb's width from the end of the longest toe to the end of the shoe.

6. The heel of the shoe should fit well and not slide.

7. The sole of the shoe should protect the foot from injury and provide cushioning.

"10 Points of Children's Shoe Fit," excerpted from the American Orthopaedic Foot and Ankle Society (AOFAS) website at http://www.aofas.org. © 1999 AOFAS. Reprinted with permission of the American Orthopedic Foot and Ankle Society.

8. The shoe should be made out of material that gives and breathes, such as leather.

9. The shoe should provide enough room for the child's foot to grow.

10. A proper-fitting shoe should not cause calluses, sores, or other deformities.

Special Considerations

- Babies and crawlers do not need shoes. They only need soft booties or socks to keep feet warm.

- Toddlers do not need shoes in a protected environment. When they do wear shoes, make sure they don't have heavy or sticky soles that can cause falls.

- Children should be measured at every store visit for shoe size, as their feet can grow very rapidly. Follow the ten points of shoe fit to avoid painful foot problems like blisters, calluses or foot deformities.

Chapter 7

Shoe Shopping Checklist

Shoes that constrict your feet can lead to a variety of painful conditions in the feet and ankles. Your first line of defense is finding shoes that fit properly. Keep the following in mind:

- Avoid pointed shoes. Instead, choose shoes that give your toes room to move. Laced shoes are a smart choice. They usually provide more toe room.

- Choose shoes with low heels. Ignore fashion trends that dictate high heels or pointed toes. When buying shoes, consider the long-term benefits of comfort and freedom from pain.

- Go for softer, flexible shoes with cushioned insoles. Steer clear of vinyl and plastic shoes.

- Buy sandals with straps.

- Don't assume that your feet are both exactly the same size. Measure both of them.

- Don't assume that you have one shoe size for your adult life. Your foot size changes as you age.

"Shoe-Shopping Checklist," from *Mayo Health Clinic Oasis*, October 19, 1998, ©1995-1999 Mayo Foundation for Medical Education and Research. Reprinted with permission from Mayo Foundation for Medical Education and Research, Rochester, MN 55905.

• Shop for shoes during the noon hour. Since your feet swell throughout the day, sizing shoes at mid-day increases the odds of finding a good fit.

Smart shoe shopping is sometimes enough to solve corns, hammer-toe, ingrown toenails, and other foot problems. But if these conditions persist, call your doctor.

Chapter 8

The Low-Down on High Heels

The big fashion news last fall was the return of spike and stiletto heels. Many met this report with dread and trepidation—another season of sore feet.

High heels hurt and can cause significant health problems including bunions, heel pain, toe deformities and painful trapped nerves. Frankly, most women are tired of wearing shoes that hurt their feet. A 1993 survey of 620 women found that the majority were dissatisfied with their shoes even though most paid between $50 and $200 for dress shoes.

"Fashion shoes are expensive and come with hidden costs," explains orthopaedic surgeon Glenn B. Pfeffer, M.D., San Francisco. "First you spend up to $200 for a pair of shoes, then you're taking taxis all over town because you cannot walk any distance in spike heels, and finally there's the medical cost of wearing these shoes."

Women have about 90 percent of the 795,000 annual surgeries for bunions, hammertoes, neuromas (trapped nerves) and bunionettes— the four most common problems linked to poorly designed and poorly fitting shoes. Approximately two-thirds of these conditions requiring surgery can be attributed to the patients' shoewear selections.

The total estimated cost for this avoidable surgery is $2 billion annually. With an average time lost from work of four weeks per person, the cost of time lost is about $1.5 billion. That's a total of 3.5 billion health care and workforce dollars lost each year to poorly fitting, poorly designed shoes.

People take an average of 10,000 strides per day, and high heels shift the force of these strides to place pressure on the ball of the foot and the metatarsal heads (bones at the base of the toes). A 3-inch heel creates seven times more stress on the forefoot than a 1-inch heel, thereby increasing the possibility of foot problems with each step on improbably high heels.

Minor missteps in spike or stiletto heels can have disastrous results, and women are twice as likely to suffer a sprained ankle while walking in heels than while more sensibly shod.

Frequent wearing of high heels can also shorten the Achilles tendon over time and cause wearers to lose range of motion in the foot and suffer other foot problems and pain as a result.

A study by the American Orthopaedic Foot and Ankle Society (AOFAS) indicates that this shortening of the Achilles tendon in high-heel wearers is responsible for the disproportionate number of American women who suffer heel pain. Women make up as much as 75 percent of the two million Americans suffering heel pain, and regular stretching of the Achilles tendon and calf muscles can often relieve the problem.

The AOFAS discourages wearing fashion shoes with a heel height greater than 2¼ inches and recommends high-heel wearers limit themselves to two or three hours in such shoes per day. "Have yourself dropped off in front of the restaurant in high heels," advises Dr. Pfeffer, "then take them off when you get back in the car."

While shoe design impacts foot health, proper shoe fit is equally important. A 1993 AOFAS survey of 386 women found that 88 percent wore shoes too small for their feet, 80 percent reported pain and discomfort and 72 percent had one or more foot deformities. The average woman in these studies had not had her feet measured in more than five years.

Forcing the foot into a shoe too small and subjecting it to daily pounding and pressure can cause deformities over time. Bunions, hammertoes, mallet toes and claw toes are often the result of poorly fitting shoes.

"Women should not only look for low, shock-absorbent heels, but also a rounded toe box that fits the shape of their foot," advises Carol C. Frey, M.D., Los Angeles.

For a dramatic demonstration of the problem of poor shoe fit, stand on a piece of paper and have a friend draw a tracing of your weight-bearing bare foot. Now take the dress shoes you most commonly wear and place them over the tracing. If your forefoot is much larger and rounder than the toe box of your shoe, you may be setting yourself up for painful foot problems in the near future.

Proper shoe fit is important and relatively easy to achieve. The AOFAS, National Shoe Retailers Association (NSRA), and Pedorthic Footwear Association (PFA) have jointly prepared a brochure, "10 Points of Proper Shoe Fit," to help consumers make intelligent and healthy shoewear selections.

Chapter 9

Socks—
Essential Equipment for
Athletes

Introduction

For the serious athlete, socks have become recognized as an essential component of footwear that can determine the difference between success or failure on the playing field. Unfortunately, for the sports medicine professional, the role of socks in preventing injury and in enhancing performance is misunderstood and often neglected in treatment protocols.

Recreational and competitive athletes can receive state-of-the-art information on sock fiber technology and construction techniques from premium sporting goods vendors and technical publications peculiar to their sport. On the other hand, health care professionals receive no formal training on the topics of footwear or hosiery, yet they are called upon regularly to give information to patients and the lay public in these unfamiliar subject areas. No wonder that physicians and podiatrists are often quoted in consumer magazines giving erroneous information about socks and footwear.

It is refreshing to see the subject of "socks" included in this comprehensive program of topics relative to the field of podiatric sports medicine.

"Socks: Hosiery—Essential Equipment for the Athlete,"American Association of Podiatric Sports Medicine Annual Meeting 1997—Lecture Highlights, by Douglas H. Richie, Jr., D.P.M. © 1997, 2000 A.A.P.S.M.; reprinted with permission of the author.

Historical Review

There were virtually no original scientific articles pertaining to hosiery published in the medical literature until 1989. Then, almost overnight, clinical researchers recognized that major advances had been made during the 1980s in the fields of fiber technology and sock construction techniques. Hosiery now appears like high-tech sports equipment with possible medical applications. A large number of studies were carried out on various patient populations, including athletes, to determine the role of hosiery in preventing pedal pathologies.

A series of articles published by Andrew Boulton and Arisites Veves at the Manchester Royal Infirmary documented the protective effect of hosiery on the feet of diabetic and arthritic patients. At the same time, Herring and Richie published their studies demonstrating the superiority of acrylic fibers over cotton fibers in preventing the frequency and severity of friction blisters in running athletes.

A significant amount of published research then followed, documenting attempts to utilize hosiery products to treat various clinical conditions. Ufer and co-workers studied the effect of hosiery to warm the feet of patients with spastic quadriplegia. Wolfe and Palladino conducted a study to determine the effect of hosiery on friction blisters and racquetball players. The effect of over-the-calf sports socks to reduce swelling in the feet and legs was reported by Brown and Brown.

The United States military, plagued with ever-increasing blister frequency in military recruits, carried out their own research documenting the ability of various sock systems to reduce friction blisters. These prospective studies demonstrated the highest level of scientific investigation attempting to determine the effect of various sock fiber combinations on the feet of a large number of human subjects engaged in marching and running.

The principles proven and validated by these studies are the foundation of this presentation. The subject areas covered are those of most interest to the sports medicine health care professional: fiber technology, friction blisters, sports specific challenges and shoe-fitting applications.

Socks and Foot Pathologies

The following foot pathologies can be directly affected by the type of hosiery worn by the athlete:

* **Toenails:** subungual hematoma, onychomycosis, onychogryphosis,

- **Integument:** friction blisters, hyperkeratoses, heloma dura/molle,

- **Infections:** dermatophyte, yeast, bacteria, viral (verruca),

- **Mechanical or Shear Induced Injury of Subcutaneous Tissue:** capsulitis, bursitis, calcaneal fat pad atrophy,

- **Mechanical or Shear Injury Against Bone Prominence:** retrocalcaneal exostosis, sesamoiditis, hallux valgus, tailor's bunion, accessory navicular, tibial crest periostitis, medial and lateral malleolar contusion

Causes

The forces involved in generating the above-mentioned tissue injuries include ground reaction forces, tangential shearing forces, and a combination of pressure and shear induced by athletic footwear.

Numerous researchers have demonstrated that ground reaction forces can approach or exceed three times body weight in a running athlete. In addition, vertical plantar pressures against the calcaneus and metatarsals are significantly increased in the running athlete as well as special patient populations with foot deformities (i.e., rheumatoid arthritis and diabetes mellitus with neuropathy).

Shearing forces result from forward or sideways momentum of the athlete whether walking, jumping, running, or lunging. Spence and Shields identified four types of dynamic forces that can be associated with running gait: vertical forces, fore and aft shear, lateral shear, and torque. Shearing force on the skin surface of the foot is exacerbated by the type of playing surface, type of footwear, type of insole, and type of sock material. Shearing forces are thought to be more damaging to the feet than ground reaction forces. The combination of abnormal pressure and shear results in the formation of friction blisters in athletes and ulcerations on the feet of patients with diabetes mellitus.

In addition to the abnormal forces generated by the specific movements of the sport, the type of footwear worn by the athlete can generate unique damaging pressure and shear in specific areas of the feet or legs. The following unique forms of athletic footwear and the various locations of potential skin or deep tissue damage are illustrated in Table 9.1.

The Fiber Story

The ability of a sock to dissipate damaging forces on the surface of the foot rests partly on the fiber composition and more significantly on the construction technique of the manufacturer. It is the lack of understanding of fiber technology that leads most health care professionals to make erroneous recommendations to their patients regarding selection for sporting activities.

Fibers that absorb moisture are termed hydrophilic while fibers repelling moisture are hydrophobic. Cotton fiber retains three times the moisture of acrylic and fourteen times the moisture of CoolMax®. When exposed to ambient air, socks composed of cotton retain moisture ten times longer than acrylic. In descending order of hydrophilic ranking, the following fibers are listed: cotton, wool, acrylic, CoolMax®, polypropylene.

Table 9.1. Unique Footwear and Potential Damage Locations

Cycling Shoe	Rigid inflexible sole, lacks padding, constant pressure on the forefoot.
Mid-High Cross-Trainers	Cut off point of shoe upper in heel counter areas often leads to pressure abrasion on tendon-Achilles.
Plastic-Shell Footwear (i.e., Ski Boots, In-Line Skates)	Hard unyielding upper material can lead to pressure points when fit is not so perfect.
Tight-Fitting Footwear (i.e., Rock Climbing Shoes, Soccer Shoes)	Certain sports mandate that footwear be tight-fitting to enhance tactile appreciation through the feet. However, this tight-fitting footwear is notorious for creating pressure lesions and blisters.
Cleated Footwear (i.e., Football, Baseball, Soccer)	Cleats of various composition create pressure points in the sole of the shoe. Also, cleated footwear enhances coefficient of friction against the playing surface dissipating significant shear force to the next movement interface within the shoe (i.e., foot—insole interface).

During initial activity, moisture absorption from the feet becomes a desirable feature. In athletic activity, perspiration output on the feet can exceed one pint per foot. A large part of this moisture may actually accumulate in the feet as it is produced elsewhere on the body surface and drips down the legs due to gravity. Nonetheless, this volume of fluid far exceeds the absorptive capacity of any sock product. Therefore, to minimize moisture accumulation on the skin surface, the sock must set up a wicking gradient to the shoe.

Ideally, a wicking gradient occurs when the shoe upper is breathable (i.e., nylon mesh) so that ambient air encourages evaporation of water vapor. More commonly, a shoe liner or upper will contain hydrophilic fibers that draw moisture from the hydrophobic sock material. Socks that are extremely hydrophobic (i.e., polypropylene) are thought to repel water so effectively that wicking cannot occur. Socks of intermediate hydrophobic range, i.e., wool and acrylic, allow movement of water but will not absorb and retain water like cotton fibers will. Degrees of hydrophobic qualities alone, however, don't determine overall wicking capacity.

The mechanical structure of the fiber and compressibility of the fiber will determine overall wicking potential. CoolMax® fibers have four channels built into their cross-sectional geometry giving a 20-percent higher perimeter area than traditional round fibers. The result is higher water/vapor transport through enhanced surface exposure for capillary action.

Natural fibers (cotton-wool) when laden with moisture, compress more easily than synthetic fibers (acrylic, CoolMax®). Thus, cotton and wool socks have a higher resistance to sweat transport of wicking. When wet, acrylic fibers swell less than 5 percent while cotton swells 45 percent and wool swells 35 percent. Swollen fibers that are compressed reduce air spaces and thus reduce moisture transport. Thus, cotton socks exhibit a 2.4 times higher resistance to moisture transport.

When combining hydrophobic qualities and mechanical fiber qualities, the fibers that wick moisture best are, from best to worst: CoolMax®, acrylic, polypropylene, wool, cotton.

In studies conducted on runners wearing synthetic fiber socks versus cotton socks, other significant differences surfaced regarding preferability of fiber composition. Cotton fiber socks, when wet, were observed to stretch and lose their shape inside the shoe. This led to bunching and wrinkling of the socks compared to acrylic fiber socks. After multiple wash-wear cycles, cotton fiber socks were noted to become abrasive leading to potential irritation on the skin surface of the athlete.

In some sport applications, the thermal-insulation quality of the fiber composition becomes critical. New synthetic fibers composed of a hollow core material known as Thermax® have been shown to effectively insulate against heat loss. Natural wool fiber socks are still preferable in the outdoor industry because of their remarkable ability to maintain heat while wet. However, the abrasive nature of 100-percent wool fiber socks has required the blending of wool into other high-tech synthetic fiber materials.

Blisters and Other Skin Injuries

Friction blisters are among the most common foot injuries affecting the athlete. Blisters on the feet are even more prevalent and debilitating in military recruits. A study performed on 357 Marine recruits at Parris Island, South Carolina, revealed a 69-percent prevalence of blisters during a four-month period of training. Blisters serious enough to warrant medical evaluation at sick call occurred in 24.4 percent of all trainees. It has been estimated that over 5,000 Basic Trainees at Lackland Air Force Base were treated for friction blisters during one calendar year in 1990.

Factors necessary for friction blisters are shear force, pressure and moderate levels of moisture. All of these forces can be mitigated by a proper sock system.

Herring and Richie investigated the role of fiber and sock construction techniques in the prevention of blisters on the feet of running athletes. Their findings demonstrated that acrylic fiber socks will have less blisters and smaller blisters than cotton fiber socks. In addition, athletes were able to determine a drier foot with acrylic socks compared to cotton.

These findings were significant only when socks were constructed with dense terry padding rather than in generic "cushion-sole" socks.

Plagued with ever-increasing frequency of blisters, the United States Military conducted three randomized prospective studies on various sock systems. The standard military issue sock is a 50-percent cotton and 50-percent wool cushion-sole sock. The three studies attempted to compare newer fiber construction techniques and double-layer technology to reduce blister frequencies.

In a study of 357 Marine recruits on Parris Island, South Carolina in 1992, the use of a CoolMax® liner with a heavily padded terry design outer sock using a wool/polypropylene blend significantly reduced blisters compared to a single-layer sock (40 percent vs. 69 percent).

Adding a CoolMax® liner to the standard sock significantly reduced sick call visits (24.4-percent standard vs. 9.4-percent standard with liner).

Another study of 1,079 soldiers in 1993 tested five sock systems on blister frequency and acceptability by soldiers. Synthetic fiber socks significantly outperformed the standard wool sock. Adding a CoolMax® liner to the wool sock significantly reduced blisters. When comparing single, extra-thick acrylic padded socks to double-layer sock systems, the double-layer system was superior owing to the shielding of the open terry loops from the skin surface and the movement interface created by the double-layer system. Three other military studies have demonstrated a blister prevention superiority of double sock systems versus single-layer socks.

Fitting

Proper fitting of athletic footwear is critical for comfort, injury prevention and performance. Fitting of shoes, particularly athletic shoes, is a lost art in the modern retail marketplace. The emergence of high-tech sports hosiery products has made the shoe-fitting process even more difficult.

Shoe and foot measurement techniques are archaic in today's modern athletic footwear industry. The Brannock measuring device was developed in 1927, long before athletic shoes were developed and long before high-sports specific hosiery products were invented. The majority of modern-day athletic footwear is manufactured overseas in third-world countries where sizing parameters vary significantly, even within the same single factory.

In 1995, the author conducted a shoe-fit study for a premium sports hosiery company. The results of this study revealed the following:

1. Measuring feet barefoot with a Brannock device successfully predicted accurate athletic shoe size only 30 percent of the time.

2. When subjects wore a standard cushion-sole sock and were measured, accuracy for shoe size improved 10 percent.

3. When measuring a subject barefoot (as recommended by the Brannock Company), and then fitting the subject with athletic shoes and thick sports specific socks, the Brannock measurement was accurate only 15 percent of the time (an 85-percent failure rate!)

4. When measuring a subject with thick sports specific sock standing on the Brannock device, the accuracy for predicting proper shoe size improved by 10 percent.

5. When wearing properly fitted shoes with a generic sports sock, adding a thick heavily padded sock demanded an increase in length of shoe 77 percent of the time.

Therefore, measuring an athlete with a Brannock measuring device has minimal value when correlating with shoe sizes of modern day athletic footwear. Still, the skill of the fitter can allow translation of the shoe size to an "adjusted size" based on a knowledge of inventory and peculiarities of brand-size characteristics. The athlete should be measured and fitted wearing the specific sock that will be ultimately worn with the footwear. This is a reversal of the normal fitting process in most athletic shoe stores where socks are purchased as an "add-on" after shoes have been fitted.

Sports Specific Applications

Sports-specific socks were pioneered by ThorLo in the early 1980s. Soon, all major sock manufacturers followed with socks packaged and presumably designed for specific sports, i.e., tennis, golf, running, etc. What began as functional differentiation for a few key sports has led to a bevy of sock packaging techniques and marketing hype with products designed for every conceivable activity. In reality, there is very little technical difference within any particular company in the design of their hosiery products for various individual sports. In the end, however, the zeal of the American public to purchase socks specific for each sport has spawned a $250,000,000 industry.

Socks should be designed specific to the shoe, rather than the sport itself. The biomechanical movement and stresses of recreational and competitive sporting activities vary greatly. Designing a sock to mitigate those stresses has resulted in very similar features, despite the varieties of foot stresses found in each sport. What carries more variation are the shoe designs and the environmental challenges of the sport. Here, sock design in the upper and fiber composition can be varied greatly to meet the demands peculiar to the sport.

Table 9.2 gives examples of sock design and fiber variations as well as the sports applications that are best suited.

Table 9.2. Construction Techniques of Athletic Hosiery

Upper Design	Sport/Activity
Over-the-calf	Baseball, Basketball, Outdoor (including liners) Ski, Snowboard, Soccer
Mid-calf	Skate
Slouch	Aerobics
Crew	Running, Golf, Tennis, Racquetball, Hiking
Mini-Crew and Roll Top	Golf, Tennis, Running

Construction	
Thin or Thin Double Layer	Outdoor (liners), Cycling, Running (racing), Skiing
Padded or Thick	Jogging, Skiing, Hiking, Tennis,
Double-Layer	Basketball

Fiber	
Acrylic	Golf, Tennis, Hiking
Acrylic/Wool	Outdoor-Cold
Acrylic/Thermax®	Outdoor-Cool
Acrylic/CoolMax®	Outdoor-Warm
CoolMax®	Running, Cycling, Liners
MicroSafe®	Therapeutic Hosiery (i.e., Diabetes)

Chapter 10

The Sporting Foot

Athletes are the fittest group of injured people in the world. The athlete's feet have served as a testing ground for new medical treatments and products in much the same way that race cars have pioneered advances for the automotive industry.

Even the non-athlete is subject to the injuries common in athletes. Just by stepping incorrectly off a curb, you can suffer an ankle sprain similar to that suffered by a basketball player coming down from a rebound. Walk excessively on a vacation in Rome and you'll experience the same overuse syndromes of tendinitis or bursitis suffered by the marathon runner who increases training mileage too rapidly.

Sixty percent of all athletic injuries occur in the lower extremity and a majority of these affect the foot. Why? Almost all sports involve running and jumping, the trauma of which is absorbed primarily by the foot. A 150-pound athlete hits the ground with about 300-450 pounds of force. In an hour's workout, an athlete's foot is subjected to approximately five million foot-pounds of force—enough force to move a five-story building!

Most feet handle these enormous pressures admirably, but any weaknesses in training, structure, or protection will invariably lead to foot pain or injury.

"Chapter 7: The Sporting Foot," by Barry H. Block, D.P.M. J.D., excerpted from *FOOT TALK* at www.foothealth.com. © 1996, Barry H. Block, D.P.M. J.D.; reprinted with permission.

Training Injuries

The most common training injuries result from overuse. Occurring when an individual exceeds the training capacity of his body, overuse injuries are most common in "weekend athletes"—those who suddenly gain enthusiasm for a new sport. Also affected are athletes who increase their training schedules too rapidly. A runner who has been training 10 miles a week and suddenly increases his mileage to 40 miles a week in anticipation of an upcoming marathon is a likely candidate, as is the tennis player who has stopped playing during the winter and goes out to play three sets his first time out.

The training injury you suffer depends on which body part is the weakest or is put under the most stress. Muscles, tendons, fascia, ligaments, bones, bursa, and joints can all become injured or inflamed as a result of overuse. Many of these syndromes end with the suffix "itis" which is Latin for inflammation. Tendinitis is an inflammation of a tendon. Arthritis is an inflammation of a joint, and so forth.

Prevention

Common sense is the key in the prevention of most overuse syndromes:

1. If you're beginning a new sport or returning to an activity after a long hiatus, start out gradually.

2. Increase your level of activity gradually. Runners, for instance, should not increase mileage by more than 10 percent a week.

3. Do the proper warm-up and stretches before working out.

4. If you are participating in an activity and experience pain, stop and call it a day. Pain is a device of your body's early warning system. If you ignore nature's warning, you may subject yourself to even further damage.

5. Set up a sensible training schedule with adequate rest days. The American College of Sports Medicine, in a policy statement, recommends vigorous exercise for at least one-half hour, three to five times a week. Studies have shown that working out more than five times a week does not lead to significant fitness or performance gains, but does lead to an increase in athletic injuries.

In general, the treatment of all overuse injuries requires Rest, Ice, Compression and Elevation—summarized by the acronym RICE.

Rest: This allows nature to heal any injured part. Depending on the severity of your injury, this can range from a decrease in activity or mileage to a complete cessation of activity. Use your best judgment.

Ice: This is the most effective way to manage most acute injuries. Ice should be applied fifteen minutes at a time to the painful or injured part, especially during the first seventy-two-hour period. Ice is preferable to heat because it also reduces swelling.

Heat and cold both cause a helpful increase in the local blood supply, but each works via a different mechanism. Heat stimulates an increase in blood flow in an attempt to cool off the skin. If, however your circulation is diminished, heat can cause an actual burn to your skin. This is one of the reasons that heating pads are not recommended for those who have cold feet. Heat increases the metabolic demands on your skin. Burning of the skin can occur when your body cannot cope with this added demand.

Cold decreases the metabolic demand on your skin and causes a reflex increase in the deep blood supply. This increase is your body's attempt to warm up the skin. While frostbite is remotely possible from the use of ice, it is certainly less likely than is the possibility of a burn from the use of heat.

The best way to make a moldable icepack is to moisten a hand towel and place it into the freezer for 45 minutes. Wrap this pack around the injured part for 15 minutes and then return it to the freezer for another 45 minutes. Continue this regimen until bedtime. Be sure to leave the icepack in the refrigerator overnight. If you leave it in the freezer, it will come out hard as a rock by morning.

Compression: This usually takes the form of an ACE bandage or tape strapping. The objective is to reduce swelling and to restrict the range of motion of the injured part. The more severe the injury, the greater the limitation of motion required. Fractures and ligament tears, for instance, generally require cast immobilization.

Elevation: This speeds up the recovery process by allowing excess fluids to drain via gravity. One of the easiest methods of nighttime elevation is to place a few large books or telephone directories under the base of your mattress. Avoid using a pillow for elevation at night, as it invariably winds up on the floor by morning.

Beyond these basics, each of the following common athletic foot injuries presents its own particular nuances.

Achilles Tendinitis

Legend has it that the Greek warrior Achilles was invulnerable, except for a small weakness at the back of his heel. As a child, Achilles was dipped from the heels in the river Styx by his mother Thetis, making him invulnerable everywhere except at the point where she held him. Achilles met his death when Paris was able to shoot an arrow into his heel.

The Achilles tendon is aptly named, because it is the weakness of many athletes, from dancers to runners. Achilles tendinitis is an inflammation of the tendinous insertion of the calf muscles (gastrocnemius and soleus) into the back part of the heel. It is a condition characterized by pain in the posterior part of the heel which can extend upward to the calf. Individuals with shortened or tight calf muscles are particularly prone to this problem. Achilles tendinitis is commonly aggravated by any of the following factors:

1. Excessive increase in activity level, especially if running up hills, climbing, or participating in any activity in which pulling of the tendon is involved. For instance, a ballet dancer can suffer this injury as a result of coming down from pointe, where the relaxed tendon is pulled taut.

2. Too great a transition in heel height. Most often affected are women who go from wearing high-heeled shoes to flat sport shoes.

3. Failure to properly stretch the Achilles tendon.

Proper stretching of the tendon is most easily done by leaning against a wall. Standing two to three feet from the wall, place both hands flat on the wall at shoulder height and lean forward at approximately a forty-five-degree angle. making sure that both heels remain flat on the ground. This stretch should be done for a minimum of three minutes before and after your activity. The tendons should be stretched slowly, by gradually increasing tension on them. Avoid bouncing, since it causes a contraction of the calf muscle.

Treatment: Treatment of Achilles tendinitis requires the basics of R.I.C.E. plus the insertion of heel lifts. A heel pad of one-half to three-quarters of an inch will relieve the pressure on the tendon and allow it to rest.

NEVER allow any physician to inject a steroid such as cortisone into an inflamed tendon. Once a common treatment, this is not only unnecessary but it is also outright dangerous. Studies have shown that when tendons are injected with steroids, their structure weakens, increasing the chance of future rupture.

If you are chronically plagued with Achilles tendinitis, see your sports podiatrist for further diagnosis and treatment.

Tendinitis can also occur on the top of your foot. This is generally due to either a tight-fitting shoe or a shoe on which the laces have been over-tightened. This type of tendinitis usually resolves itself once a change to a properly fitting shoe is made.

Bursitis

A bursa is a balloon-like sac which cushions a tendon as it moves over a joint. When overuse occurs, these sacs fill with fluid and become painful and inflamed.

There are numerous bursae in the foot, any of which can become irritated due to overuse. The first mode of treatment after the basic R.I.C.E. is the use of a non-steroidal anti-inflammatory medication such as aspirin. Protective padding at the bursa site is also helpful, particularly when the bursa is located behind the heel. Padding provides protection from shoe irritation. Chronic bursitis may require physical therapy and possibly the use of injectable steroids.

Arch Pain (Plantar Fasciitis)

The plantar fascia is a ligamentous band which runs under your arch from the heel to the ball of your foot. This band helps to support your arch and prevent it from collapsing under the weight of your body.

Running and jumping put an additional strain on the fascia, often causing it to become irritated, and resulting in a dull aching pain. This condition can also affect non-athletes, particularly those who are heavy. This is due to the additional downward pressure of extra body weight which stretches the plantar ligaments.

A solidly built shoe with a rigid heel counter (see Choosing a Running Shoe) can often prevent this condition. Strapping is both a good preventive and therapeutic measure.

The most effective long-term solution to plantar fasciitis is the wearing of an orthotic, a custom-made shoe insert, which helps support your arch. Orthotics, which are made by your podiatrist, are more effective than the over-the-counter devices commonly sold in sporting goods stores (which are only sold by size). Each foot has its own "prescription" and unless you're extremely lucky, the over-the-counter device won't fit properly.

Heel Spurs

This painful condition of the heel has affected athletes from Joe DiMaggio to Billie Jean King and is somewhat related to plantar fasciitis. A spur is a piece of bone which has been gradually pulled off the bottom of the heel near the origin of the plantar fascia. This tearing occurs when the plantar fascia is over-stretched, such as when the arch is put under great stress. Heel spurs are also common in heavy non-athletes.

Heel spurs require the same prevention and treatment as plantar fasciitis: R.I.C.E., strapping, a supportive shoe, and orthotics. When the pain in the heel is acute, injection of a steroid into the heel bursa may be indicated.

Foot surgery for the removal of the heel spur is a last resort, when all other conservative measures have failed. Why? The skin around the heel has a very poor blood supply. Heel spur surgery prematurely ended the brilliant career of baseball's Joe DiMaggio because his surgeon elected to perform the now-obsolete "Griffith" procedure, which involved making a large incision around DiMaggio's heel that never healed properly.

Today's modern procedures such as endoscopic plantar fasciotomies involve a tiny incision and are far less traumatic.

Sever's Apophysitis [Sever's Disease]

Children aged eight to 14 often suffer heel pain due to a disruption of the growth plate at the back of the heel. This condition, known as apophysitis, is most common in children who run and jump a lot, particularly ballet dancers and gymnasts. The back of the heel is the last part of the foot to ossify (mature). The stresses, put on the heel by jumping cause the growth plate to be pulled, resulting in pain.

Taping and cushioning of the heel are two good preventive measures. Apophysitis usually subsides after the child reaches his fifteenth or sixteenth birthday. If your child is suffering from this condition, you may want to temporarily modify his athletic program until the problem is resolved. A child gymnast for instance, might be restricted from vaulting for a few months.

Fractures

A fracture of the foot or ankle is one of the most violent and dramatic sports injuries. Fractures are usually easily diagnosed. Severe pain, swelling, and discoloration (due to underlying bleeding) rapidly follow the initial trauma. Often a loud cracking sound can be heard at the time of the fracture. Suspected fractures should be examined and x-rayed as soon as possible by a podiatrist or orthopedist. This is also true of stubbed or broken toes. A popular misconception is that broken toes will heal themselves without treatment. This is not always the case. Hall of Fame pitcher "Dizzy" Dean was struck in the toe by a hot line drive during the 1937 all-star game. The resulting fracture forced Dean to alter his delivery and ultimately ruined his pitching arm.

If a broken toe is not taped properly, it may heal crookedly, necessitating additional surgery at a future date.

Treatment of a foot fracture will require immobilization of the injured part. Major fractures require plaster casting. Minor fractures such as broken toes need only taping. Some fractures will require a combination of taping and a wooden shoe.

Stress Fractures

Less traumatic is the stress or fatigue fracture. This type of fracture falls into the category of overuse injuries and occurs when a bone is stressed past its tensile limits. If you bend a paper clip back and forth many times, it will eventually weaken. So it is with a bone that is bent or pounded excessively (particularly on hard surfaces).

Unlike a traditional fracture, a stress fracture is difficult to diagnose. There is no severe pain and discoloration. Instead, dull aching pain, tenderness, mild swelling, and some redness are often present. The characteristic complaint of the athlete with a stress fracture is that of foot or leg pain which gets worse during activity and feels better during rest periods, only to feel worse when activity is continued.

Stress fractures are often misdiagnosed because initial x-rays are almost always negative. Only after 21 or more days after injury (when the body has laid down calcium in an attempt to heal the fracture) are x-rays positive. Treatment of a stress fracture requires a combination of rest and immobilization. Stress fractures generally heal in four to eight weeks.

Shin Splints

This is a catchall expression for many conditions which cause pain in the lower front part of the leg. Shin splints is an overuse syndrome of one or more muscles which originate on the leg and insert into the foot. The two basic conditions often found are anterior and posterior shin splints.

Anterior Shin Splints: The anterior muscles are located on the outside front part of the leg. They act to slow down and prevent the foot from slapping the ground These muscles can become irritated when an athlete begins to train on hills or changes from a flatfooted to a toe-running style. Anterior shin splints are often predisposed by a relative weakness of the front leg muscles. Activities such as running tend to build up the calf muscles more than the anterior leg muscles.

Studies have shown that when the calf muscles become more than four-and-a-half times stronger than the anterior leg muscles, the development of shin splints is likely. Prevention of anterior shin splints is accomplished by exercising these muscles. If you religiously exercise them, you will gradually build them up and avoid the muscle fatigue and inflammation of anterior shin splints.

The exercise that is most effective in building up these muscles is dorsi-flexion of the foot. In a sitting position, stretch the front part of your foot up toward your leg, as if trying to touch your shin with your toes. This exercise should be done in three sets of ten repetitions each day. After the first week, you may begin to add a one pound weight per week for the next five weeks. You needn't use standard weights. A few books in a pail can be hung over your foot. Treatment of anterior shin splints consists of R.I.C.E. plus the avoidance of hill running or hard surfaces.

Posterior Shin Splints: This type of shin splints is an irritation of the posterior tibial muscle at its origin in the lower inside pad of the leg. This is a deep muscle which inserts into the arch area and helps support the foot. When the foot excessively pronates (the arch flattens), this muscle is stressed, causing fatigue and pain.

Supportive shoes, strapping, and/or orthotic shoe inserts generally resolve this type of shin splint.

Ankle Sprains

This condition borders on being both a training and a structural injury. Ankle sprains are certainly among the most commonly suffered injuries of athletes They are more common in individuals with a large range of ankle motion. If you can easily invert your feet (turn the soles toward each other) your chances of a sprain are increased.

Sprains are not easy to prevent. Most occur when your foot plants in an incorrect position. If you have a tendency to sprain your ankles often, stable low heeled shoes, strapping. and elastic ankle supports can be helpful.

The treatment for an ankle sprain depends on the severity of the injury. A minor ligament pull requires little treatment. If after a few minutes, you can hop on the injured foot without pain, it's safe for you to return to your activity.

If you can't bear weight without pain you will need R.I.C.E. and a further work-up. In a moderate ankle sprain, a tear often occurs in the lateral talo-fibular ligament. Tears of this nature should not be taken lightly. Because of the poor blood supply to this area, ligament injuries may take even longer to heal than bone fractures.

In severe ankle sprains the calcaneal-fibular ligament may be severed. Treatment of this type of sprain ranges from casting to surgery (to re-sew the torn ligaments).

Structural Injuries

Limb Length Difference

Foot, knee, leg, hip, and back pain felt on one side of the body can often be the result of a difference in the length of the limb and studies have shown that approximately nine out of ten individuals have a measurable limb length difference. A shortened limb can be hereditary or may stem from back problems such as scoliosis (a curvature of the spine).

There are some simple ways of detecting limb length difference. When you have your clothes hemmed do you have to take up one side more than the other? Look in the mirror. Is one shoulder higher than the other? Inspect the bottom of a well worn sneaker. Is one side more worn than the other? Chances are the longer limb is hitting harder and wearing out the sole faster.

In most cases, because the longer limb hits harder and therefore transmits more force to that side, pain doe to a limb length difference will be present in that longer limb. A limb length difference can also result if one foot pronates (collapses) more than the other. This collapsing tends to shorten the foot and limb.

Limb length problems are more severe in the athlete than the non-athlete. A quarter inch difference may not cause any symptoms in the non-athlete, but the athlete with that same quarter-inch difference will experience pain because he is contacting the ground with two to three times the force of the non-athlete. His or her quarter-inch shortage becomes in effect a one-half to three-quarter inch shortage. Runners have been known to actually limp without even knowing it. Have a friend observe you as you run. Are your arms swinging symmetrically or is one arm swinging faster to compensate for balance?

Structural limb length differences are easily managed through the use of either a heel lift or an orthotic insert.

Functional Limb Length Difference

Functional limb length differences result from running on uneven surfaces such as an indoor banked track. In this situation, the inner foot is subjected to greater force than the outer foot. Running on the beach exerts this type of pressure (the average beach slopes about 14 degrees) as can running on the street, since most roads are banked for drainage. The logical solution to functional limb problems is to alternate directions when running, thus equalizing the force on both limbs.

Knee Pain

Knee pain associated with athletic participation; is often caused by structural foot problems. Many times an athlete comes into my office complaining of both foot and knee pain, very often not making the connection between these problems.

The knee is basically a hinge joint designed to move only in an up and down direction flexion/extension). The smooth operation of the knee assumes that the foot will be stable to the ground. If the foot pronates (collapses) the leg rotates inward causing the knee to move from side to side (obliquely). This abnormal motion causes the cartilage under the kneecap to wear unevenly, resulting in the common and painful knee injury, chondromalacia patellae, often referred to as "runner's knee." Chondromalacia patellae responds well to orthotic inserts which prevent the foot from excessively pronating.

Protection-Based Injuries

Blisters

Almost everyone has experienced the painful and annoying lesions resulting from excessive friction and pressure on skin commonly known as blisters. While they may be considered a minor affliction by some, you

62

can be sure that Jimmy Connors doesn't agree. During the 1979 Grand Prix Master's tennis tournament, a painful foot blister forced him to default and cost him an almost certain $100,000 first prize. You may never find yourself in Connors' position, but taking proper care of your blisters will prevent the pain and disability of an infected blister.

Prevention: To prevent blisters, you have to eliminate friction. One of the prime sources of friction is a shoe which fits improperly. If you find that your shoes are causing friction, you can modify them by making slits above the area of the blister formation.

Spenco Second Skin® is an over-the-counter product which can be applied to the areas on your foot which chronically form blisters. If your skin is either too dry or too sweaty, you will also have a tendency to form blisters. If your skin is dry, apply a thin coat of petroleum jelly to your foot before activity. If your foot tends to sweat, a little cornstarch added to your shoe and/or sock may be helpful.

Treatment: Small blisters require the least care. Apply ice to them for a few minutes, then cover them with a bandage. Never remove the blister's overlying skin. This acts as a barrier against bacteria and aids in the prompt healing of the blister.

For large and painful blisters, more care is required:

1. Sterilize a new sewing needle, either by cleaning it with 70-percent isopropyl alcohol, heating it with a match, or by placing it in a pressure cooker for a few minutes.

2. Clean the area around the blister with an antiseptic such as alcohol or Betadine®.

3. Make many small punctures in the blister to allow fluid to escape. Blot this fluid with a small piece of sterile gauze.

4. Apply a topical antibiotic ointment such as Mycitracin® or Bacitracin® to the blister site.

5. Cover the blister with a protective pad.

6. If the blister contains blood or becomes infected, see your doctor.

Black-and-Blue Toenails

This condition, technically known as subungual hematoma, is a painful and unattractive condition of the nails which is caused by the accumulation of blood under the nails, and occurs when the nails bang against the shoe during activity.

Prevention: Prevention of this condition requires the selection of a shoe with adequate length and toe box height. If this condition happens to you often, try buying the next size shoe or a style with a higher toe box. Existing shoes can be salvaged by making a slit in the upper at the point where the nail contacts. With your shoes on, make a mark at the point where you feel the offending nail. Now remove the shoe and make a vertical slit where you made your mark. Keeping your nails as short as possible is another effective method of preventing black toenails.

Treatment: Painful hematomas should be drained. You can do this yourself in much the same way you would drain a blister that is, by using a sterile pin to make several holes in the nail, but a podiatrist or other physician can usually perform the procedure less painfully and more effectively.

How to Choose an Athletic Shoe

Confused about buying a good pair of athletic shoes? No wonder! Sales of athletic shoes have soared in the last decade and there are currently hundreds of different styles and shapes available. This is not only attributable to the increased number of people engaged in physical activity, but also to the new social acceptability of these shoes for casual wear. From blue suede leather to day-glow orange nylon mesh, athletic shoes have become a staple of every fashionable wardrobe.

The evolutionary root of today's training shoe was a croquet shoe used by the upper class around the turn of the twentieth century. This shoe has subsequently undergone modification to produce cleated soccer, football, baseball, and golf shoes, spiked sprinting shoes, high topped basketball, boxing, and wrestling shoes, as well as the ever-popular tennis sneaker.

The term sneaker became popular because its quiet rubber sole made it possible to "sneak up" on someone without being heard.

Most sports medicine authorities agree that the basic training shoe is the most versatile general sports shoe. Following the 1960 Olympic games, German athletic companies began advertising these shoes for sale to the general public. The Olympic Committee frowned on the practice of portraying athletes wearing name brand shoes and there was quite an uproar about athletes accepting compensation for this type of endorsement. The idea, however, was successful. Thus started the fierce competition among manufacturers to capture an increasing share of a rapidly growing market. Athletic shoes became the "chic" thing to wear during the 1979 New York City Transit strike. Now it seems that everybody from supermarkets to high class boutiques is selling training shoes.

Unfortunately, many of these shoes have numerous shortcomings. No shoe can be expected to fit all feet or perform best for all sports. If you specialize in an individual sport, you should purchase a shoe designed for that sport. The characteristics of a specific sport shoe will be determined by the motions used in that sport.

Activities such as running and jogging most often involve unidirectional motion (straight ahead). Tennis, racquetball, and ping pong require a great deal of lateral motion. Basketball, soccer and football involve both unidirectional and lateral motion.

The more linear your sport, the stiffer the sides of your shoes should be. The more lateral the sport, the more twist should be possible in the shoe. A simple way to test this characteristic is to hold the shoe in your hand and twist it as if you were wringing out a towel. A tennis shoe should twist easily; a running shoe should not.

Fitting Variables

Each shoe company uses its own lasts (models of the foot) over which they construct their shoes. One company's shoe may fit you comfortably, while another company's same size shoe will not. There may be no shoe which fits your foot perfectly. Only comparative fittings of different styles and sizes will assure you of the best possible fit. Some companies such as New Balance produce athletic shoes both in wide and narrow widths. The shoe last type will also be a factor.

Last Type

Two types of construction are commonly used in the manufacture of an athletic shoe; board lasting and slip lasting. You can determine the method used by examining the inside bottom of the shoe.

Board lasted shoes have a cardboard insert glued into the bottom of the shoe which adds greater rigidity to the shoe. Slip lasted shoes have no board, making the shoe somewhat lighter and less supportive. If you examine a slip lasted shoe carefully, you will notice the

65

stitch marks where the bottom has been sewn together. Slip lasted shoes are generally lighter and less expensive for the shoe manufacturer to produce.

The choice of which last type you should choose depends on the amount of support and shoe stability you need and the amount of weight you are willing to tolerate. Board lasted shoes are best for support and stability, but somewhat heavier than slip lasted shoes.

Last Shape

Two basic last shapes are available; straight and curved (inflare). The last shape is an important factor in determining whether your shoe will fit properly, yet few people ever bother to check whether a particular shoe or sneaker matches the shape of their foot. Many people buy shoes by brand name or on the recommendation of a friend or athletic magazine. I'm often asked, "What is the best shoe?" Unfortunately, there is no one best shoe for everyone. A particular Nike might be best for your foot, while a particular Adidas or Reebok might be best for your friend.

You can compare your foot shape to the sole by placing the bottom of the shoe against the bottom of your foot. Does your foot match the shape closely? An efficient method for doing this is to make a tracing of your foot before visiting the local sporting shoe store. Cut out the tracing and bring this model of your foot to the store. Now you can rapidly compare this tracing to any of the dozens of available shoes on display to find out which brands and models match most closely. With the high cost of athletic shoes, it pays to select wisely.

Quality Control

Most sport shoes are mass produced, often in Korea, Taiwan, and Hong Kong. Quality control can often be a problem. Examine each pair of shoes carefully before you buy them. Look for obvious defects such as loose stitching, or improperly glued parts. Next place the shoes on a flat surface. if you can rock the shoe from side to side, find another pair. Look at the counter of the shoe. It should be perfectly level.

Heel Height

The heel height of an athletic shoe is another variable in your fitting. Athletes with short calf muscles or a history of Achilles tendinitis should look for the highest heel available. Many athletic shoe manufacturers are now incorporating a heel lift into their shoes. If you can't easily touch your toes from a standing position, you should benefit from increased heel height.

Heel Counter

The heel counter is found in the back part of the shoe. It functions to provide support for the heel bone on ground contact. The counter should be as rigid as possible. You can test the counter strength by holding the shoe flat in your hand and attempting to bend the counter forward with three fingers. If the counter bends easily, look for a better shoe.

Shock Absorption

A good training shoe should provide as much protection to your foot as possible. The shock absorption layer is usually found directly above the bottom or wear layer Some companies use different colors to distinguish each sole layer. The shock absorption layer should provide good cushioning, without completely collapsing. It may be difficult to determine how good a shoe absorbs shock without running in it. Some athletic magazines run such tests on shoes, and it may be a good idea to contact them if you aren't certain about the particular shock absorption of a specific model.

Sole Flexibility

The front part of the sole (where the foot bends) should be flexible. Take the shoe in one hand and with the other hand attempt to flex the sole upward. Keep in mind that your legs must undergo the same effort and motion during running. Too stiff a sole means wasted effort. If you can't flex the sole easily, the sole is not flexible enough.

Toe Box

Look for a shoe with a high toe box. Adequate space in the front part of the shoe provides room for the toes to flex during the propulsive phase of running. If the toe box is too low, the toes bang and scrape against the top of the shoe, leading to blisters, broken toenails, and black and blue toes. This is particularly important if you wear a sports orthotic.

Inner Cushioning

The shoe must also have ample inner cushioning. This provides for proper shock absorption within the shoe. Put your hand into your shoe and press down on the sole. There should be some give. Many athletic shoe manufacturers add Spenco-type inner soles for this purpose.

Arch Supports

Many athletes are concerned with arch support, but what most shoe companies advertise as arch supports (small foam pads) are not functional. How much support can sponge rubber provide to a 150-pound athlete? Recently some shoe companies have included "orthotic type" foam inserts in their running shoes. While these are better than foam arch supports, they still are a long way from being functional orthotics. There is simply no way to mass produce an arch support that will fit everyone's arch. If you require arch support you should see a sports oriented podiatrist who will probably rip out the prefabricated arch from your shoe and replace it with something more substantial.

Cost

You don't always get what you pay for. Athletic shoes currently are priced from about $25 to well over $100, and the most expensive shoe is not always the best one for you. On the other hand, don't be baited by sales, particularly of unknown brands. Consider your shoes important equipment. Find the shoe with the best features and which feels most comfortable.

Replacing Worn Sports Shoes

After a while, your once new athletic shoes will begin to look old and you'll want to replace them. The question is "when?" Because many athletic shoes cost over $100 a pair you'll want to make them last as long as possible.

The first parameter to look at is sole wear. A worn sole is not by itself reason enough to replace a shoe. Most athletic shoe stores as well as shoe repair outlets are equipped to resole your shoes, generally at a small fraction of the cost of a new pair. If you check the classified sections of any running or tennis magazine, you will also find similar services.

The sole layers of many sports shoes are color coded to indicate which is the wear layer (usually the black layer on the bottom) and the shock absorption layer (usually the lighter colored layer above the wear layer). When you notice that the colored layer is beginning to show through, it's time to replace or rebuild the sole. Rebuilding can be accomplished by applying a product such as ShoeGoo® to the sole.

If the heel counter is shot, be prepared to buy a new shoe soon. You may be able to extend the useable life of the shoe somewhat by adding a plastic M-F Heel cup or a Tuli® Heel cup (both available in most sporting goods stores). A breakdown in the heel counter indicates a decrease in the total structural integrity of the shoe.

If the upper part of the shoe begins to separate from the sole, there's not much you can do. Start shopping!

If you are happy with your old pair of shoes, it makes sense to replace them with the same model. This is sometimes difficult because athletic shoe companies tend to believe that "new is always better." European manufacturers are sometimes wiser.

Karhu, a Finnish company has produced the same model (#2323) for at least 10 years. It was a superior shoe when it was first introduced, and it remains so today, despite the numerous "improvements" of other shoe manufacturers.

Chapter 11

Picking the Right Foot Protection

A safety consultant has opined that there is no one footwear product that can be used in a variety of work sites. A worker must match his shoes or boots to the requirements of a specific workplace by knowing the dangers, responsibilities and environmental conditions linked to that workplace. The consultant noted that not enough employers and workers know the proper type of footwear to use. He observed that many company footwear programs select shoes or boots that protect against only one or two dangers when there are actually many other hazards in the workplace.

Safety consultant Michael Ziskin brings some order, and science, to the selection of safety footwear. Michael Ziskin practices what he preaches when it comes to selecting and wearing safety footwear. Ziskin, a consultant who specializes in personal protective equipment in industry and on hazardous waste sites, owns no fewer than five pairs of safety footwear: general-purpose steel-toe-work shoes; liquid-proof construction boots with cleated soles; insulated steel toe shoes for cold weather; chemical-resistant steel toe and shank work boots with chevron soles; and boots for fire fighting. He is planning to buy another pair of boots, with a nonconductive fiberglass toe.

Few safety footwear users face the diversity of hazards that Ziskin does, but his approach to footwear selection has broad application. "There is no all-purpose, super-product," said Ziskin, founder and

"Are You Picking the Right Foot Protection?" in *Occupational Hazards,* Vol. 59, No. 8, Pg. 43(2) August 1997, by Gregg LaBar. © 1997 Penton Publishing Inc.; reprinted with permission.

president of Field Safety Corp., Guilford, Conn. "You have to know the specific hazards, the tasks and environmental conditions, and find shoes or boots that match them."

Unfortunately, not enough employers and employees give foot protection its due or know how to select the right kind of equipment, according to Ziskin. The "Achilles' heel" of many foot protection programs, he said, is selecting footwear that protects against only one or two hazards when multiple hazards are present.

The National Safety Council estimates that U.S. workers suffer some 180,000 disabling foot and toe injuries each year. According to the Bureau of Labor Statistics, employees in construction, transportation and public utilities, and wholesale trade are at the greatest risk of foot and toe injuries.

OSHA Requirements

OSHA's (Occupational Safety and Health Administration) personal protective equipment (PPE) standard (29 CFR 1910.132) requires hazard-specific protective equipment and employee training in its use, limitations, maintenance, and disposal.

The section on foot protection (1910.136) requires protective footwear "where there is a danger of foot injuries due to falling or rolling objects, or objects piercing the sole, and where...exposed to electrical hazards."

Non-mandatory Appendix B of the PPE standards requires employers to "match the protective devices to the particular hazard." Relative to footwear, it offers recommendations for:

- Impact protection when carrying or handling materials such as packages, objects, parts or heavy tools.

- Compression protection for work involving manual material handling carts, bulk rolls and heavy pipe.

- Puncture protection from sharp objects such as nails, wire, tacks, screws, large staples, scrap metal, etc.

In addition, where needed, safety footwear should protect against chemicals, electricity and slips and falls.

According to Ziskin, the OSHA standard is a good starting point but "never really points you to the right product." He said manufacturers can help with information about what hazards their footwear are designed for, but employers must determine how the products will be used and how they will interact with job tasks and work environments.

"Footwear selection can be a struggle once your eyes are opened. The more you know about the limitations of products, the less you know about how they will perform in specific work situations," said Ziskin, who plans to use his position as chair of the American Industrial Hygiene Association's Protective Clothing and Equipment Committee to address such problems.

Expert Advice

For several years, Ziskin has been concerned about the "guinea pig" or "trial-and-error" approach to selecting personal protective equipment. As long as there are no major accidents, employers and employees assume they have selected the right equipment and it is being used properly, Ziskin explained. An accident, however, often triggers a knee-jerk reaction to purchase "better" equipment.

Ziskin prefers a systematic approach that evaluates the hazards up front and anticipates potential changes in the work environment. He recommends that company programs emphasize:

Engineering controls and work practices: It is a mistake, Ziskin said, to equate foot protection with safety footwear. Foot protection can be achieved by means in addition to safety shoes and boots. For example, maintenance and housekeeping can control foot hazards such as sharp objects and chemical leaks. In another example, using a better ladder may help prevent slips and falls, regardless of what shoes are worn.

Good work practices can minimize the risks even in the most dangerous situations, according to Ziskin. He is working on a Superfund site, for example, that is an abandoned metal fabrication shop. The floor of the shop is covered with water and oil, which poses a major risk for slips and falls. Slip- and oil-resistant safety footwear will be required, but employees will not start the bulk of the project until the work area is cleaned up. Ziskin said the preparation includes sucking up the water, scraping off the oil and washing down all surfaces.

Slip-resistant footwear alone would be the easy solution but probably fall short in controlling the risks, Ziskin said.

Multiple hazards: Most safety footwear is designed for one or two types of hazards, not multiple hazards. It is generally for "either low-hazard conditions or very specific high hazards," Ziskin explained.

The typical steel toe work boot or shoe, for example, protects against impact from the top and penetration to the sole. Where chemical hazards are present, however, a specialized boot made of rubber, PVC or neoprene (depending on the chemical) is needed. Where there are electrical hazards, a fiberglass toe replaces the steel toe.

Ziskin warned that relative risks and hazards can change. On a construction site, for example, trenching work poses the risks of trench collapse and engulfment. As a result, footwear for that situation should be cleated and allow for quick escape. When workers are 30 feet off the ground on that site, however, protection should focus on preventing slips and falls.

Some employers or employees may be tempted to choose footwear that is "the best that money can buy" to avoid the burden of hazard assessment. Not only is that approach costly, Ziskin said, but also it can be ineffective because even the best non-specialized products cannot account for all possible hazards.

Documentation: A formal process for recording how hazards are evaluated and PPE selected makes legal and safety sense, Ziskin said. This documentation should also cover how employees were trained and otherwise prepared to wear PPE. He emphasized that the documentation and training include information on when footwear becomes worn out and not as protective.

In the event of an OSHA inspection, Ziskin said, documentation will be crucial to proving the existence of an effective program, even if an inspector finds an occasional worker not wearing the appropriate foot protection. Good documentation also makes it easier to reassess hazards, Ziskin said.

Human factors: According to Ziskin, "There is an incredible number of barriers to wearing personal protective equipment properly. It generally makes work harder, slows you down and is less comfortable."

To minimize employee opposition, Ziskin advocates employee involvement in footwear selection. He recommends that employers make comfort one of the key elements in product evaluation. Even if a protective, comfortable product is not available at an affordable price, Ziskin insists, employees will appreciate the concern and will not use discomfort as an excuse for ignoring PPE requirements.

More Attention Needed

Ziskin's basic message is that foot protection is an unheralded safety and health issue. Hand protection and glove use get more attention, according to Ziskin, pointing in particular to the extensive

74

chemical permeation and degradation data available for gloves. There is little such information for foot protection, he pointed out, and "it's tougher to test shoes. Do you test the top of the shoe, the sole or the sides?"

Ziskin does not have those answers, but he believes more must be done to ensure that footwear protects against the specific hazards present and anticipated.

"Don't forget what shoes and boots are for," Ziskin said. "They are supposed to protect the part of the body that is in most direct contact with contaminants and hazards. These are things—chemicals, sharp things, rolling objects, heavy loads—that we generally would not put our hands near."

Ziskin believes the "the collective experience of the user community"—including some of the unfortunate "guinea pigs" mentioned earlier—will help employers improve their foot protection efforts.

Five Questions for Footwear Selection

Answering these five questions should give employers the information they need to select the appropriate foot protection, according to safety consultant Michael Ziskin.

1. What are the hazards (e.g., impact, penetration, compression, chemical, heat, electrical)?

2. What are the employees' work tasks?

3. What are the environmental influences (temperature, mud, steep slopes, wind, precipitation, lightning, distance off the ground)?

4. What is the worst thing that could happen?

5. What are the key human performance factors (equipment fit, ease of movement, comfort, fatigue, employee training, morale, behavior)?

Chapter 12

Foot Pain Prevention

Preventing Foot Problems in Childhood

The first year in a person's life is important for foot development. Parents should cover their baby's feet loosely, allowing plenty of opportunity for kicking and exercise. The child's position should be changed several times. Staying too long on the stomach can strain the feet. Children generally walk between 10 and 18 months; they should not be forced to start walking early. Wearing just socks or going barefoot indoors helps the foot develop normally and strongly and allows the toes to grasp. Going barefoot outside, however, increases the risk for injury and other conditions, such as plantar warts. When outdoors, shoes should be light, flexible, and made of natural materials that "breathe". (Children's feet perspire greatly.) Footwear should be changed every few months as the child's feet grow. Footwear should never be handed down. High impact sports can injure growing feet, and parents should be sure that their children's feet are protected if they engage in intensive athletics.

Foot Care

Toenails should be trimmed short and straight across. Filing should be straight across as well using a single movement, lifting the file

"What Are the General Preventative Measures for Foot Pain?" from the website at http:///www.webmed.com. Copyright © 1999, Nidus Information Services, Inc.; reprinted with permission.

before the next stroke. The file should not saw back and forth. A cu- ticle stick can be used to clean under the nail. Skin creams can help maintain skin softness and pliability. Taking a warm foot bath for 10 minutes two or three times a week will keep the feet relaxed and help prevent mild foot pain from fatigue. Adding one-half cup of Epson salts increases circulation and adds other benefits. Taking foot baths only when feet are painful is not as helpful. A pumice stone or loofah sponge can help get rid of dead skin. Hiking or strenuous walking can cause blisters. To prevent them, one study reported that treating feet with antiperspirants before setting out may be helpful. Reflexology is an Oriental massage therapy that manipulates hands and feet. A pleas- ant exercise using this method can be done while taking a bath. Use the thumb, index and middle finger to rotate each toe in a circular motion. Then, make a fist and rotate it slowly around the bottom of the foot. Finally, gently twist each foot as if ringing wet clothes, mov- ing the top and bottom in opposite directions.

Foot Care for People with Diabetes

Daily foot care is extremely important for people with diabetes who are at risk for nerve damage and poor blood flow to the feet. Preven- tive foot care could reduce the risk of amputation in people with dia- betes by 44% to 85%. Patients should make a daily inspection and watch for changes in color or texture, odor, and firm or hardened ar- eas, which may indicate infection and potential ulcers. When wash- ing the feet, the water should be warm (not hot) and the feet and areas between the toes should be thoroughly dried afterward. Moisturizers should be applied, but not between the toes. Corns and calluses should be gently pumiced and toenails trimmed short and the edges filed to avoid cutting adjacent toes. Patient should not use medicated pads or try to shave the corns or calluses themselves. People with diabe- tes should avoid high heels, sandals, thongs, and going barefoot. Shoes should be changed often (three times a day if possible). They should not wear tight stockings or any clothing that constricts the legs and feet. A new hand-held device that uses a nylon fiber brush may en- able the physician to identify nerve damage that can lead to ulcers by pressing it against several points on the foot and eliciting the patient's response to the pressure.

A person with diabetes should check with a specialist in foot care for any problems. Hospitalization and intravenous antibiotics for up to 28 days may be needed for severe foot ulcers in diabetic patients. In one study, intravenous therapy using ofloxacin or penicillin for only seven days followed by an oral antibiotic was adequate treatment. A number of treatments (Dermagraft, Apligraf, Regranex) are now available that stimulate new cell growth and help heal skin ulcers or use cultures of human skin cells, although their benefits are still unproven.

Granulocyte-colony stimulating factor, or G-CSF (filgrastim, Neupogen, Amgen) is showing promise as an effective alternative to antibiotics. One small study shows that treatment with human nerve growth factor (NGF) may safely prevent and reverse some of the nerve damage caused by diabetes. One study indicated that administering hyperbaric oxygen (given at high pressure) promoted healing and helped prevent amputation. There was no follow-up however, and more research is needed. According to a new study, the wearing of magnet-laden socks seems to reduce or eliminate the pain associated with diabetes induced foot disorders. Well-fitted shoes are the best way to prevent nearly all problems with the feet. They should be purchased in the afternoon or after a long walk, when the feet have swelled. The shoe should have adequate cushioning, one-half inch of space should be left between the largest toe and the tip of the shoe, and the toes should be able to wiggle upward. A person should stand when being measured, and both feet should be sized, with shoes bought for the larger-sized foot.

Women who are used to wearing overly pointed-toe shoes may assume that tight-fitting shoes are normal, hence increasing the risk for many foot disorders. New shoes should have padding, a flexible sole, and should always feel comfortable right away without requiring a period of breaking-in. Ideally, the shoe would have a removable insole. Elderly people wearing shoes with thick inflexible soles also may be unable to sense the position of their feet relative to the ground, significantly increasing the risk for falling. Some experts recommend that older people wear thin hard soles. More research is needed to determine if thick soles are actually responsible for foot injury in younger adults who engage in high-impact exercise.

If shoes do require breaking-in, moleskin pads should be placed next to areas on the skin where friction will occur. Shoes purchased for exercise should be specifically designed for a person's preferred sport. The heel area should be strong and supportive (but not too stiff) and the front of the shoe flexible. As soon as the heels show noticeable wear, the shoes or heels should be replaced. If a person insists on wearing high-heeled shoes, the heel should be wedge-shaped. (Even in these cases, the heel height should not be extreme.) People should avoid extreme variation between exercise footwear, street, and dress shoes. Shoes should be changed during the day. The way shoes are laced can be important for preventing specific problems. Laces should always be loosened before putting shoes on. People with narrow feet should buy shoes with eyelets farther away from the tongue than people with wider feet. This makes for a tighter fit for narrower feet and looser for wider. If, after tying the shoe, less than an inch of tongue shows, then the shoes are probably too wide. Tightness should be adjusted both at the top of the shoe and at the bottom. Where high arches cause pain, eyelets should be skipped to relieve pressure.

Although people believe that foot-binding is a problem limited to Chinese women of the past, it should be noted that fashionable high-heels are designed to constrict the foot by up to an inch. High heels are the major cause of foot problems in women and one study suggests that wearing high-heels may even lead to arthritis of the knee. Fortunately, according to a recent survey, nearly half of working women now wears flats; about one quarter wears pumps less than 2 1/4 inches in height and another quarter wears athletic shoes. Only 3% reported wearing shoes with heels higher than 2 1/4 inches. Women who insist on high-heels should at least look for shoes with wider toe room, reinforced heels that are relatively wide, and cushioned insoles. They should also reduce the amount of time they spend wearing high-heels. The American Orthopaedic Foot and Ankle Society now awards a Seal of Approval to women's shoes that they determine are healthy.

Correct Walking and Exercise

In addition to wearing proper shoes and socks, a person should also walk often and correctly to prevent foot injury and pain. The head should be erect, back straight, and the arms relaxed and swinging freely at the side. A person should step out on the heel, move forward with the weight on the outside of the foot, and complete the step by pushing off the big toe. A person should prepare for long hikes by putting moleskin pads on the heel and other parts of the foot that might be rubbing on the shoe. At the end of a hike, the foot should be checked for irritation and redness. Gentle stretching and heel lifts after warm-up and before running can help prevent Achilles tendinitis and heel pain.

Insoles and Orthotics

Insoles: Insoles are flat cushioned inserts that are placed inside the shoe; they can be obtained in athletic drug stores. They are designed to reduce shock, provide support for heels and arches, and resist moisture and odor. Most well-known brands of athletic shoe have built-in insoles. Dr. Scholl's is the most popular insole, but many others are now available, including Pedifix, Sorbothane, Implus, Footfit and Kiwi. Prices for these insoles range from $5 to $20. The Spenco orthotic arch support is a high-end insole that can be molded by putting it into boiling water for two minutes. It is sometimes recommended by health practitioners. In general, over-the-counter insoles offer enough support for most people's foot problems. Shoe stores that specialize in foot problems often sell customized, but more expensive, insoles.

The thickness of socks must be considered when purchasing insoles to be sure they do not squeeze the toes up against the shoes. Women who have worn high-heels for prolonged periods and have developed short, tightened Achilles tendons should consider heel cushions, which are inserted inside the shoe and should be at least one-eighth inch high but not more than one-quarter inch. People respond very differently to specific insoles and what may work for one person may not for another.

Orthotics: For severe conditions, such as fallen arches or body-structural problems that cause imbalance, podiatrists or physicians may need to fit and prescribe orthotics, or orthoses, which are insoles molded from a plaster of Paris cast of an individual's foot. Orthotics are usually categorized as rigid, soft, or semi-rigid. Rigid orthotics are often used to prevent excessive pronation (the turning in of the foot) and are useful for people who are very overweight or have uneven leg lengths. Some experts warn that rigid orthotics may cause sesamoiditis or benign tumors that form from pinched nerves. Soft orthotics are made from a light weight material and are often beneficial for people with diabetes or arthritis. They need to be replaced periodically, and because they are bulkier than rigid orthotics, they may require larger shoes. Semi-rigid orthotics are usually made of layers of leather and cork reinforced by silastic. They are often used for athletes, in which case they are designed for a specific sport. The cost of examinations, casting, and x-rays is high but may be covered by some insurance plans.

Before seeking prescription orthotics, people with less severe problems should consider testing the lower-priced over-the-counter insoles. One study found that 72% of people reported less foot pain from store-purchased insoles compared to 68% of those who had them custom made.

Chapter 13

Orthotics

About This Text

The Board for Accreditation of Prescription Foot Orthotic Laboratories (BAPFOL) Technical Standards Document was developed by the Technical Standards Committee in conjunction with feedback from membership of the Prescription Foot Orthotic Laboratory Association (PFOLA). Terminologies and definitions were arrived at by a combination of previously developed definitions in medical publications, and discussions involving individuals who have contributed to the development of the foot orthotic field for many years. These discussions, and their subsequent conclusions, were subject to on-going examination and feedback from a large cross-section of the foot orthotic industry to assure the broadest possible input.

This document is not a static document. Rather, it is subject to expansion and revision, as needs and understanding within the industry make such revisions necessary. BAPFOL continues to ask for input into the evolution of these standards from both the foot orthotic industry, and from those in the medical field who utilize custom, prescription foot orthotics.

"Technical Standards Document," Prescription Foot Orthotic Laboratory Association , © 1998 Board for Accreditation of Prescription Foot Orthotic Laboratories (BAPFOL); reprinted with permission. All information supplied here is intended to be for the purposes of education and does not state or imply the "only" or "correct" approach to the given topic. Biomechanics and foot orthoses manufacturing are both evolving disciplines, and the information presented herein will evolve as does the discipline.

Functional Foot Orthosis

Functional Foot Orthosis (as relates to custom foot orthosis)—An orthotic device that is contoured to the plantar, medial, lateral and posterior aspect of a replication of the foot to control or reduce abnormal motion or abnormal position of the foot and to control the abnormal motion or abnormal position of the lower extremity that is affected by the position and/or motion of the foot. When applicable, modifications such as wedgings or postings are utilized to control foot motion or position.

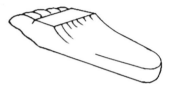

Figure 13.1. *Rigid Functional Orthosis*

Rigid Functional Orthosis—A functional foot orthosis made to maximally prevent abnormal motion or abnormal position of the foot and leg during gait. This device is made from a rigid material that displays minimal flexibility during use, given that this flexibility is a function of the thickness of the material, the intrinsic rigidity of the material, the size of the orthotic plate, the weight of the patient, and the degree of instability of the foot.

Semi-Rigid Functional Orthosis—A functional foot orthosis used to partially control abnormal motion or abnormal position of the foot and leg during gait. This device is made from a material that displays moderate flexibility during use, given that this flexibility is a function of the thickness of the material, the intrinsic rigidity of the material, the size of the orthotic plate, the weight of the patient, and the degree of instability of the foot.

Accommodative Orthosis—An orthotic device that supports the foot but does not attempt to align the joints of the foot during stance or gait.

Fashion Shoe Orthosis—Any orthosis fabricated for a typical fashion shoe or dress shoe and specifically designed to fit the shape of the shank of the shoe. These devices can be fabricated from rigid, semi-rigid, or soft materials.

Diabetic Orthosis—A removable orthotic insert that provides total foot contact with multiple density materials that are suitable with regard to the patient's condition. This device is made to disperse weight as evenly as possible throughout the plantar aspect of the foot and to reduce pressure from pre-ulcerative or ulcerative areas.

Heel Stabilizers

Heel Stabilizer—A foot orthosis that incorporates not only the plantar pedis but also the medial and lateral aspects of the rearfoot and/or midfoot. These devices are made to following specifications:

* **Type A Heel Stabilizer**

  * **Deep Heel Seat**—To a height just inferior to the lateral maleolus.

  * **Lateral Flange**—To just proximal to the base of the fifth metatarsal.

  * **Medial Flange**—To the mid-point of the first metatarsal shaft.

  * **Distal Plantar Edge**—Ending at the mid-point of the first ray medially and just proximal to the base of the fifth metatarsal laterally.

* **Type B Heel Stabilizer**

  * **Deep Heel Seat**—To a height just inferior to the lateral maleolus.

  * **Lateral Flange**—To just proximal to the base of the fifth metatarsal.

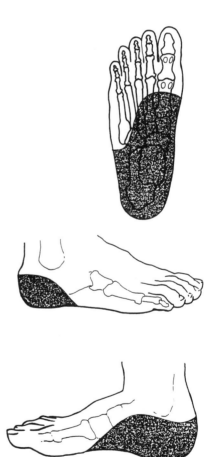

Figure 13.2. *Type A Heel Stabilizer.*

85

- **Medial Flange**—Full medial flange extending onto the first metatarsal shaft.

- **Distal Plantar Edge**—To the bisection of the first and fifth metatarsal heads.

- **Type C Heel Stabilizer**
  - **Deep Heel Seat**—To a height just inferior to the lateral maleolus.

  - **Lateral Flange**—To the mid-shaft of the fifth metatarsal.

  - **Medial Flange**—Full medial flange extending onto the first metatarsal shaft.

  - **Distal Plantar Edge**— To the bisection of the first and fifth metatarsal heads.

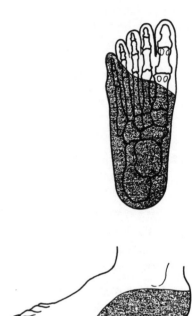

- **Type D Heel Stabilizer;** promotes out-toeing
  - **Deep Heel Seat**—To a height just inferior to the lateral maleolus.

  - **Lateral Flange**—To just proximal to the base of the fifth metatarsal.

  - **Medial Flange**—To the mid-point of the first metatarsal shaft.

  - **Distal Plantar Edge**— Ending at the mid-point of the first ray medially and at the end of the fifth toe laterally.

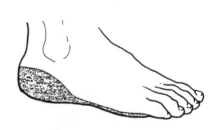

Figure 13.3. *Type D Heel Stabilizer.*

86

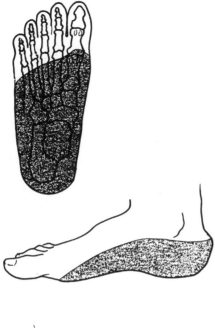

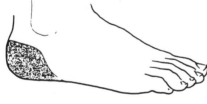

Figure 13.4. Type E Heel Stabilizer.

- **Type E Heel Stabilizer;** promotes in-toeing

  - **Deep Heel Seat**—To a height just inferior to the lateral maleolus.

  - **Lateral Flange**—To just proximal to the base of the fifth metatarsal.

  - **Medial Flange**—To the mid-point of the first metatarsal shaft.

  - **Distal Plantar Edge**—Ending at the mid-point of the fifth metatarsal ray laterally and at the sulcus of the hallux medially.

Gait Plates

Gait Plate—A foot orthosis that is designed to induce in-toe or out-toe. Gait plates should include the following shapes:

- **To induce in-toe:** Cut proximal to the fifth metatarsal head and extended distal from the first metatarsal head to the sulcus of the first toe.

- **To induce out-toe:** Cut proximal to the first metatarsal head and extended distal from the fifth metatarsal head to the end of the fifth toe.

Understanding Orthotic Concepts

Calcaneal Bisection—A line drawn on the posterior aspect of the heel that bisects the calcaneus into equal medial and lateral portions. This line is either perpendicular, everted, or inverted to the leg.

Frontal Plane Relationship of the Forefoot—A relationship established by projecting the Calcaneal Bisector onto an imagery line drawn parallel to the plantar aspect of the all metatarsal heads when the subtalar joint is placed in its neutral position and both axes of the midtarsal joint are fully pronated (locked). In some instances, the line across the metatarsal heads is modified by elevated or depressed metatarsal heads. The forefoot frontal plane relationship may be perpendicular (neutral forefoot), inverted (varus), or everted (valgus).

Forefoot to Rearfoot Relationship on Positive Representation of the Foot—When a positive representation of the foot is placed on a transverse plane, the line that bisects the posterior heel (the laboratory equivalent of the Calcaneal Bisector) will be inverted, everted, or perpendicular to the floor. The position of the heel bisector in relation to the floor is determined by the frontal plane relationship of the forefoot.

Balanced Forefoot (neutral forefoot)—The correction of an abnormal forefoot (valgus or varus frontal plane relationship)

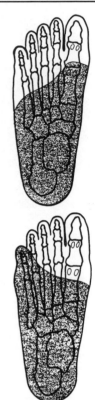

Figure 13.5. Gait Plate to induce in-toe (top); to induce out-toe (bottom).

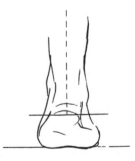

Figure 13.6. Calcaneal Bisection.

so that the forefoot-to-rearfoot relationship is perpendicular, or neutral. This correction is accomplished by adding an intrinsic or extrinsic forefoot post.

Intrinsic Forefoot Post—Changing the angulation of the forefoot platform to invert or evert the positive representation of the foot.

Forefoot Platform—A flat plane created across the metatarsal heads on a positive representation of the foot. At its proximal aspect, the forefoot platform blends into the plantar aspect of the foot at the metatarsal shafts, and is constructed so that the platform extends proximal to the proximal aspect of the first and fifth metatarsal heads. The distal leading edge of the orthotic device either meets the plane of the platform, or extends onto the plane of the platform. The leading edge of the finished device ends just proximal to the first and fifth metatarsal heads.

Extrinsic Forefoot Post—Material added to the distal portion of the plantar aspect of the orthosis to increase the distal edge contact area and to stabalize, invert or evert the device.

Extrinsic Rearfoot Post—Material added to the inferior surface of the heel of the orthotic shell to increase the contact area and to stabilize, evert, or invert the orthosis at heel contact.

Heel Lift—Material added to the inferior surface of the heel of the orthosis to increase the thickness of the orthotic and elevate the heel relative to the supporting surface.

Intrinsic Rearfoot Post: Shell Grind Method—The inferior surface of the heel of orthotic shell is ground to increase the contact area and to stabilize, evert, or invert the orthosis at heel contact.

Intrinsic Rearfoot Post: Medial Heel Skive Method—The plantar surface of the medial heel area of the positive representation of the foot is flattened to stabilize, invert, or evert the rearfoot on the orthosis.

Medial Arch Fill—The addition of fill to the positive representation of the foot that is primarily medial to the medial slip of the plantar fascia. This addition turns the medial edge of the orthotic shell away from the arch of the foot.

Full Heel Expansion—Fill added to the lateral border and lateral/posterior/medial heel of positive representation of the foot to allow for soft tissue expansion upon weight bearing.

Half Heel Expansion—Fill added to the lateral border and lateral/posterior heel of positive representation of the foot to allow for soft tissue expansion upon weight bearing.

Lateral Flange—An increase in height of the orthosis on the lateral side of the foot starting lateral to the heel and continuing distally at variable length usually not beyond the fifth metatarsal head. The height is variable to the prescription, but no higher than just inferior to the lateral malleolus. An increase in the height of the orthosis on the lateral side of the foot starting lateral to the heel and continuing distally at variable length beyond the 5th metatarsal base and usually not beyond the 5th metatarsal head.

Figure 13.7. Lateral Flange.

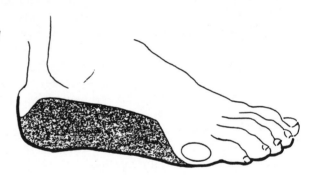

Lateral Clip—An increase in the height of the orthosis on the lateral aspect of the foot starting proximal and lateral to the center of the heel and ending distally at the proximal aspect of fifth metatarsal base. The height is variable to the prescription, but no higher that just inferior to the lateral malleolus.

Medial Flange—An increase in the height of the orthosis on the medial side of the foot starting medial to the heel and extending distally with increasing height, with the apex near the navicular, and then decreasing in height to end along the first metatarsal shaft. The height of the flange is variable to the prescription.

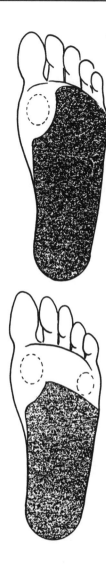

Heel Cup Height—The vertical distance between the heel contact point of the positive representation of the foot and the circumscription line of the heel cup on the positive representation of the foot.

1st Metatarsal Cut Out: A. Complete removal of material under first metatarsal head in sulcus length orthotic shell. B. Cut out of orthotic shell just proximal to first metatarsal head in metatarsal length orthotic shell.

1st Ray Cut Out—Cut out of rigid shell beginning proximal at the first metatarsal base and angled to the lateral aspect of first metatarsal head.

Soft Tissue Supplement—Soft, cushioning material that augments the foot's natural cushioning.

Top Cover—Any material used on the top of the orthosis to cushion, finish or give the orthosis better wear resistance. Examples: neoprene = cushioning; leather = finish; vinyl = resistance to perspiration.

Extension—Any non-rigid material added to the orthosis extending its length beyond the metatarsal heads.

Figure 13.8. *1st Metatarsal Cut Out. Top: Complete removal of material under first metatarsal head in sulcus length orthotic shell. Bottom: Cut out of orthotic shell just proximal to first metatarsal head in metatarsal length orthotic shell.*

Pressure Accommodation—A method of relieving pressure from a localized area on the medial, lateral, plantar or posterior aspect of the foot to the surrounding areas. This is generally accomplished by suspending a particular area of the foot by creating a cut out or a concave pocket under a localized area.

Metatarsal Pad—Tear shaped modification to the orthotic or a positive representation of the foot to raise the metatarsal heads. Typically, it begins proximally at the metatarsal bases and gradually thickens and widens till just proximal to metatarsal heads, where it thins in height and narrows in width, ending distally at the metatarsal heads.

Scaphoid Pad—A pad that is plantar and medial to the longitudinal arch and gives extra support to medial arch area. The pad is applied to the dorsal surface of the orthotic shell.

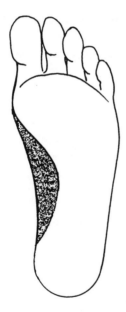

Figure 13.9. Scaphiod Pad.

Cuboid Pad—A pad that is plantar to the cuboid bone. This pad raises the cuboid relative to the supporting surface. The pad is applied to the dorsal surface of the orthotic shell.

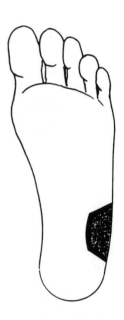

Figure 13.10. Cubiod Pad.

Neuroma Pad—A dome shaped pad placed in the metatarsal interspace or on the shaft of the metatarsals. It starts at the proximal third of the metatarsal shafts and:

- **A.** If it is placed in the interspace, it slopes and ends at the metatarsal heads.

- **B.** If it is placed on the shaft of the metatarsal, it slopes and ends under or just proximal to the metatarsal head.

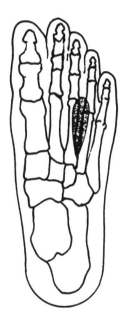

Figure 13.11. Neuroma Pad.

Heel Cushion—Resilient material used to cushion the heel such as sponge rubber, polyurethane foam, or neoprene. The material is applied to the dorsal surface of the orthotic shell, usually from the posterior aspect of the heel to the base of the fifth metatarsal.

Heel Spur Accommodation—An oval, concave, or horseshoe type depression in the heel area of the orthotic shell. It is positioned plantar to the medial tubercle of the calcaneus and is used to disperse weight off of the area and to increase shock absorption to the inflamed area.

Morton's Extension—Material added under the first metatarsal head and in some cases the proximal and distal phalanx of the hallux.

Orthosis Arch Fill—Material added to the plantar aspect of medial arch of the orthosis to give extra support and/or resilience to the orthotic shell.

Bottom Cover—Material added to the bottom of the orthotic shell to finish the orthosis and protect it from wear. Common materials are leather, suede, vinyl, neoprene, and polyurethane foams.

Chapter 14

Using Shockwaves to Treat Feet

Claire Page has coped for two years with a sharp pain in her right heel that throws off her beloved golf game. "It's been very painful over the summer," the 56-year-old Londoner said.

The semi-retired medical secretary, has plantar fasciitis, an inflammation of the fibrous band of tissue that helps maintain the arch of the foot. The condition, better known as heel spurs, is a common problem aggravated by all weight-bearing sports.

But recently, Page was among the first patients to take part in a clinical trial investigating a new treatment—shock waves—for plantar fasciitis. For about 20 minutes, doctors at London's Fowler Kennedy Sport Medicine Clinic used a device invented to destroy kidney stones to send about 3,800 high-energy shock waves through her foot. London is the only Canadian site for the six-center international study that will involve a total of 150 patients. The other centers are in Atlanta, Detroit, Boston, and two sites in Germany.

Principal investigator Ned Amendola, an orthopedic surgeon at the Fowler Kennedy center, said 25 patients will be enrolled in London. Half the patients in the randomized study will receive shock-wave therapy, the other half a placebo. Amendola, who oversees the trial but doesn't administer treatment, doesn't know which patients get the real thing.

London was chosen as the Canadian site by Dornier Medical Systems Inc. of Kennesaw, Ga., after the U.S. Food and Drug Administration approved the trial. It will investigate the safety and efficacy of pain relief using shock-wave treatment. Amendola said traditional treatments, including use of splints, cortisone injections and even surgery, provide slow relief if any at all.

In Germany, where shock-wave treatment has been used for orthopedic purposes since 1993, the method has an 80-percent success rate with heel spurs, said Holly Pavliscsak, a clinical monitor with Dornier. Shock-wave treatment has also been applied to problems such as shoulder tendinitis, tennis elbow and golf elbow, although none of these applications are yet approved in the United States.

Amendola sees the plantar fasciitis study as a way to determine if the treatment is effective for pain relief—a finding that could open the technology to other orthopedic applications.

If Page received the actual therapy as opposed to a placebo, Pavliscsak said she should feel some pain relief within 72 hours and within three months, should experience noticeable relief. Most people with plantar fasciitis have similar symptoms: pain when they get out of bed or after long periods of sitting, standing or activity.

Amendola said a patient is given a local anesthetic to freeze the foot so there's no pain as shock waves are applied. The rationale is that the heel pain involves tissue the body can't heal, and shock waves jump-start the healing process. The procedure is only done once. If it's proven effective, Amendola said it would mark a huge improvement in treating a common but often debilitating problem. Anyone wanting information about the study should call 1-800-992-3674.

Chapter 15

Foot Surgery

Foot surgery has undergone tremendous changes in the past few decades. In the first half of the twentieth century the emphasis was on correcting the physical manifestation of the problem with little effort made toward addressing the forces behind the deformity—in much the same manner that a mechanic may replace a tire with uneven wear without realigning the wheels.

This tendency contributed to unacceptably high failure and recurrence rates in foot care. Also a factor was the lack of sophisticated instruments available. As recently as 1970 many surgeons were still utilizing modified hammers and chisels to perform foot surgery. Today, most foot surgery is performed with high-speed power equipment that enables the surgeon to make precise bone incisions.

Today's foot surgery focuses on getting the patient walking as soon as possible, sometimes immediately after surgery. This is in sharp contrast to foot surgery of the past, which too often left the patient immobilized for long periods of time. Still, the decision to have foot surgery is not one to be taken lightly. If you are considering having foot surgery, keep the following information in mind:

Almost all foot surgery is elective. You should have your foot operated on only after you have tried more conservative therapies. A heel spur, for example, will often respond to strapping, steroid injections, or to the wearing of orthotic devices (customized sole inserts), so you owe it to yourself to try these therapies first. Do what is best for you, not what is most expedient for the surgeon.

However, in the case of certain conditions, such as painful bunions or hammertoes, the conservative option, such as wearing a molded shoe, may be unacceptable to you. If this is the case, surgery may be the only alternative.

Avoid "same day" surgery. Most foot conditions develop slowly. This gives you the time to make a careful, sound decision. Don't let yourself be pressured while you're "in the chair." If you have doubts, go home and sleep on it. You may also want to get a second opinion. Most health insurance companies will be more than happy to send you to a qualified doctor, often at no charge to you.

The only type of surgery that should be performed during your first visit is minor skin surgery, such as the removal of an infected ingrown toe nail or the removal of a skin tumor such as a wart. Occasionally emergency surgery is necessary, as in the diagnosis of osteomyelitis (bone infection), but this is a rare occurrence. There is no valid reason why corrective bone surgery can't be scheduled at your convenience.

Elect a time that is best for you. Since foot surgery is elective, plan to have it done when you will be least inconvenienced. Swelling results from most foot surgery and necessitates the wearing of a surgical shoe for a few weeks. If you have to attend a wedding, you'll probably want to delay the procedure until after the festivities. If your job requires the wearing of stylish shoes, you may want to delay the surgery until your vacation.

Weather may also be a factor in the choice of your surgery date. Most people who live in a cold climate prefer to have their feet operated on in warmer weather because it is easier to fit a swollen foot into a sandal than a winter boot.

Cosmetics alone is not a good reason to have foot surgery. You may consider your foot problem unattractive but, unless you model your feet for a living, it's usually best to leave them alone. Good reasons for having foot surgery are to relieve pain, to help you walk better, or to help you fit into normal shoes.

Select the best foot surgeon available. Find out the qualifications of your surgeon. Every podiatrist or orthopedist is legally permitted to operate on your feet, but the training and experience of individuals varies widely. While there is no one criterion by which to judge an individual's competence, you should look for the following attributes: a) completion of a surgical residency; b) board certification; c) hospital surgical privileges; d) satisfied patients; and e) a good reputation among other specialists.

A doctor who over-advertises to obtain surgical patients should be considered suspect—a top foot surgeon needs only his or her track record as his advertisement. Your surgeon should not be offended if you ask for a second opinion or a copy of your X-rays. There are first-rate surgeons in every large city, so invest the time and energy to seek these individuals out. You deserve the best.

Foot surgery is not painful. Many procedures can be performed under local anesthesia. Your foot can be numbed with a Novocaine-like substance: Marcaine® is popularly used because it keeps the foot pain-free for about twelve hours. More extensive foot surgery is usually done under general anesthesia.

If you are in pain after the anesthetic wears off, many analgesic tablets, ranging from aspirin to narcotics, are available to keep you pain free.

Allow time for your foot to heal. Modern surgical techniques now allow you to walk on an operated foot shortly after surgery. But don't expect to be running a marathon the following week. Nature needs time to fully heal the foot and this can vary with the individual. Some "fast healers" return to work a few days after surgery. Others need a week or more to recover. The duration and extent of the surgery are also factors. In general, the more extensive the surgery, the longer the recovery time.

The foot's healing process occurs in two stages. In the first phase, known as the "primary" healing stage, the body actively heals the incisions. This period lasts three to four weeks and you will be aware of the process. In the "secondary" healing stage, your body gradually remodels the bones which have been operated on. This stage can take from several months to several years, and you will rarely be aware of the underlying changes. Gradually you will be able to resume all normal activities but you may occasionally feel a funny numbness, twinge, tingling or other sensation. When these disappear, you know that the healing process is complete.

Office Versus Hospital Surgery

Where to have your surgery is an often-controversial subject. Simply put, minor foot surgery should be performed in a doctor's office and major foot surgery should be performed in a hospital. But there are complicating factors. Some surgeons' offices now contain operating suites as elaborate and well prepared as those in hospitals. And some procedures previously thought of as being major, are now considered minor. So, where your procedure should be done depends ultimately on how much support care you need.

Most doctors' offices are not equipped for such ancillary services as general anesthesia, attending physicians, or nursing. Nor are they equipped for overnight stays. If your surgery is extensive, if you have a medical problem such as a heart condition, or if you have no one to care for you at home, you will be better off in a hospital. If your procedure is minor, you are in good health, and you have someone to take care of you at home, you're better off having your surgery performed in a well-equipped doctor's office.

Conventional Versus Minimal Incision Surgery

Two distinct techniques of foot surgery are currently being utilized and there is a great deal of controversy over the advantages and disadvantages of each method.

Conventional foot surgery is the predominant style used by hospital-based surgeons. In this technique, the surgeon makes a lengthy incision over the area to be operated on and proceeds to "open up" the area. The surgeon can then visualize the internal structures and proceeds to cut and remove bone using power drills and saws. Scalpel blades are often used to cut and reposition soft tissue structures such as tendons and capsules. This type of surgery is often referred to as "open" surgery.

Minimal incision surgery is performed predominantly in doctors' offices. In this technique a small incision is made over the involved area. A small dental-type drill is used to "grind off" bone. This method is often referred to as "closed'" surgery since the surgeon cannot visualize the actual bone.

It is this inability to literally see the bone which fuels the vigorous opposition of many surgeons to "closed" surgery. They argue that due to the comparatively "blind" technique many unidentified structures are cut. This argument has somewhat lessened with the advent of portable imaging devices such as the Lexiscope®. Opponents also point out that often necessary ancillary procedures such as the insertion of a joint implant or repositioning of tendons and joint capsules are simply not possible with minimal incision surgery.

Minimal incision surgeons contend that their technique offers the following advantages:

1. It can be performed in a doctor's office, thus saving considerable expense to the patient.

2. The patient does not have to remain in the hospital overnight. He may immediately ambulate, and often return to work within days.

3. The scar is usually smaller. Minimal incision surgeons also argue that with the use of X-rays during the actual surgery, they do know what structures they are cutting. It is probable that advances in technology, which will improve the ability of the "closed" surgeon to see the structures he or she is cutting, will in turn enhance the scope and safety of procedures. The photon image intensifier, which acts like a portable fluoroscope to make the underlying bones "visible," is just one of the many devices holding such promise.

The technique performed on your foot will depend on both the training of your surgeon and the severity of your foot condition. Small procedures such as the elimination of bone spurs on the toes are most easily corrected by minimal incision surgery. Major foot deformities involving the replacement of joints can only be corrected using "open" techniques. There are some conditions such as metatarsal deformities and minor bunion operations in which either technique can be utilized.

Soft Tissue Procedures

These procedures do not involve the cutting of bone. They range from the simple removal of a wart to the more complicated removal of a deep nerve tumor (neuroma).

Wart Surgery

As discussed, warts are benign skin tumors caused by a virus infection. They are commonly found on the bottom surface (plantar) of the foot and therefore are usually referred to as plantar warts. Technically warts are known as verrucae and papillomas. Surgical excision of a wart is indicated in cases when the growth is large, or when non-surgical therapy such as the use of acid has not been successful.

The surgeon first applies local anesthesia to numb the wart area and then uses an instrument known as a curette to "scoop out" the entire growth. No sutures (stitches) are needed to close the wound, and usually no significant scar results. Sometimes a cauterizing agent such as phenol is used to help prevent the wart from recurring. This procedure is not debilitating. The area where the procedure was performed may feel sore for a few days, and there may be some bleeding, but you should he able to return to your job the next day.

Nail Surgery

Nail surgery is also a relatively minor procedure. The most common indications are chronically ingrown and infected nails, in which case a small section of the side of the nail is usually removed. If you have a history of repeated infections of the same nail, the growth portions (nail root and matrix) at the back of the nail may also be removed. This can be accomplished by surgically removing these "growing" sections.

More commonly a caustic phenol solution is applied to these areas to prevent regrowth. The result is that the major portion of the normal nail will continue to grow, while the offending ingrown section will not. This procedure is both simple and highly effective. Occasionally, however, the offending portion of nail will regrow and the procedure will have to be repeated. In some cases of severely deformed or fungus-infected nails, it may be necessary to remove the entire nail. Again, you and your doctor will make the decision as to whether the procedure should be temporary or permanent (removal of the entire growth plate).

Permanent removal of a nail is not as drastic as it sounds. Your toenails serve little function and you can do very well without them. After this procedure is performed, a "nail-like" tough skin forms where the nail originally was. This can be covered with nail polish or an artificial nail.

Removal of a nail portion is not debilitating. You may, however have to wear loose-fitting shoes for a few days after the procedure.

Morton's Neuroma

Morton's neuroma is a fairly common benign nerve growth usually developing between the third and fourth metatarsals and most often found in women. It is caused by the irritation of branches of the medial and lateral plantar nerve as they cross between the metatarsal bones.

Wearing tight shoes pushes the metatarsals together squeezing the tumor between them, and this friction causes the nerve to enlarge.

102

Symptoms of a neuroma vary but may include a sharp, tingling or burning sensation that radiates to the toes.

The conservative treatment of a neuroma includes injections of steroid into the neuroma as well as changing to wider shoes. If these measures are not successful, surgery may be necessary.

The procedure for neuroma removal requires an incision over the neuroma site. The surgeon then must carefully dissect and remove the entire tumor. Often the ligaments attaching the adjoining metatarsals are cut. This allows these metatarsals to separate and helps prevent recurrence of the tumor. Neuroma removal can be performed in either an office or hospital. This procedure requires sutures and you will have to wear loose shoes or sandals for about two weeks afterward.

Toe Procedures

Most toe procedures are designed to eliminate painful corns. These accumulations of extra skin develop because of excessive friction on the skin of the toe as it gets pressed between the bone on the inside and the shoe on the outside. This is usually caused by two structural conditions: most commonly, the tendons of the toe gradually contract causing the toe to "buckle up" and rise. As the "knuckle" of the toe rises higher it is likely to rub against the top of the shoe. thereby causing a corn. When this condition occurs at the middle of a toe it is known as a hammertoe. Mallet toe results when the buckling occurs at the end of the toe.

The second condition that may cause a corn is the presence of a bone spur on a toe. A bone spur—technically known as an "exostosis"—is a calcium deposit that forms on an area of bone subject to great friction. Bone spurs usually form at the ends and the sides of toes. The most common location for this type of corn is on the outside of the little toe, where friction against tight shoes is the greatest.

Corns due to bone spurs can also occur in between the toes as the skin gets rubbed between two toe bones. These corns become soft and rubbery due to the presence of moisture between the toes and are known as "soft" corns. Another place that corns caused by bone spurs are likely to occur is at the end of a toe. Occasionally these bone spurs occur underneath a nail causing a painful condition known as a subungual exostosis.

"Soft Tissue" Toe Surgery—Tenotomy

A tenotomy is a simple procedure available for the correction of a hammertoe. Tenotomies are useful only in hammertoe cases where the problem is being caused by a contracted (tightened) tendon. The tendons going to your toes are located just below the skin. Look down at the top of your foot. If your tendons are tight, you can probably see them as "cordlike" structures. In a tenotomy, the surgeon uses a tiny blade to sever a tight tendon on the top of your foot, beyond your toes. Occasionally the tendon on the bottom of the toe is also cut. Sometimes the surgeon will also perform a capsulotomy in which he cuts the joint capsule just below the tendon as well.

Tenotomies are only useful when a hammertoe deformity is "flexible." By "flexible," we mean that the toe can be manually straightened. When a hammertoe has progressed to the point where the "knuckle" joint becomes rigid, a tenotomy to relax the tight tendon will be of little value. If you have a hammertoe, reach down and try to straighten the toe. If you can easily straighten the toe, a tenotomy may be indicated. If the toe is "stiff" and unbending, a tenotomy (or capsulotomy) by itself will be virtually useless. If your corn is a result of a bone spur, it is also unlikely that you will benefit from a tenotomy.

Perhaps the most compelling limitation to the tenotomy is that its benefits tend to be temporary. After the procedure you will need to stretch the corrected toe daily for many months to prevent the tendon from reshortening.

Bone Procedures for Toe Problems

The most effective long-term cures for corns due to hammertoes and bone spurs are procedures that either straighten the toe or remove the offending spur. When the corn occurs near the "knuckle" or joint, a procedure known as an arthroplasty is performed using either the open or closed technique. In the open method, an incision is made on the top of the toe and a section of bone at the raised area of the "knuckle" is removed. In the closed method, a small incision is made on the top or the side of the toe and a burr is inserted into the bone, and rotated by a dental-type drill. The excess bone is pulverized into bone paste, which is then squeezed out of the small hole on the top of the toe.

The advantage of the closed technique is that only a tiny scar will remain after the toe has healed. The advantage of the open method is that there is less chance of subsequent stiffening of the joint. In the open procedure, the offending bone is cleanly removed from the joint space. In the closed or minimal incision technique, bone paste can be left in the joint and this paste can regrow to form bone, which may result in a stiff or arthritic joint. Each procedure takes about thirty minutes and can be performed in a doctor's office under local anesthesia. If you have this procedure done on a Friday, expect to be back to work on Monday (albeit in loose or cut-out shoes).

As in any procedure performed on the foot, it is important that no pressure be put on the operated area. Your doctor may give you wooden "post-op" shoes, or you may choose to wear loose fitting sneakers or an old pair of shoes with a hole cut in the top. If the weather is warm, sandals are also acceptable. Whatever you select, remember that no pressure is to be put on the healing wound for several weeks.

Surgery for "Spurs" on Toes

Bone spurs are actually calcium deposits that result from increased pressure or friction on bone. The body "lays down" this calcium for protection in the same way that the skin develops callus to protect itself from excessive force. Technically known as an exostosis, this is basically a permanent condition, which cannot be helped by reducing the amount of calcium in your diet.

Bone spurs can occur anywhere on your foot. You may be able to feel them as small lumps and bumps. Often these lumps are painless. If this is the case, leave them alone. Sometimes they may result in corns, particularly when they develop on the outside of the little toe or between the toes, where they result in "soft" corns. Surgery is indicated when you can no longer get relief from wider shoes. A subungual exostosis occurs when a bone spur develops underneath a toenail. Surgery is indicated for this painful condition when you can no longer get relief from wearing a shoe with a higher toe box (the part of the shoe above the toes).

In the case of a simple exostosis, in which there is no joint involvement, closed surgery can be used to easily grind off the extra bone. This procedure is done in an office under local anesthesia and usually requires no sutures. An exostosis can also be removed via open surgery. Ultimately it is up to your surgeon to choose the method, but it is important for you to be aware of the options.

Metatarsal Surgery

The metatarsals are the "long" bones of your feet. The "ball" of the foot is the area located below the front part of the metatarsal bones. Metatarsal problems range from the bunion, which is the deformity occurring at the first metatarsal, to a "tailor's bunion," which is found on the fifth metatarsal. Plantar-flexed or "dropped" metatarsals are a condition that often results in painful callus formation on the bottom of the foot.

Bunion Surgery

A bunion is a deformity found at the first metatarsal-phalangeal joint, behind your big toe. It is a condition that develops slowly and results from the gradual dislocation of the metatarsal-phalangeal joint that has become "unstable" during the propulsive phase of walking (a time when the joint should be stable). As the deformity progresses, the big toe itself will shift toward the outside of the foot. In severe cases, the big toe will actually overlap or underlap the second toe. Bunions are often painful and they can make shoe fitting very difficult. Contrary to what many people believe, tight shoes do not cause bunions, but they will aggravate them and accelerate their development. The tendency for bunion formation is hereditary and surgery is the only way to correct them. Exercises, splints, and other devices look good on paper but they just don't work. The forces causing a bunion are simply too great for any known device to correct. Orthotics designed to stabilize the foot during gait are custom-made inserts which fit into your shoes. While these devices do not correct a bunion, they may be useful in providing relief and slowing down bunion development.

If your bunions don't hurt and you don't have difficulty finding shoes, there is no need for surgery. You should, however, see a podiatrist about having orthotics made to counteract deforming foot forces. If your bunions are painful, bunion surgery is indicated.

Most of the recent advances in foot surgery have been directed at bunion surgery. In the past, emphasis was placed on the removal of the "exostosis" or lump, and straightening of the big toe. The reasoning was "if the toe looks straight, it will function properly." Each surgeon had his own favorite procedure. Today, we know that there are many different types of bunions and that no single procedure will give the best results. Your surgeon must first X-ray your foot to determine the type of joint you have. He or she will then measure the various angles of your foot. Only then can it be determined which procedure is best for your bunion. Procedure selection is very important. No matter how expertly the surgery is done, your results are only as good as the procedure selected.

In a "simple" bunion, where the toe is straight, only the exostosis need be removed. This procedure can be done either in an open or closed manner. Most bunions, however, are not simple and require either cutting of capsular tissue, or cutting of bone (osteotomy). These procedures are generally best done using the open technique. in which there is less chance of traumatizing the first metatarsal-phalangeal joint.

Depending on the nature and severity of the bunion, your surgeon and you will decide whether to perform the procedure in an office or hospital and whether to have the operation done under local or general anesthesia. If you have bunions on both feet, you'll want to decide whether or not to have them corrected at the same time. Each choice has its own advantages and disadvantages.

You'll initially have a longer recuperation time when you have both feet operated on at the same time, but you may feel that this is preferable to having one foot operated on and then having to go back and do the other foot later. The recovery period from bunion surgery will vary depending on the specific procedure and your body's healing rate. Most people can walk satisfactorily within a few days after surgery. Again, you will have to wear modified footgear until the post-op swelling subsides. Some people need a couple of months to return to normal shoes. Don't expect to be a "cripple" after bunion surgery, but don't expect to go dancing the week after either.

If you work at a desk job, expect to return to work the week after surgery. If you have a walking job or have both feet operated on at the same time, your disability time will probably be two weeks or more. Keep in mind that these are general guidelines which your surgeon may modify. Don't be misled by advertisements for "lunch-hour" bunion surgery—you may turn out to be "the slowest healer" the doctor has ever had!

Prevention of bunion recurrence. After bunion surgery you must take measures to prevent the recurrence of this deformity. The best way to do this is with orthotic devices, which act to control the faulty biomechanics responsible for the instability of the first M-P joint.

"Bunion-Like" Conditions

The joint involved in bunion formation (the first metatarsal-phalangeal or M-P joint) assumes more weight than any other foot joint in the propulsive phase of gait, and is more likely to be affected by osteoarthritis, a condition resulting from excessive "wear and tear" in which extra bone is deposited near the joint. This extra bone restricts the motion of the joint and causes severe pain during walking.

While bunions result from a gradual dislocation of the joint, painful bunion-like conditions can occur in which there is no dislocation of the first M-P joint. In these cases, the big toe and joint will look straight, but will hurt when moved. In the early stages of osteoarthritis of the big toe joint, a small bone spur forms at the top or side of the joint. This spur causes a limitation of motion, creating a condition referred to as hallux limitus. If left untreated, eventually the condition progresses to the point where there is virtually no motion left in the joint. This is referred to as hallux rigidus.

The early stages of hallux limitus should be treated with physical therapy to maintain as much range of motion as possible. When normal ambulation is no longer possible, surgery is necessary to "remodel" the joint. This is an open procedure in which the excess bone surrounding the joint is excised and it is often necessary to replace the entire joint with an artificial implant.

After this procedure it is important that vigorous physical therapy be instituted to maintain normal joint motion. Osteoarthritis can also affect the lesser metatarsals. In these cases. therapy and treatment parallel that of osteoarthritis of the first M-P joint.

Tailor's Bunion

A tailor's bunion or "bunionette" is a bunion-like condition of the fifth M-P joint (the area behind the little toe). It derives its name from the old belief that tailors developed this condition as a result of working at their sewing machines with their legs crossed and the outside of their feet touching. This condition is caused by faulty foot mechanics and, like a conventional bunion, tends to be hereditary.

Two procedures are commonly used to correct the tailor's bunion. In some cases, an angulated incision is made in the bone, which is then slid inward. Other times the front or side part of the bone is removed. Regardless of which method is elected, this is generally a highly successful procedure, and post-op ambulation and healing are rapid.

Surgery for "Dropped" Metatarsals

Ideally, all five metatarsal bones should hit the ground at the same level. Often, however, one or more metatarsals can be structurally lower than the others. This condition is referred to as plantar-flexed or "dropped" metatarsals. The increased pressure of one metatarsal hitting the ground with more force than the others often results in the formation of a painful callus-like lesion known as an intractable plantar keratoma (IPK).

The conservative treatment of an IPK involves using an accommodative orthotic with a built-in depression below the dropped metatarsal. While this device will not correct this condition, it will allow the dropped metatarsal to functionally hit the ground at the same level as the other metatarsals. In an older, less effective treatment, metatarsal pads were placed behind the affected bone. The theory was that these pads "raised" the dropped metatarsal.

Experience has shown, however that it is better to let a plantarflexed metatarsal drop harmlessly into a small hole, than to attempt to "lift" it. When conservative therapy has not been successful, surgery is indicated. This highly successful procedure, known as an osteotomy, involves surgically raising the dropped metatarsal. This can be accomplished easily using either the open or closed method. In both cases, an incision is made into the metatarsal causing a precise surgical fracture. The patient is allowed to walk immediately in wooden post-op shoes that "float" the fractured bone and let it heal in a new raised position. Healing from an osteotomy takes about three weeks.

Heel Spur Surgery

A heel spur is a painful bone formation on the heel caused by the gradual "pulling off" of bone from the heel by the stretching of the ligaments of the arch. These ligaments originate in the heel and terminate in the metatarsal bones. Surgery is indicated only after all other conservative treatments have been unsatisfactory.

Heel spur surgery is performed through a small incision on the inside back part of the foot. It is no longer considered absolutely mandatory to remove the entire spur. Often detaching ligaments attaching to the spur (the plantar fascia) is sufficient to make this condition asymptomatic.

Major Foot Surgery

Major foot surgery is also available for the correction of foot deformities such as flatfeet, high arched feet, clubfoot, and ankle instability. Many of these procedures require the use of wires, screws and extensive casting to fixate bones. This type of surgery should therefore not be considered as "ambulatory." The procedures for these "reconstructive" surgeries are complex and are best discussed with your own surgeon.

What to Expect after Surgery

Foot surgery is unique—in what other type of surgery are you required to walk on a healing wound? The foot, though, is a sturdy structure that responds well to this challenge, and most foot surgery heals uneventfully. But you should be prepared for any of the following possible post-op complications:

Post-op Swelling (edema). Some swelling should be expected following your operation. Generally, the more extensive the surgery, the greater the swelling will be. Elevating your feet will help reduce this swelling. One way you can do this is to place a large book such as an encyclopedia or Sears catalog under the base of your mattress. Remember that the more you're on your feet after surgery, the longer it will take for the swelling to go down. Most edema should be gone after one month. Some residual swelling, however, may remain for the next few months. This residual swelling should not be painful, but may restrict you from wearing tight-fitting shoes.

Black and blueness. This is a normal sequela of surgery and results from small internal bleeding in the wound site. Sometimes this discoloration may even appear in other parts of the foot. Bunion surgery, for example, might result in black and blue adjoining toes. Post-op discoloration will gradually fade and completely disappear within a month.

Soreness. This will also vary with the extent of surgery and your own pain threshold. Many people require little or no pain medication after surgery-often the application of ice is sufficient. Others use aspirin or Tylenol®. If you are in discomfort, your surgeon can prescribe medication ranging from codeine to stronger narcotics. Generally it makes sense to take as little medication as needed following surgery. Still, you don't have to be a hero. Take as much medicine as you need to feel comfortable. The soreness you feel after surgery will peak in about forty-eight hours and will decrease every subsequent day.

Infections. Your foot surgery was performed under sterile conditions, so the risks of infection are minimal. Keeping your bandages clean after surgery will also decrease the chances of an infection developing, but unfortunately, even under the best of conditions infections may occur. Fortunately, modern antibiotics make infections much less of a problem than they once were. Be aware of the "cardinal" signs of an infection: throbbing pain, increased temperature, redness, swelling, pus.

Infections take a few days to develop. If you notice any of these signs, call your doctor immediately. The sooner an infection is detected, the faster it can be resolved.

Numbness. This is a normal post-operative finding that results from the cutting of small nerves during surgery. You may experience "funny" feelings such as a pins-and-needles sensation or an occasional sharp pain. These feelings are signs that your wound is healing and that the nerves are regenerating. Normal feeling should return to the operated part of your foot within a few months.

Part Two

Foot Conditions

Chapter 16

Athlete's Foot

What's the Problem?

Athlete's foot is the most common term to describe a fungus condition involving the skin of the feet and toes. Another term is *Tinea pedis*. However, that means a ringworm type infection and the term is misleading, since the organisms that cause it are not worms, but are fungus spores technically known as dermatophytes. A more appropriate name is dermatophytosis. The three names above really mean the same thing.

The patient first notices an itching sensation, usually between the toes. The skin in that area may have small blisters and be peeling. A less itchy form of athlete's foot can appear as a dry, red peeling condition on the bottom of the foot.

How Does It Feel?

The skin may be red with scaling and there may be small blisters containing a sticky, clear fluid around the area. The skin may have a stinging or burning feeling. The area between toes may show peeling with cracks and redness and maceration (moist, white wrinkled area). Generally there is considerable itching.

"Athlete's Foot—Skin Fungus Infection, Dermatophytosis, Tinea Pedis, Ringworm," by Dennis White, DPM, from the Podiatry Online website at http://www.footdoc.com, © 2000 by Dennis White; reprinted with permission.

Let's Do a Test!

If home treatment is unsuccessful, laboratory tests are indicated. Some scrapings from the skin are examined under the microscope and others are sent for a culture to determine which type of fungus is responsible. In some resistant cases, a secondary bacterial infection may develop and can be very serious.

How Did This Happen?

The fungi organisms that cause athlete's foot are microscopic and grow like small plants, surviving on the protein called keratin in dead skin. The source of the fungus is usually from the soil, an animal such as a dog, cat or rodent, or possibly from another person. Many people actually have the fungus on their skin but unless certain conditions are present, athlete's foot will not develop. These conditions include injury such as bruising or breaks in the skin. Areas of the body where moisture accumulates favor growth of these organisms, like between the fourth and fifth toes. The fungi thrive in a dark, warm, moist environment, which is often the case inside our shoes and socks. People who go barefoot all the time have little or no incidence of this problem. We don't know why some people develop this problem and others do not. Many times only one member of a family will have dermatophytosis, even though bathrooms and showers are shared. There may well be an individual predisposition to develop it.

What Can I Do for It?

At home, dust anti-fungal powders in your socks and shoes every day. Apply an over-the-counter cream two to three times daily. Wash canvas shoes frequently and change socks at least every day. People with diabetes or circulatory problems should take especially good care of their feet. If it persists over two weeks, consult your podiatric physician.

What Will My Doctor Do for It?

First of all, they will examine you to determine if you have a fungus and not some other skin condition. After diagnosing the type of fungus, more effective topical preparations or possibly oral medications may be prescribed. If a secondary bacterial infection is present, culture and sensitivity tests may be necessary and antibiotics may

116

be utilized. Although fungus infections have sometimes been very difficult to manage, new medications have been developed that are quite successful. Treatment should continue for a period of time after the symptoms have cleared to make sure it is gone.

Can I Prevent It from Happening Again?

The best offense is a good defense! Use powder in shoes and socks. Do not wear synthetic or nylon socks that trap perspiration. Wear cotton to absorb moisture. Dry feet thoroughly, particularly between toes (consider a hair drier on low heat). Change socks and wash shoes periodically. Use your topical medicine and if it doesn't improve, check with your foot and ankle specialist right away.

Chapter 17

Ingrown Toenail

Although an ingrown toenail does not constitute an emergency, it is a fairly common problem and can be extremely painful. The great toe is almost exclusively affected, and the condition may be complicated by bacterial or fungal infection. Depending on the extent of impingement and infection, management of ingrown toenails may involve conservative measures or minor surgery.

Problems with ingrown toenails seem to occur principally among persons in two age groups. Acute bacterial infection associated with an ingrown toenail occurs more frequently among younger patients (aged 10 to 20 years) of both sexes. Inflammation and infection frequently develop following trauma, such as stubbing the toe, improper nail trimming (in a curve, rather than straight across), and picking or tearing the toenails. As the injured or torn nail grows outward, impingement of its edge may lead to infection.

An increase in the incidence of ingrown toenails occurs during the fifth and sixth decades, particularly among women. With advancing age, the toenail can become deformed; the subsequent thickening and hypertrophy are associated with chronic fungal infection. Incurring of the outer edges causes significant discomfort. Bacterial infection is uncommon in this scenario.

Here I describe several procedures that can be performed in the office; I will explain the pros and cons of each. I will also outline my

"Ingrown Toenails: Office Procedures that Relieve Pain—Steps that Prevent Recurrence," by Michael Coughlin in *Consultant*, Volume 38, November 1998, p. 2761(9). © 1998 Cliggott Publishing Co.; reprinted with permission.

method of placing a digital nerve block. A brief review of the anatomy of the toenail sets the stage.

The Normal Toenail and Nail Bed

The toenail is composed of three layers of overlapping keratinized cells: a thin, stiff, brittle dorsal layer, a thicker, softer middle layer; and a thin deep layer that probably is derived partly from the nail bed.[1] Despite its apparent density, the nail is actually 10 times more permeable to water than the adjacent skin. This permeability enables successful treatment with topical agents that are effective against some mycotic infections.

The toenail grows 0.01 to 0.05 mm/d; growth is more rapid in younger persons. Replacement of an injured or avulsed nail can take three to six months. Accordingly, recurrent in-grown toenails often become symptomatic three to six months after an initial avulsion procedure.

The toenail is supported by the nail unit: the proximal nail fold, the nail bed, the nail matrix, and the hyponychium. The epithelial surface of the nail bed has undulating ridges that interdigitate with the toenail's under-surface, creating a firm attachment as the nail grows distally. The proximal nail fold (including the cuticle), the lateral nail folds, and the hyponychium constitute the epithelial borders of the toenail. The hyponychium forms a seal between the distal toenail and the nail bed.

The nail matrix is the main germinative area of the nail unit. It extends proximally from the distal aspect of the lunula for the entire width of the nail. Thus, when you are excising the matrix region, always resect beyond the proximal margin of the lunula to avoid recurrent growth.

The matrix extends proximally 5 to 8 mm above the edge of the cuticle to a point near the insertion of the long extensor tendon and the interphalangeal joint. (This anatomic fact is important; if infection follows a toenail ablation, it may extend into this joint.) The lunula produces the middle layer of the nail; the eponychium contributes the thin outermost layer.

Distally, the nail matrix is contiguous with the nail bed. There is germinative potential in the proximal nail fold tissue and in the upper layers of the nail bed as well.[2] These areas may be factors in occasional postoperative recurrent nail growth following attempted toenail ablation.

The toenail gives stability to the distal soft tissue of the toe, which frequently becomes elevated following ablation of the nail. As a new nail grows outward, it often impinges against the soft tissue, leading to nail deformity or an ingrown toenail.

The orientation of the nail matrix cells and the longitudinal grooves of the nail bed result in typical distal growth of the toenail. Injury to the toenail matrix or plate may result in elevation of the nail, detachment, or abnormal growth.

How an Ingrown Toenail Develops

The term "ingrown" toenail is unfortunate, because it implies that the nail edge grows laterally into the adjacent soft tissue. Actually, this tissue becomes inflamed and hypertrophied, and the edge of the toenail impinges on it. When the nail plate penetrates the soft tissue, inflammation and infection frequently follow.

Normally, there is a 0.5- to 1-mm space between the lateral nail fold and the lateral margin of the nail. The nail fold, which is lined with a thin layer of epithelium, is sufficiently wide to avoid irritation from the nail. The space is reduced with trauma, compression from shoes or tight stockings, or other extrinsic pressure. Reactive swelling leads to epithelial hyperplasia and permanent soft-tissue hypertrophy. Finally, the toenail margin cuts into the lateral nail fold, resulting in a foreign-body reaction and secondary infection.

Ingrown toenails may be classified according to the magnitude of inflammation and infection:

- Stage 1—Swelling and erythema along the lateral nail border. The toenail edge may be embedded in the lateral nail fold.

- Stage 2—Increased pain, drainage, development of actual infection.

- Stage 3—Chronic infection, with development of granulation tissue; hypertrophy of the adjacent soft tissue.

Assessment

A detailed family history may reveal nail problems or familial factors. Genetic disorders, especially those associated with collagen abnormalities (e.g., Darier's disease, nail-patella syndrome, and pachyonychia congenita), can cause dermatologic and nail disorders. Trauma and mycotic infection are common causes of toenail abnormalities, but hematologic, endocrine, hepatic, renal, pulmonary, and gastrointestinal disease can also significantly change the texture, shape, color, thickness, or growth rate of the toenail.[3]

Vascular insufficiency may cause conditions other than ingrown toenail (e.g., fungal infections leading to elevation of the toenail). Inspect the foot and leg for signs of other skin abnormalities, such as blisters, ulcers, rashes, and lesions.

An x-ray film of the involved toe is sometimes helpful in evaluating a recurrent toenail infection. X-ray studies may also help in assessing osteomyelitis of the phalanx and, on occasion, in diagnosing a subclinical subungual exostosis.[4] The latter condition may lead to chronic toenail elevation, ulceration, and/or infection.

Conservative Treatment

Prophylactic measures. Loose-fitting stockings and shoes with a roomy toe box may decrease extrinsic pressure on the toenail. Correct toenail trimming may prevent impingement on adjacent soft tissue. Tell patients to cut toenails straight across; trimming nails in a curve down to the lateral margins promotes nail "spikes" and impingement on the adjacent soft tissue.[5]

General measures. Once inflammation or infection has occurred, conservative measures may help alleviate symptoms. Tell patients to decrease activity, such as running and other sports; this may reduce inflammation. Soaking the foot in tepid, soapy water three times daily often reduces erythema. Massaging the inflamed area will promote drainage. Use of a broad-spectrum, first-generation cephalosporin may counter an early infection.

Elevating the nail edge. If the impingement is not severe, you may be able to reduce it by elevating the advancing edge of the toenail, displacing the soft tissue as the nail slowly grows outward.[6] A digital nerve block is usually necessary for the initial procedure in the office.

After the anesthetic has taken effect, tear a wisp of cotton from a cotton-tipped wooden applicator. Break the wooden stick spirally, and use the sharp point to wedge the cotton beneath the edge of the ingrown toenail. Tell patients to paint the inflamed area with alcohol two or three times daily to help resolve the inflammation. Often, they must return to the office for a re-packing, after which they can do this at home.

Emphasize that it may take three months until the toenail grows beyond the lateral toenail fold and that the packing must remain in place for that period. (Obviously, the more the toenail has been cut back, the longer it will take to re-grow.) Instruct patients to soak the toe for 15 minutes every other day, then remove the cotton with fine tweezers and repack it as you have done. Tell them to cut the re-grown nail transversely and to avoid picking and tearing it.

With stage 2 and 3 infections, when the nail plate has penetrated deep into the adjacent soft tissue, excision of the lateral nail margin can quickly alleviate symptoms. Whether a diagonal or longitudinal section of nail has been removed, patients must also be counseled about the technique of elevating the advancing nail edge. Failure to do this guarantees a high rate of recurrence of infection.

Nail debridement. Chronic mycotic infection may result in an elevated and deformed toenail, but it may not need to be removed. Simple debridement, using a hand clipper and power nail sander, may reduce the nail's size. It may be trimmed back to its attachment to the nail matrix and bed. Proper nail care every few months thereafter may be sufficient to avoid pain and subsequent infection.

Surgical Treatment

Triangular excision of the nail. When there is acute inflammation and infection, excision of a triangular segment of the edge of the nail may reduce severe symptoms. After removal of this portion, however, the adjacent soft tissue may hypertrophy and fill the space. As the remaining nail advances distally, it may then impinge on the elevated and thickened lateral and distal soft tissue, leading to recurrent episodes of infection. Thus, the patient must keep the growing edge of the nail elevated with cotton packing, as described above.

Some physicians advocate cutting a V-shaped wedge from the center of the nail, in the belief that this will decrease the lateral soft-tissue impingement. I find that this treatment is largely ineffective.

Nail edge (partial nail plate) avulsion. For patients with chronic bacterial infections (stages 2 and 3) following toenail impingement in the lateral nail fold, a partial nail plate avulsion is indicated. For this, as well as all following procedures, first place a digital anesthetic block and cleanse the toe with an iodine-povidone solution.

Elevate the outer edge of the nail plate by advancing a small Freer's elevator beneath the nail to a level proximal to the cuticle. Using a small bone cutter or scissors, cut the nail edge longitudinally. Remove the narrow nail section with a hemostat. Inspect the lateral nail fold to make sure that no nail remains in it. Cover the toe with a compression gauze dressing.

Give patients an analgesic agent, to be used as needed. Although acute infections usually resolve rapidly after nail edge resection, your preference and/or the severity of the infection will determine the need for a systemic antibiotic. Tell patients to remove the dressing twice daily and soak the foot in a tepid Epsom salt solution (1 tablespoon of Epsom salts per basin of water) to help reduce inflammation. A fresh dressing should be applied after soaking. Once drainage subsides, no dressing is required.

Follow-up care is key to avoiding recurrent infection. As the growing nail advances, patients must keep the nail edge elevated with cotton, as previously described, until it grows past the end of the lateral nail fold. Instruct patients in proper toenail trimming techniques.

Complete nail plate avulsion. In extensive (stage 3) or paronychial infection, a complete nail plate avulsion may be necessary. Although this helps resolve an acute infection, it removes soft-tissue support of the distal phalanx. As the new nail grows, it frequently impinges on the distal soft tissue. Because of the high rate of recurrence following complete toenail avulsion, reserve this procedure for those with severe infections (stages 2 and 3).[7]

After the initial preparations, use a small Freer's elevator to lift the entire nail to a point proximal to the cuticle. Grasp and remove the elevated nail with a hemostat. The initial bleeding is usually controlled with a compression dressing. Aftercare is the same as for partial avulsion.

Tell patients to start tepid soaks in Epsom salt baths after 24 hours to help diminish inflammation. Again, use of antibiotics depends on your preference and the severity of the infection. Patients must change dressings daily until drainage subsides. The toe may be painted with alcohol to diminish drainage. Instruct patients about maintaining elevation of the distal and lateral nail margins for several months during nail re-growth, to prevent recurrent infection.

Complete toenail avulsion has a poor long-term success rate, probably because patients fail to comply with follow-up care. Reported rates of recurrent infection are as high as 86%.[8,9] Both partial and complete toenail avulsion may require further procedures—partial or complete onychectomy (ablation)—to prevent recurrent infection.

Partial Onychectomy

Nail edge ablation (partial onychectomy, or Winograd's procedure[10]) can be performed only after complete resolution of an acute infection.

Following nail edge avulsion, a four- to six-week wait may be required for the infection to subside.

After obtaining anesthesia and cleansing the toe, use a Penrose drain as a tourniquet around the base of the toe. Make an oblique incision at the apex of the nail plate and a longitudinal incision along the lateral nail fold, excising the lateral cuticle and eponychium. Resect the matrix down to the phalanx and laterally to include the nail fold in this region. Some physicians carry the excision just to the distal edge of the lunula, while others (believing there is significant germinative tissue in the nail bed) continue the incision along the lateral nail fold as well. (I carry out the latter procedure.) In other cases, only the proximal and lateral nail matrix in the area of the lunula is resected. Excise all matrix from the cortex of the distal phalanx.

Approximate the skin edges with interrupted sutures, and apply a gauze compression dressing. Have the patient return after 24 hours to have this dressing changed. Although fairly brisk bleeding occurs initially, it usually subsides within 48 hours. Remove the sutures after two or three weeks. Nail re-growth varies following this procedure, but it usually occurs in fewer than 10% of patients.

Complete Onychectomy

In the case of a severe toenail deformity or when significant deformity results from a chronic mycotic infection, a complete toenail ablation (Zadik's procedure [11,12]) may be indicated. If the patient has an acute bacterial infection, avulse the toenail first, and carry out ablation after the infection has subsided. With chronic nail infection or a mycotic infection with deformity, avulsion and ablation may be performed at the same time.

After the usual preparations and placement of a tourniquet, make oblique incisions at each apex of the nail plate. Excise the entire cuticle, eponychium, and proximal nail matrix, extending into the lateral nail folds. Leave the toenail bed in place; its removal would leave a large area deficient of any soft-tissue coverage. Carry out a loose skin closure with interrupted sutures.

Apply a gauze compression dressing, to be changed after 24 hours. The initial brisk bleeding usually subsides in 24 hours. Remove sutures two to three weeks following surgery. After a few days, patients can apply a desiccating agent on the operative area to reduce drainage.

Warn patients that there may be a minor re-growth of nail tissue from germinative tissue along the course of the nail bed. A recurrence rate as high as 30% following complete onychectomy has been reported.[3,8]

This rarely presents a problem, but re-excision occasionally becomes necessary when recurrence is significant.

Phenol Matrixectomy

Surgical ablation can be avoided with an alternative procedure involving use of phenol (carbolic acid).[7] After placing an anesthetic block, partially or completely avulse the affected toenail, as necessary. After partial avulsion, curette the toenail edge.

Spread a protective coat of petroleum jelly on areas adjacent to the exposed matrix, and sponge the matrix dry with cotton swabs. Dip a swab into a fresh 88% phenol solution and make two or three brief applications to the matrix; follow each application with an alcohol rinse to dilute the acid.

Phenol matrixectomy is technically easy and often causes less postoperative pain than the other procedures described.[13] Nevertheless, a high rate of recurrence (from 3% to 20%) has been reported because of difficulty in ablating the proximal and peripheral nail matrix.[4,10]

Syme's Amputation

Occasionally, when a more extensive excision is necessary or a more reliable procedure is desired, a Syme's amputation of the distal phalanx is performed. Following preparation of the toe and application of a tourniquet, make an elliptical incision to excise the nail matrix and bed, the lateral and proximal nail folds and cuticle, and the skin adjacent to the distal phalanx. Then excise the distal half of the distal phalanx; this enables closure of the distal plantar skin to the dorsal skin. Apply a compression gauze dressing, to be changed daily until drainage subsides.

The patient is allowed to walk, wearing a postoperative shoe or a sandal until the swelling subsides. Remove the sutures three weeks after the surgery. In comparison with onychectomy and phenol matrixectomy, Syme's amputation carries a decidedly lower recurrence rate (4% to 12%).[4,10] This quality renders it desirable to many patients, but some (especially women) consider the procedure cosmetically unacceptable.

References

1. Dockery GL. Nails, fundamental conditions and procedures. In: McGlamary ED, ed. *Comprehensive Textbook of Foot Surgery.* Baltimore: Williams & Wilkins; 1987:3-37.

2. Johnson M, Comaish J, Shuster S. Nail is produced by the normal nail bed: a controversy resolved. *Br J Dermatol.* 1991;125:27-29.

3. Coughlin MJ. Toenail abnormalities. In: Mann RA, Coughlin MJ, eds. *Surgery of the Foot and Ankle.* St Louis: Mosby-Year Book Inc; 1993:1033-1071.

4. Coughlin MJ. Abnormalities of the toenail. In: DeLee JC, Drez D, eds. *Orthopaedic Sports Medicine: Principles and Practice.* Philadelphia: WB Saunders Company; 1994:1878-1891.

5. Johnson KA. Ingrown toenails. In: Johnson KA, ed. *Surgery of the Foot and Ankle.* New York: Raven Press; 1989:83-100.

6. Ceh SE, Pettine KA. Treatment of ingrown toenail. *J Musculoskeletal Med.* 1990;7(5):62-82.

7. Mann RA, Coughlin MJ. Toenail abnormalities. In: Mann RA, Coughlin MJ, eds. *Videotextbook of Foot and Ankle Surgery.* St Louis: Medical Video Productions; 1991:56-66.

8. Pettine KA, Cofield RH, Johnson KA, Bussey RM. Ingrown toenail: results of surgical treatment. *Foot Ankle.* 1988;9:130-134.

9. Dixon GL. Treatment of ingrown toenail. *Foot Ankle.* 1983;3:254-260.

10. Winograd AM. A modification in the technique of ingrown nail. *JAMA.* 1929;91:229-230.

11. Murray WR. Onychocryptosis. *Clin Orthop.* 1979;142:96-102.

12. Zadik FR. Obliteration of the nail bed of the great toe without shortening the terminal phalanx. *J Bone Joint Surg.* 1950;32:66-67.

13. Kuwada G. Long-term evaluation of partial and total surgical and phenol matrixectomies. *J Am Podiatr Med Assoc.* 1991;81:33-36.

—by Michael Coughlin

Dr. Coughlin is clinical professor of orthopedic surgery at Oregon Health Sciences University, Portland. He is an orthopedic surgeon in Boise, Idaho, specializing in surgery of the foot and ankle and is a past president of the American Orthopaedic Foot and Ankle Society.

Chapter 18

Onychomycosis

In Brief

Onychomycosis is a particular concern for active people because they're exposed to fungi in locker rooms and because hot, sweaty feet enable the infection to flourish. A thorough physical exam and potassium hydroxide exam of debris from the nail plate can help rule out look-alike conditions and provide information that will guide drug therapy. Treatment with the new generation of onychomycosis medications—itraconazole, fluconazole, and terbinafine hydrochloride—is costly but produces impressive cure rates. Active patients need detailed instruction about preventive measures to avoid recurrence.

At one time, onychomycosis was thought of as a nuisance or a cosmetic problem that affected few people. The infection, now thought to be far more widespread, causes discomfort and embarrassment for millions of people and puts them at risk for such complications as bacterial cellulitis and subungual hematoma.

Before new antifungal medications were developed, healthcare professionals clipped and groomed infected nails, and the infection required long-term treatment. The failure rate was high. Now, however, with a correct diagnosis and the use of effective, albeit expensive, oral antifungal agents, onychomycosis can be cured in up to 90% of patients.

"Diagnosing and Treating Onychomycosis," by Mark P. Seraly, MD with Mark L. Fuerst in *The Physician and Sports Medicine*, Vol. 26, No. 8, August 1998. © 1998 The McGraw-Hill Companies. Reproduced with permission of McGraw-Hill, Inc.

Who is at risk for onychomycosis?

By one estimate, onychomycosis occurs in 8.7% of Americans,[1] but because of underreporting, the prevalence could be as high as 20% to 25% of the population, especially in patients aged 40 to 60. A number of factors contribute to the infection's increasing prevalence. Onychomycosis is more common in older adults because exposure to trauma increases and immunity decreases with age; the infection is rare among children. People with hyperhidrosis of the feet are at increased risk because of moisture and maceration of the skin.

Immune-suppressed people are also at increased risk of acquiring tinea pedis and onychomycosis; this includes those with solid-organ and bone marrow transplants, those who have human immunodeficiency virus (HIV) infection, and those receiving cancer chemotherapy.

Certain activities put patients at risk for fungal nail infection. Footwear that promotes sweaty feet, such as athletic shoes and boots, presents a risk. Walking barefoot in areas of frequent contamination, such as communal showers, swimming pools, and bathing facilities and on hotel carpets, also can lead to infection. Fitness enthusiasts are at risk on both counts.

What medical and psychological problems are associated with onychomycosis?

Older people who have it are at increased risk of infectious bacterial cellulitis from maceration and skin breakdown, because the skin's resistance against such infections decreases with age. Distorted nail plates may also lead to a risk of bacterial infection. Other medical problems associated with onychomycosis are discomfort from thickened nails, subungual hematoma, allergic urticaria, and eczematous dermatitis—also called a dermatophytid eruption. Also, in older patients who have arthritis, distorted nail plates from onychomycosis may exacerbate pain from underlying joint disease by altering gait patterns.

Onychomycosis also has a psychological impact. Patients may avoid fitness centers or swimming pools because they are embarrassed about the appearance of their feet and concerned about spreading the infection.

What are the signs and symptoms of onychomycosis?

Generally, toenail onychomycosis begins as a result of a chronic tinea pedis infection. Most commonly, the fungus migrates under the distal nail plate, causing a nail-bed infection that causes discoloration at the distal end of the plate and subungual debris or scaling that distorts the nail plate. With time and trauma, the plate can become brittle and crumble, which can make activity painful.

What are the clinical variants of onychomycosis?

There are four classic clinical variants.[2] The most common, distal onychomycosis, leads to a subungual infection at the hyponychium, where the nail bed distally attaches to the nail plate. Once the nail bed is altered by onychomycosis, debris caused directly by fungal infection begins to lift the nail plate, altering the natural protective barrier. This can result in mixed infections with bacteria such as pseudomonads or *Proteus* organisms, *Candida* species, and molds such as *Aspergillus* species, *Scopulariopsis brevicaulis*, or *Scytalidium hyalinum*.

The second most common form, white superficial onychomycosis, is often associated with distal onychomycosis. This type generally occurs only when dermatophytes directly invade the dorsal nail. The nail plate becomes white (leukonychia mycotica) and brittle. The toenails are more commonly involved than fingernails.

The third form is proximal subungual onychomycosis. This is the least common variant and is a marker for an HIV infection. The dermatophyte enters the nail plate at the proximal nail fold, creating subungual debris and separating the proximal plate from the nail bed.

The fourth form is *Candida* onychomycosis, which causes onycholysis, or a separation of the nail plate from the nail bed. This infection causes a yellowish white subungual debris and paronychia, or a boggy, red pustular eruption at the lateral nail fold, which is often confused with a bacterial infection. This type of onychomycosis is more common on the fingernails, particularly among those who do work that keeps their hands wet, such as dish washing.

Another variant is total dystrophic onychomycosis, in which all of the nail plates have been destroyed by dermatophyte. This is most commonly seen among patients who have acquired immune deficiency syndrome with CD4 levels below 450.

How do you differentiate onychomycosis from other nail dystrophies?

Approximately 50% of nail plate dystrophies are caused by fungus. The remaining 50% are caused by a variety of disorders. These include inflammatory skin diseases such as psoriasis and lichen planus; bacterial paronychia that mimics onychomycosis; contact dermatitis, particularly among people who use nail cosmetics with nickel, formaldehyde resin, or acrylic monomers; phototoxic reactions (photo-onycholysis) to oral antibiotics such as tetracycline; and anxiety disorders.

Psoriasis of the nail plate can present as dorsal pitting onycholysis and subungual debris. Looking for characteristic psoriatic plaques on the scalp, elbows, knees, and buttocks helps differentiate onychodystrophy from onychomycosis.

Early in the disease course, lichen planus can be confused with onychomycosis, especially among nondermatologists. Lichen planus of the nail plate is associated with nail plate thinning, longitudinal ridge formation, splitting, and matrix scar formation, which produces an "angel wing" deformity. The presence of violaceous flat-topped papules on the wrists or ankles and white lacy lines (Wickham's striae) on the buccal mucosa helps differentiate lichen planus from fungal onychomycosis.

Onychodystrophy from external irritants typically causes an eczematous dermatosis on the skin surrounding the nail plate, which is generally not seen in patients who have onychomycosis. Photo-onycholysis from tetracycline and tetracycline family members is often painful and acute in onset, unlike *Candida* onychomycosis, which is asymptomatic and slowly progressive.

What tests are used to diagnose onychomycosis?

Physicians need to document the fungal infection. The simplest, most cost-effective test is the potassium hydroxide (KOH) examination. Using a small curette or No. 15 scalpel or blade, the examiner removes the crumbly subungual debris, then obtains a sample of the scale by firmly scraping the undersurface of the affected nail plate, cutting as close to the leading edge of the infection as possible. It is important to obtain a deep specimen.

The scales are placed on a slide with one drop of 10% to 20% KOH solution for 30 minutes. A variety of KOH preparations with and without dyes are available and can demonstrate the presence of hyphae by direct microscopy. Hyphae with a "boxcar" appearance confirm dermatophyte onychomycosis.

Based on recent epidemiologic data[3,4] more than 90% of the fungi that cause onychomycosis are dermatophytes, such as *Trichophyton*, *Epidermophyton*, and *Microsporum*. The most common one is *Trichophyton rubrum*. About 8% of cases are caused by nondermatophyte molds, and less than 0.07% are caused by yeast (*Candida albicans*).

132

A positive KOH test determines that the patient's onychodystrophy is caused by a fungal organism, and no follow-up culture is necessary unless it is required by the patient's insurance provider for reimbursement. If the KOH test is negative, a nail culture is performed to help identify the genus and species of the invading pathogen, which will help guide treatment decisions. Nail cultures help the clinician distinguish dermatophyte-induced onychomycosis from yeast and nondermatophyte-related onychomycosis. This information can be helpful when selecting the most appropriate oral antifungal agent. Nail plate cultures fail to isolate the pathogen in up to 30% of cases. Therefore, if the culture is negative but onychomycosis is strongly suspected, a second culture should be performed. If the second culture is negative and the clinical suspicion is still high, consider doing a nail plate biopsy.

How do you treat onychomycosis?

Two traditional therapies—griseofulvin and ketoconazole—are no longer used because of poor success rates, ranging from 15% to 30% for infected toenails. The two medications (particularly ketoconazole) carry the potential for significant toxicity and are expensive—patients who have toenail onychomycosis require 10 to 18 months of daily therapy for a complete cure.

Currently, three newer oral antifungals—itraconazole, terbinafine hydrochloride, and fluconazole—are suggested All three are safe and effective. Both itraconazole and terbinafine bind to the keratin in the nail plate, itraconazole for nine months and terbinafine for two to four months. In contrast, fluconazole levels drop quickly because the drug does not bind well to lipids or keratin. Patients generally need to be on fluconazole longer than the other two medications, usually until there is complete clinical and onychomycologic cure, which may take 10 to 18 months.

It takes a full month for skin cells to turn over. That is why athlete's foot treatments generally require about one month of antifungal creams. Onychomycosis treatment generally takes longer, and can be slower in patients who have poor peripheral circulation.

Itraconazole. Itraconazole has a broad spectrum of activity, being effective against dermatophytes, *Candida*, and nondermatophyte molds.[5] Typical therapy involves 200 mg of itraconazole daily for 12 weeks, or it can be given as pulsed therapy: 400 mg daily for seven days with a three-week medication break. Treatment is repeated twice for a total of three pulses for toenails and repeated once for a total of two pulses for fingernails. An efficacy study[6] of three months of itraconazole pulse therapy with follow-up at 12 months showed that the drug was effective in the treatment of toenail onychomycosis with complete cure in 64% of patients, marked improvement in 88%, and mycologic cure in 64%.

Used alone, itraconazole is not cardiotoxic, but its use with astemizole, terfenadine, or cisapride can cause high plasma levels of these agents and can cause cardiotoxicity and life-threatening arrhythmias. Other drug interactions are possible when itraconazole is taken with cyclosporine, tacrolimus, digoxin, lovastatin, simvastatin, phenytoin, rifampin, H2 blockers, didanosine, isoniazid, midazolam hydrochloride, triazolam, or diazepam. Itraconazole should be used cautiously in patients who are on sulfonylureas or warfarin.

The most common side effects include elevated liver enzymes, nausea, and rash.

Terbinafine hydrochloride. Terbinafine, shown in clinical studies to be active against *T. rubrum* and *T. mentagrophytes*, is prescribed at 250 mg daily for 12 weeks. In efficacy studies[7-10] of terbinafine 250 mg/d for 12 weeks, between 50% and 74% of patients were completely cured, 71% to 100% had marked improvement, and 76% to 88% were mycologically cured.

There are no major drug interaction concerns with terbinafine and no known interactions that are even clinically significant. Because of this, and because this agent is fungicidal, does not activate the cytochrome P450 system, and does not have active metabolites, it is the treatment of choice.

The most frequently reported side effects include gastrointestinal symptoms, elevated liver enzymes, rashes, urticaria, pruritus, and taste disturbances. Some patients have experienced severe cutaneous reactions from oral terbinafine, including Stevens Johnson syndrome, toxic epidermal necrolysis, and allergic urticaria.[11]

Fluconazole. Onychomycosis is an off-label indication for fluconazole, which is indicated for treatment of oropharyngeal and esophageal candidiasis, systemic candidal infections, and cryptococcal pneumonia. In addition to dermatophytes, fluconazole has been shown to be effective against *Candida*[12,13] and some molds (*Bipolaris* species and *Rhodotorula rubra*).[13] As an onychomycosis treatment, fluconazole has no generally accepted standard dose, duration of therapy, or recommendation on pulse therapy vs daily therapy against dermatophytes and *Candida*.

A study[14] of fluconazole at 150 mg/wk for three to 12 months showed that six months after stopping therapy, 72% of patients were clinically cured, 87% had marked improvement, and 79% were mycologically cured, with a relapse rate of 11%.

Drug interactions are possible when fluconazole is taken with cisapride, terfenadine, astemizole, phenytoin, rifabutin, rifampin, midazolam, triazolam, or tolbutamide.

The most common side effects of fluconazole include elevated liver enzymes, gastrointestinal complaints, headache, and skin rash.

How do you monitor these patients?

In general, systemic toxicity is uncommon with oral antifungal agents. I order a liver function test (LFT) to screen for hepatotoxicity and bone marrow toxicity. Approximately one in 50,000 to 250,000 patients who are treated for onychomycosis with fluconazole or itraconazole has the potential for serious liver toxicity. With terbinafine, the risk of hepatotoxicity is less. Since some drug interactions can occur, it is important to take a good medication history before initiating oral antifungal therapy.

For itraconazole and terbinafine, I do a baseline liver panel, and repeat this at weeks six and 12 of treatment. For fluconazole, there is no generally accepted recommendation; for most patients, I follow the same protocol as with the other drugs. If LFTs are abnormal at baseline, I do not initiate oral antifungal therapy. If LFTs become abnormal during the course of therapy, I discontinue the oral antifungal agent.

At the baseline exam, I explain the treatment benefits and risks, including side effects such as headache. Once blood is drawn, I nick the proximal border of the infected nail plate with a scalpel to mark the area of infection. At weeks six and 12, I remeasure the distance from the mark to the proximal nail fold adjacent to the cuticle. (Clearing starts where the new nail appears at the proximal nail fold.) I ask about side effects and repeat the blood tests.

I ask patients to return at nine months for re-examination. At that visit, I emphasize maintenance therapy and review prevention measures. If the infection appears to be recurrent, I reculture the nail plate.

Because of the nature of newer oral antifungals, which bind to the nail plate for at least several months, I don't retest the nail plate or nail bed for infection for at least six to nine months after discontinuation of the oral antifungal.

How successful is treatment?

The treatment failure rate is estimated at 10% to 20%. If the patient has a true positive KOH test and takes the medication as prescribed, the medications generally don't fail. There are no long-term data for any of the oral antifungal agents on the duration of cure following clearance of onychomycosis. Patients who comply with preventive measures reduce their chances of reinfection.

What is the role of topical therapy?

Currently, there are no topical therapies for treating onychomycosis. Some agents are being studied, including amorolfine 5% lacquer. In isolated, single-nail-plate disease, it has shown some efficacy.

The only way to cure onychomycosis is to use oral antifungal agents and to prevent reinfection.

What can patients do to speed healing and prevent recurrences?

There is no generally accepted algorithm on preventing reinfection. I suggest that patients use a topical antifungal cream once a week if they have a history of fungal infection of the toes or toenails. Imidazole cream or terbinafine are fine for maintenance, or I suggest using Zeasorb-AF (Stiefel Laboratories, Coral Gables, Florida), which is a superabsorbent powder that contains miconazole. This is particularly good for athletes who sweat because it keeps moisture off the skin and reduces maceration. Antifungal sprays are helpful to use in boots, shoes, and athletic shoes.

Patients should wear thongs in bathing facilities, gyms, locker rooms, and showers and on hotel carpets. Athletes should wear polypropylene socks under white cotton socks to wick moisture away from the skin. Foot powders can be used to absorb moisture and keep skin clean and dry.

Prevention is important because treatment is expensive. One course of antifungal therapy can cost from $450 to $1,000. Health maintenance organizations will generally cover the cost and treatment of onychomycosis, but many require a positive culture and/or documentation of patient discomfort before allowing antifungal treatment.

References

1. Elewski BE, Charif MA: Prevalence of onychomycosis in patients attending a dermatology clinic in northeastern Ohio for other conditions, letter. *Arch Dermatol* 1997;133(9):1172-1173.

2. Zaias N: The Nail in Health and Disease, ed 2. Norwalk, CT, Appleton & Lange, 1990, pp 106-119.

3. Kemna ME, Elewski BE: A U.S. epidemiologic survey of superficial fungal diseases. *J Am Acad Dermatol* 1996;35(4):539-542.

4. Elewski BE: Large-scale epidemiological study of the causal agents of onychomycosis: mycological findings from the Multicenter Onychomycosis Study of Terbinafine, letter. *Arch Dermatol* 1997;133(10):1317-1318.

5. Piérard GE, Arrese JE, De Doncker P: Antifungal activity of itraconazole and terbinafine in human stratum corneum: a comparative study. *J Am Acad Dermatol* 1995;32(3):429-435.

6. De Doncker P, Decroix J, Piérard GE, et al: Antifungal pulse therapy for onychomycosis: a pharmacokinetic and pharmacodynamic investigation of monthly cycles of 1-week pulse therapy with itraconazole. *Arch Dermatol* 1996;132(1):34-41.

7. Arenas R, Dominguez-Cherit J, Fernandez LM: Open randomized comparison of itraconazole versus terbinafine in onychomycosis. *Int J Dermatol* 1995;34(2):138-143.

8. Brautigam M, Nolting S, Schopf RE, et al: Randomised double blind comparison of terbinafine and itraconazole for treatment of toenail tinea infection: Seventh Lamisil German Onychomycosis Study Group. *BMJ* 1995;311(7010):919-922 [published erratum in BMJ 1995;311(7016):1350].

9. Goodfield MJ: Short-duration therapy with terbinafine for dermatophyte onychomycosis: a multicentre trial. *Br J Dermatol* 1992;126(suppl 39):33-35.

10. van der Schroeff JG, Cirkel PK, Crijns MB, et al: A randomized treatment duration-finding study of terbinafine in onychomycosis. *Br J Dermatol* 1992;126(suppl 39):36-39.

11.   Gupta AK, Lynde CW, Lauzon GJ, Mehlmauer MA, et al: Cutaneous adverse effects associated with terbinafine therapy: 10 case reports and a review of the literature. *Br J Dermatol* 1998;138(3):529-532.

12.   Assaf RR, Elewski BE: Intermittent fluconazole dosing in patients with onychomycosis: results of a pilot study. *J Am Acad Dermatol* 1996;35(2 pt 1):216-219.

13.   Smith SW, Sealy DP, Schneider E, et al: An evaluation of the safety and efficacy of fluconazole in the treatment of onychomycosis. *South Med J* 1995;88(12):1217-1220.

14.   Montero-Gei F, Robles-Soto ME, Schlager H: Fluconazole in the treatment of severe onychomycosis. *Int J Dermatol* 1996;35(8):587-588.

— by Mark P. Seraly, MD with Mark L. Fuerst

Dr. Seraly is an assistant professor and director of clinical services in the department of dermatology at the University of Pittsburgh Medical Center in Pittsburgh. Mr. Fuerst is a medical writer in Brooklyn, New York.

Chapter 19

Skin Disorders of the Feet

In Brief

Skin disorders of the foot are common in patients who exercise. Knowing the causes, diagnostic indications, and treatment of seven common skin conditions—friction blisters, calluses, corns, talon noir, tennis toe, plantar warts, and tinea pedis—can help physicians manage these disorders in active patients.

Exercise and sports participation enhance physical and psychological well-being, but often involve wear and tear on the feet that can cause pedal aches and pains and injury. Skin disorders are among the most common sports-related foot problems. If managed improperly, conditions such as friction blisters or tinea pedis can impede regular exercise. Physicians who know how to assess and treat common cutaneous conditions of the feet can help minimize discomfort, speed recovery, and prevent recurrence so patients can continue to be active.

Friction Blisters

The skin is well adapted to a wide range of mechanical trauma. However, mechanical irritation such as sudden, intense friction or repetitive rubbing to which the skin has not adapted can cause cell

"Skin Disorders of the Foot in Active Patients," by Craig G. Burkhart, MD, MSPH, in *The Physician and Sports Medicine*, Vol. 27, No. 2, February 1999. © 1999 The McGraw-Hill Companies. Reproduced with permission of McGraw-Hill, Inc.

necrosis within the epidermis, leading to a separation of the epidermal layers that fills with fluid—the classic friction blister.

Individuals whose feet are prone to friction blisters can minimize blister formation by keeping their feet as dry as possible. Helpful steps include the use of foot powders such as Zeasorb (Stiefel Laboratories, Inc, Oak Hill, New York), frequent changes of socks, wearing acrylic socks[1] or two pairs of socks,[2] and wearing sandals or non-occlusive shoes when not exercising.

Another useful product is moleskin. Cut slightly larger than areas of intense friction or sensitive skin, it can help prevent blister formation. Liquid adhesives such as Mastisol (Ferndale Laboratories, Inc, Ferndale, Michigan) promote adherence of moleskin to the foot. Alternatives to moleskin are the "liquid" bandages such as New Skin (Medtech Laboratories, Inc, Jackson, Wyoming), which dries to form a tough protective covering on the skin.

Once a blister forms, it is sterile as long as it remains intact. Nevertheless, it is prudent to aspirate lesions that are more than 5 mm in circumference.[3] Unroofing the blister is not recommended, since this increases discomfort and the risk of infection. Appropriate bandages, including an antibiotic ointment and either moleskin or gauze, should be applied over the roof of the intact blister.

Footwear should be examined to see if seams or rough areas correspond to the sites of blisters. Placing nonskid cushions or non-slip insoles in the shoe may prevent excessive foot movement during exercise.[4]

Calluses

Calluses are the skin's adaptation to frequent, low-intensity friction. They form through increased cell cohesion, reduced shedding, and a thickening of the outer epidermal layer of dead skin. The resulting indurated areas generally form over bony prominences and have accentuated normal skin lines throughout (Figure 19.1). Calluses are usually not painful and, in fact, can benefit athletes, since the hardened skin protects areas subjected to repeated pressures.

If calluses become painful, treatment should reduce pressure and trauma to the foot. The first step is to make sure shoes fit properly. Shoe inserts that provide cushioning, such as gel insoles or Spenco Polysorb (Spenco Medical Corporation, Waco, Texas) reduce direct pressure to the metatarsals and heels of the feet, diminishing the development of calluses. Using full-sole inserts, however, may require patients to purchase shoes a half size larger than normal to make room for the insert.

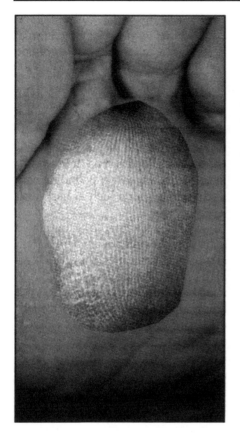

Figure 19.1. A callus over the metatarsals shows characteristically accentuated skin lines. Figure 19.1. Courtesy of Craig G. Burkhart, MD, MSPH.

Treatment can also include softening calluses with keratolytics such as a salicylic acid ointment or lotion (e.g., Pansol—Baker Cummin Dermatological Pharmaceutical, Miami) or a lactic-acid product (e.g., Lac-hydrin—Westwood Pharmaceuticals, Inc, Buffalo).[5] Another effective measure is to soak calluses in warm water and remove the softened keratin with an abrasive such as a pumice stone.[6] For most athletes, however, calluses are normal adaptations to external forces and need not be softened, padded, or scraped.

Corns

There are two types of corns: hard and soft. Hard corns, the more common variety, appear on the lateral surface of the toes and on the plantar surface of the foot overlying the distal metatarsal heads and are typically surrounded by callused skin.[7] They are horny indurations and thickenings of the stratum corneum that form a conical, deep central core pointing toward the dermis. They are surrounded by semiopaque thickening of the dead skin layer that is best seen after the surface keratin is pared (Figure 19.2).

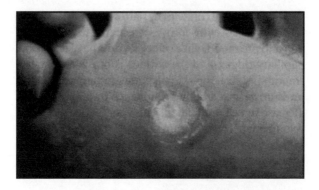

Figure 19.2. *A corn has a semiopaue, glossy center that is revealed when the superficial dead keratin is pared away. Figure 19.2. Courtesy of Craig G. Burkhart, MD, MSPH.*

Soft corns are hyperkeratotic, sodden lesions that occur between the toes, usually between the fourth and fifth digits (Figure19.3). These corns are grayish-white and soft to palpation and have a slightly sour odor. They are caused by the overriding of adjacent phalanges or by the apposition of phalangeal condyles by narrow shoes.

Like calluses, corns form as a response to friction and pressure. Unlike calluses, corns have no papillary ridges, and the surface is burnished smooth because the skin responds to pinpoint pressure against a bony prominence by a rapid increase in cell production. This causes the development of layers of immature cells that never form a competent dead-skin layer as in a callus. Corns are tender on direct pressure.

Factors that contribute to corn formation include structural problems such as osteoarthritis, hammertoe, pes cavus, and hallux valgus. Corns on the dorsa of the toes and on the lateral side of the fifth toe are aggravated by tight-fitting shoes.

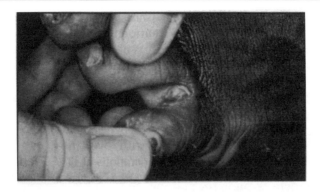

Figure 19.3. *Soft corns usually occur interdigitally, most commonly between the fourth and fifth digits, and are often caused by wearing narrow shoes that pinch the toes. Figure 19.3. Courtesy of Craig G. Burkhart, MD, MSPH.*

The treatment of most corns consists of decreasing the size of the hyperkeratotic growth and relieving or eliminating pressure on the affected area of the foot. Patients can reduce corn size by daily home treatment with over-the-counter preparations of 17% salicylic acid. Once or twice a week, the white, dead superficial tissue should be pared away with a pumice stone, nail file, or other debriding instrument. Patients should be carefully instructed to stop applying the keratolytic agent in the event of irritation or tenderness and to scrape away only nonsensitive tissue.

Paring corns in diabetic patients requires special care, since these patients often have no cutaneous pain in the foot as a result of peripheral vascular and neurologic changes. Debriding of corns in the elderly must also be done carefully to minimize the risk of infection. In both cases, corns should be pared gently after they have been soaked in water.

Pressure can be relieved by placing donut-shaped corn or gel-type pads, cotton balls, or lamb's wool over the corn. In addition, shoes should be sufficiently wide to prevent pinching of the toes or accentuation of pain. Other options include shoe padding or a leather metatarsal bar[6,8] that attaches to the outer sole of the shoe proximal to a painful plantar corn[9] or under the arch of the foot,[6] thereby shifting the body weight off the lesion. As a general rule, however, accommodative orthoses or orthotic shoes work better than metatarsal bars.

143

Talon Noir

Talon noir, or black heel, is an asymptomatic diffuse or speckled bluish-black patch that usually appears as a linear or irregular configuration on the back or side of the heel. It is typically seen in adolescents whose feet pound on hard surfaces in jumping sports such as basketball and volleyball.[10]

The pigmentation is caused by extravasated blood in the upper dermis and epidermis from ruptured superficial capillaries. Shaving the superficial layer of the stratum corneum (Figure 19.4) will demonstrate puncta of pigment and will help rule out plantar warts and acral lentiginous melanoma.[6,11] No treatment is necessary besides reassurance, although the use of a felt heel, gel-type pad,[4,12] or air- or gel-cushioned athletic shoes may eliminate the condition.

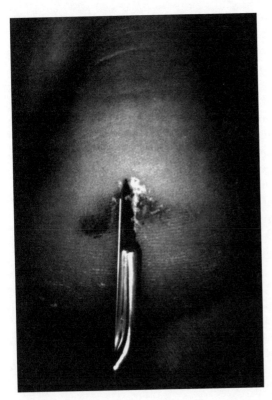

Figure 19.4. Talon Noir can be diagnosed by paring the superficial layer of stratum corneum to demonstrate the puncta of black pigment of extravasated red blood cells from the dermal papilla.. Figure 19.4. Courtesy of Craig G. Burkhart, MD, MSPH.

Tennis or Jogger's Toe

Subungual hematoma of the first and/or second toe is associated with activities such as tennis, squash, jogging, walking, hiking, mountain climbing, and skiing.[4,6,13,14] It occurs when the foot slips and the toes repeatedly jam against the front of the shoe. The resulting hemorrhage can lead to onycholysis and loss of the nail. When swelling is sufficient, pain can be severe enough to limit activity.

In most cases, patients can continue to exercise if the injured toe has adequate room to dorsiflex, which may require cutting a slit in the shoe over the affected toe. In cases of extreme pain, using a heated paper clip or a CO_2 laser, if available, to puncture the nail over a fresh hematoma instantly relieves the pain and may prevent avulsion of the nail. However, this procedure carries the risk of damaging the nail vascular matrix and is rarely necessary,[4,6] since tennis toe usually heals on its own.

Prevention requires properly fitted shoes that allow some forward foot slippage without the jamming of toes—usually about one-half inch between the end of the longest toe and the end of the shoe. Keeping nails properly trimmed, tying laces tightly, and wearing shoes that have a side-to-side strap[4] to reduce forward movement of the foot during exercise can also be helpful.

Tinea Pedis

Fungal infections of the feet are common among athletes and in the general population. Tinea pedis is rare in children under 10, but occurs frequently in adolescents and in males more than females.

Tinea pedis has three clinical forms. Intertriginous involvement of the toe webs is the most common (Figure 19.5). This type appears as a scaly, peeling eruption, with or without erythema, that may develop white maceration and soggy scaliness with fissuring. A second form is the moccasin distribution (Figure 19.6), which affects the entire plantar surface with hyperkeratotic scaling and minimal erythema. The last variant is an acutely inflammatory eruption, with vesicles and bullae, usually located on the midsole of the foot.

The fungi that cause tinea pedis, found in high levels on swimming pool decks and in locker rooms, are ubiquitous. The body's natural immune system allows them to inhabit the skin without infection. However, people have varying degrees of natural immunity to the organisms, and moisture can create an environment conducive to fungal invasion.

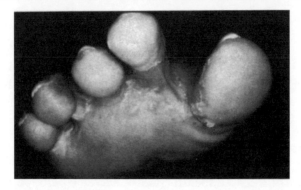

Figure 19.5. Tinea pedis most often occurs inter-digitally as a scaly, peeling, sometimes erythematous eruption. Figure 19.5. Courtesy of Craig G. Burkhart, MD, MSPH.

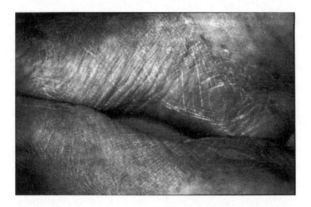

Figure 19.6. The moccasin distribution of tinea pedis, one of the three clinical forms of the infection, involves the entire plantar surface. Figure 19.6. courtesy of Craig G. Burkhart, MD, MSPH.

An essential element of prevention and treatment of fungal infection is keeping the feet dry. Patients should dry between the toes after a shower, apply foot powder daily, change socks if they become moist, wear nonocclusive shoes, and go barefoot when possible.

Treatment also includes the application of antifungal cream in the evenings. The allylamines (terbinafine, naftifine) are slightly superior to the imidazoles (miconazole, econazole, clotrimazole) but are more expensive. However, any of these medications will be effective in most cases. They may be applied a second time during the day, but keeping feet dry with powder usually yields better results.

In stubborn or severe cases, patients should take a 10-day course of oral terbinafine (a 250-mg tablet daily), itraconazole (two 100-mg tablets daily), or griseofulvin (250 mg daily), while continuing to use an antifungal cream.

Prevention and Intervention

Educating our active patients about pedal skin problems is important because many of these conditions can be prevented or minimized. However, when hygienic steps such as keeping the feet dry, wearing properly fitted shoes, and paring calluses or corns are inadequate, physicians need to step in with other measures to limit the effects of these disorders so that patients can remain active.

References

1. Herring KM, Richie DH Jr: Friction blisters and sock fiber composition: a double-blind study. *J Am Podiatr Med Assoc* 1990;80(2):63-71.

2. Basler RS: Skin injuries in sports medicine. *J Am Acad Dermatol* 1989;21(6):1257-1262.

3. Cortese TA Jr, Fukuyama K, Epstein W, et al: Treatment of friction blisters: an experimental study. *Arch Dermatol* 1968;97(6):717-721.

4. Levine N: Cutaneous injuries to the feet with sports participation. *J Dermatol Allergy* 1981;4(6):14-18.

5. Montgomery RM: Tennis and its skin problems. *Cutis* 1977;19(4):480-482.

6. Pharis DB, Teller C, Wolf JE Jr: Cutaneous manifestations of sports participation. *J Am Acad Dermatol* 1997; 36(3 pt 1):448-459.

7. Bart B: Skin problems in athletics. *Minn Med* 1983;66(Apr):239-241.

8. Sheard C: Simple management of plantar clavi. *Cutis* 1992;50(2):138.

9. Montgomery RM, Locascio WV: Padding and devices for foot comfort. *Arch Dermatol* 1966;93(6):739-746.

10. Wilkinson DS: Black heel: a minor hazard of sport. *Cutis* 1977;20(3):393-396.

12. Ganpule M: Pinching trauma in black heel. *Br J Dermatol* 1967;79:654-656.

12. Ayres S Jr, Mihan R: Calcaneal petechiae, letter. *Arch Dermatol* 1972;106(2):262.

13. Gibbs RC: "Tennis toe," letter. *Arch Dermatol* 1973;107(6):918.

14. Scher RK: Jogger's toe. *Int J Dermatol* 1978;17(9):719-720.

15. Jablonska S, Orth G, Obalek S, et al: Cutaneous warts: clinical, histologic, and virologic correlations. *Clin Dermatol* 1985;3(4):71-82.

16. Jablonska S: Warts, in Demis DJ (ed): *Clinical Dermatology*, vol 3. Philadelphia, Lippincott-Raven, 1996, pp 1-20.

17. Dachow-Siwiec E: Technique of cryotherapy. *Clin Dermatol* 1985;3(4):185-188.

— by Craig G. Burkhart, MD, MSPH

Dr. Burkhart is a clinical assistant professor in the Department of Medicine at the Medical College of Ohio in Toledo and at Ohio University College of Osteopathic Medicine in Athens, Ohio.

Chapter 20

Diagnosing and Treating Foot Odor

Foot odor is seldom discussed around the water cooler. But many people suffer from this embarrassing and at times frustrating problem, particularly active people whose feet sweat a lot. Fortunately, foot odor can usually be controlled with simple measures (Table 20.1.)

Odor Origins

Foul feet can often be traced to bacteria. The warm, moist environment inside shoes—especially athletic shoes—promotes bacterial growth on the feet. Two of the most common sources of stench are corynebacteria and micrococci. Successful treatment of foot odor depends on eradicating these organisms. This means that odor-fighting measures like activated-charcoal shoe inserts and foot powders don't get to the root of the problem.

Helpful Home Remedies

Several home remedies can help decrease foot bacteria. The most practical and long-lasting approach to eliminating odor is to avoid the warm, moist conditions required for bacterial growth. Scrub your feet thoroughly when bathing, preferably with an antibacterial soap. After rinsing, dry your feet thoroughly—a blow dryer can help. You can also apply an underarm antiperspirant containing aluminum chlorhydrate or aluminum chloride to your feet. Spray formulas are generally the easiest to apply. It helps to go barefoot or wear socks or sandals by themselves whenever possible, thus allowing air to reach the feet more easily.

Socks should be made of cotton or other absorbent materials, and they should be changed frequently. You can take an extra pair of socks to work or school for changing during the day. Wear socks whenever you wear shoes.

Table 20.1. Foot Odor Treatment at a Glance

Washing

• Wash briskly with antibacterial soap, including between the toes
• Dry skin well (a hair dryer may help)

Footwear

• Wear absorbent socks and change them frequently
• Wear shoes that "breathe"
• Allow shoes to air out at least 24 hours after use
• Over-the-counter products
• Antiperspirants can decrease moisture
• Tea soaks may help
• Benzoyl peroxide 5% or 10% gel applications may decrease bacteria

Prescription Agents

• Drysol (aluminum chloride hexahydrate 20%) at bedtime
• Drionic* device for reducing perspiration
• Erythromycin 2% or clindamycin 1% solution twice a day

When to Consider Other Treatment

• If above measures fail to cure foot odor in a few weeks
• If the odor is accompanied by skin changes

*General Medical Co., 1935 Armacoast Ave., Los Angeles, CA 90025; (310) 820-5881

Shoes that have a noticeable odor are best thrown out if practical, although some can be salvaged by washing with a soapy detergent and bleach. Alternate shoes so that they can air out between uses, at least 24 hours if possible. Look for shoes that "breathe," or ventilate, well, which depends on their construction and materials. Leather usually breathes well, but ask a salesperson about the breathability of specific shoes.

Sweating and odor may be reduced by soaking your feet daily in black tea, which contains tannic acid. One method is to brew two tea bags in one pint of boiling water for 15 minutes. Then add the tea to two quarts of cool water and soak your feet for 20 to 30 minutes. Some people report great improvement after seven to 10 days of daily tea soaks.

Prescription-Strength Relief

If these measures fail to eradicate the odor within a few weeks, it may be time to see a doctor, who can prescribe stronger remedies. One very effective agent is aluminum chloride hexahydrate 20% solution (Drysol). Initially, it should be applied to the feet overnight for three to seven nights, until perspiration is noticeably decreased, and one to three times weekly thereafter. Wrapping the feet with plastic wrap during overnight application aids in effectiveness. Drysol should not be applied to broken or irritated skin because the active ingredient and its alcohol solvent may cause further discomfort. Applying a skin lotion in the morning may minimize the irritating effects of Drysol.

Another method of reducing sweating is the use of electric-current devices. These machines pass a small electrical current through the skin and effectively diminish perspiration. Such devices can stop sweat for several weeks.

Antibiotics applied to the skin are occasionally necessary to cure foot odor if drying measures fail. Erythromycin 2% or clindamycin 1% solutions are effective in killing most odor-producing bacteria on otherwise healthy feet, and they can be applied at morning and bedtime. Alternatively, benzoyl peroxide 5% or 10% gel may be applied in a similar fashion, and unlike erythromycin and clindamycin, it is available without a prescription. Keep in mind, though, that benzoyl peroxide may bleach colored fabrics.

If these measures fail to vanquish foot odor in three to four weeks, or if your skin appears abnormal, you may be dealing with other, possibly more serious, skin problems. Athlete's foot infected by bacteria is common and requires more aggressive treatment, which may include different antibiotics. Pitted keratolysis (care-a-TOL-a-sis) is an innocuous but foul-smelling infection that causes small pits in the weight-bearing areas of the feet in addition to a distinct, pungent odor. Fortunately, it usually responds to the medical treatment described above because pitted keratolysis is caused by the same bacteria that are responsible for most cases of foot odor.

Remember: This information is not intended as a substitute for medical treatment. If you have health concerns, consult a physician.

—by Michael L. Ramsey, MD

Dr. Ramsey is an associate in the Department of Dermatology at Geisinger Medical Center in Danville, Pennsylvania, a fellow of the American College of Dermatology, and an editorial board member of *The Physician and Sportsmedicine.*

Chapter 21

Clawtoes and Hammertoes

Introduction

Clawtoes and hammertoes are a fairly common condition in cultures that wear shoes. In most cases, these problems can be traced to improper SHOES!

Anatomy

The hammertoe deformity usually consists of a hyperflexion deformity of the proximal interphalangeal (PIP) joint. Hyperflexion simply means too much downward bend at the joint. The PIP joint is the joint between the first bone of the toe and the second bone of the toe. Clawing of the lesser toes is a combination of the hammertoe deformity, plus hyperextension of the metatarsal phalangeal (MTP) joint. Hyperextension simply means too much upward bend at the joint. The MTP joint is the joint that makes up the ball of the foot.

Causes

Clawtoes are usually the result of a shoe that is too short. In many people, the second toe is actually longer than the great toe, and if shoes are sized to fit the great toe, the second (and maybe even the third toe) will have to bend to fit into the shoe. Shoes that are pointed make matters even worse. Combine pointed shoes with high heels, and the foot is constantly being pushed downhill into a wall—and the toes are squished like an accordion all the time.

There are nerve problems that can cause the development of clawing of the toes. Some of these conditions are genetic and run in families; some are the result of injury to the nerves that go to the muscles that move the toes. Clawing of the toes develops because the nerve problem leads to a muscle imbalance in the foot. People who have an exceptionally high arch have an increased chance of developing clawtoes as well.

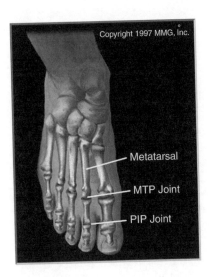

Figure 21.1. The human foot.

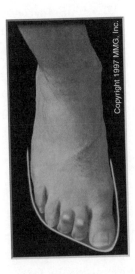

Figure 21.2. Shoe is too short

154

Symptoms

Eventually, toes that are squished day after day become fixed in that position and will not straighten out. When this occurs, pressure builds in three places:

- at the end of the toe
- over the PIP joint
- and under the MTP joint

This causes painful calluses to develop due to pressure from the shoe.

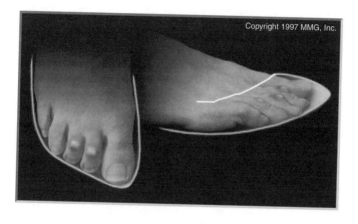

Copyright 1997 MMG, Inc.

Figure 21.3. *Calluses develop.*

Diagnosis

Diagnosis of these two conditions is obvious from the physical exam. In some cases it is important to check to make sure no other nerve problems are to blame for the condition—and special tests may be required.

Treatment

Treatment depends on how far along the process is. Early in the process, simply switching to shoes that fit properly may stop the process and return the toes to a more normal condition. If the condition is more advanced, and the toes will not completely straighten out on their own—a contracture may exist.

Pressure points and calluses caused by the contractures can be treated by switching to shoes which have more room in the toe, or by placing pads over the calluses to relieve the pressure. If all else fails, surgery may be suggested to correct the alignment of the toe.

One of the most common procedures to correct the contracture of the PIP joint in both hammertoe and clawtoe deformities is an arthroplasty of the PIP joint. In this procedure an incision is made over the PIP joint. The end of the proximal phalanx is then removed to shorten the toe and relax the contracture around the joint. The toe is then either held with pins, or sutures, in the straight position until a false joint develops.

If clawing is a problem, then the MTP joint may also have to be released to relieve the contracture of this joint and allow the proximal phalanx to come into the correct position.

After surgery, you will usually be fitted with a post-op shoe. This shoe has a stiff, wooden sole that protects the toes by keeping the foot from bending. The metal pins are usually removed after two or three weeks.

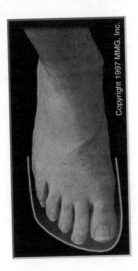

Figure 21.4. Proper shoe fitting.

Chapter 22

Bunions

Introduction

Hallux valgus is a condition which affects the joint at the base of the big toe. The condition is commonly called a bunion. The bunion actually refers to the bump that grows on the side of the first meta-tarsophalangeal (MTP) joint. In reality, the condition is much more complex than a simple bump on the side of the toe. Interestingly, this condition almost never occurs in cultures that do not wear shoes. Pointed shoes, such as high heels and cowboy boots, can contribute to the of hallux valgus. Wide shoes, with plenty of room for the toes, lessen the chances of developing the deformity and help reduce the irritation on the bunion if you already have one.

Anatomy

The term hallux valgus actually describes what happens to the big toe. Hallux is the medical term for big toe, and valgus is an anatomic term that means the deformity goes in a direction away from the mid-line of the body. So, in hallux valgus, the big toe begins to point to-wards the outside of the foot. As this condition grows worse, other changes occur in the foot that make the problem worse. The bone just

---

"Bunion/Hallux Valgus" excerpted from *A Patient's Guide to Foot and Ankle Problems*, from the Orthopaedic Patient Education website at http://www.nyorthopaedics.com. © 1998 Medical Multimedia Group; reprinted with permission.

157

Figure 22.1. Typical bunion.

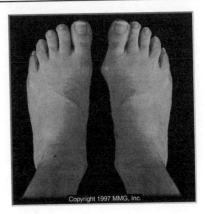

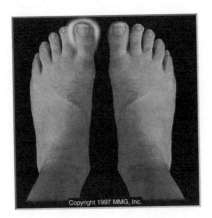

Figure 22.2. Hallux

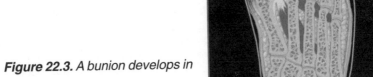

Figure 22.3. A bunion develops in response to pressure.

above the big toe, the first metatarsal, usually develops too much of an angle in the other direction. This condition is called metatarsus primus varus. Metatarsus primus means first metatarsal, and varus is the medical term that the deformity goes in a direction towards the midline of the body. This creates a situation where the first metatarsal and the big toe now form an angle with the point sticking out at the inside edge of the ball of the foot. The bunion that develops is actually a response to the pressure from the shoe on the point of this angle. At first the bump is made up of irritated, swollen tissue that is constantly caught between the shoe and the bone beneath the skin. As time goes on, the constant pressure may cause the bone to thicken as well, creating an even larger lump to rub against the shoe.

Causes

Many problems that occur in the feet are the result of abnormal pressure or rubbing. A simple way of understanding what happens in the foot due to abnormal pressure is to view the foot simply. Our simple model of a foot is made up of hard bone, covered by soft tissue, that we then put a shoe on top of. Most of the symptoms that develop over time are because the skin and soft tissue are caught between the hard bone on the inside and the hard shoe on the outside. Any prominence, or bump, in the bone will make the situation even worse over the bump. Skin responds to constant rubbing and pressure and rubbing by forming a callous. The soft tissues underneath the skin respond to the constant pressure and rubbing by growing thicker. Both the thick callous and the thick soft tissues under the callous are irritated and painful. The answer to decreasing the pain is to remove the pressure. The pressure can be reduced from the outside by changing the pressure from the shoes. The pressure can be reduced from the inside by surgically removing any bony prominence.

Symptoms

The symptoms of hallux valgus usually center around the bunion. The bunion is painful. The severe hallux valgus deformity is also distressing to many, and becomes a cosmetic problem. Finding appropriate shoewear can become difficult, especially for women who desire to be fashionable, but have difficulty tolerating fashionable shoewear. Finally, increasing deformity begins to displace the second toe upward, and may create a situation where the second toe is constantly rubbing on the shoe.

Diagnosis

Diagnosis begins with a careful history and physical examination by your doctor. This will usually include a discussion about shoewear, and the importance of shoes in the and treatment of the condition. X-rays will probably be suggested. This allows your doctor to measure several important angles made by the bones of the feet to help determine the appropriate treatment.

Treatment

Treatment of hallux valgus nearly always starts with adapting the shoewear to fit the foot. In the early stages of hallux valgus, converting from a pointed toe shoe to a wider box toe shoe may arrest the progression of the deformity. The pain that arises from the bunion is due to pressure from the shoe. Treatment focuses on removing the pressure that the shoe exerts on the deformity. Wider shoes reduce the pressure on the bunion. Bunion pads may reduce pressure and rubbing from the shoe. There are also numerous devices, such as toe spacers, that attempt to splint the big toe and reverse the deforming forces.

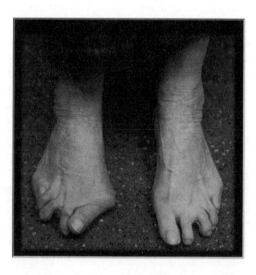

Figure 22.4. Bunions can cause increasing deformity.

If all conservative measures fail to control the symptoms, then surgery may be suggested to treat the hallux valgus condition. There are well over 100 surgical procedures described to treat hallux valgus. The basic considerations in performing any surgical procedure for hallux valgus are:

- to remove the bunion
- to re-align the bones that make up the big toe
- to balance the forces so the deformity does not return

In some very mild cases of bunion formation, surgery may only be required to remove the bump that makes up the bunion. It is more likely that re-alignment of the big toe will also be necessary. The major decision that must be made, is whether or not the metatarsal bone will need to be cut and re-aligned as well. The angle made between the first metatarsal and the second metatarsal is used to make this decision. The normal angle is around 9-10 degrees. If the angle is 13 degrees or more, the metatarsal will probably need to be cut and realigned.

There are two basic techniques used to cut and re-align the first metatarsal. In some cases, the far end of the bone is cut and moved

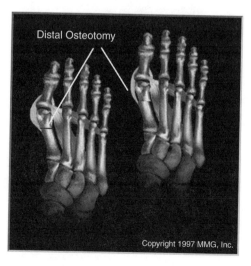

Figure 22.5. *Distal Osteotomy*

laterally (distal osteotomy). This effectively reduces the angle between the first and second metatarsal bones. The bone is held in the desired position with a metal pin. Once the bone heals, the pin is removed.

In other situations, the first metatarsal is cut at the near end of the bone (proximal osteotomy). The bone is re-aligned and held in place with metal pins until it heals. Again, this reduces the angle between the first and second metatarsal bones.

Re-alignment of the big toe is then done by releasing the tight structures on the lateral side of the first MTP joint. This includes the tight joint capsule and the tendon of the adductor hallucis muscle. As you can see, this muscle tends to pull the big toe inward. The toe is realigned and the joint capsule on the medial side of the big toe is tightened to keep the toe straight. Once the surgery is complete, it will take about eight weeks before the bones and soft tissues are healed.

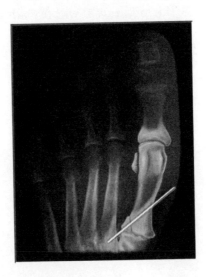

Figure 22.6. Proximal Osteotomy

This material is a resource of the Orthogate Project.

Chapter 23

Burning Feet

If your feet burn and sting almost constantly, you may have a condition called "burning feet." Burning feet are common in people more than 65 years of age. Discomfort ranges from mild irritation to severe pain. The disorder may be temporary. Possible culprits include irritating fabrics, poorly fitted shoes, a fungal infection such as athlete's foot or an encounter with a toxic substance like poison ivy.

The cause often is difficult to pinpoint. Generally it's not serious, but burning feet can signal a significant problem. For example, the following characteristics could suggest a nerve or blood vessel disorder:

- Burning, along with prickling sensation, accompanied by weakness or change of sensation in your legs;
- Burning associated with nausea, diarrhea, loss of urine or bowel control, or impotence;
- Occurrence in family members; and
- Persistence of the condition.

If the condition persists, you may have what's called a peripheral neuropathy (pe-RIF-er-ul nu-ROP-ah-thee). Your peripheral nerves connect your brain and spinal cord (central nervous system) to your sense organs, skin, muscles, glands and internal organs. Peripheral

"Burning Feet: A Common Problem with Many Causes," *Mayo Clinic Health Oasis*, June 5, 1997. © 1999 Mayo Foundation for Medical Education and Research. Reprinted with permission from Mayo Foundation for Medical Education and Research, Rochester, MN 55905.

163

neuropathy refers to damaged or diseased peripheral nerves. If the burning sensation is due to nerve damage, more than 100 causes may underlie the problem. The most common causes are:

- Diabetes mellitus;
- Inherited disorders;
- Poor nutrition due to fad dieting or alcoholism;
- Use of certain medications;
- Exposure to poisons such as arsenic or lead;
- Chronic kidney failure; and
- Liver disease.

In diagnosing this ailment, your physician will first rule out a superficial irritant or a blood vessel disorder; then he or she will consider a nerve disease and its underlying cause. A neurologist may help make the diagnosis. If your doctors can determine the cause, long-term relief is sometimes possible. Restoring an adequate diet may be enough to allow nerves to heal. Peripheral nerves heal, but they heal slowly, and it can take months for symptoms to subside.

Regardless of the cause of your symptoms, here are self-help measures you can try:

- *Socks*—Choose nonirritating socks made of cotton or a blend of cotton and synthetic fibers.

- *Shoes*—Select shoes made from natural materials that breathe. A good fit is important because it helps distribute your body weight evenly. A specially fitted insole also may help. Make sure the insole is in good condition.

- *Activities*—Reduce or eliminate activities that aggravate your condition. For example, avoid standing in one place for long periods. If you must stand still, try to take frequent breaks.

- *Foot bath*—Cool your feet in cold, but not icy, tap water for 15 minutes twice a day.

- *Rest*—Get enough sleep.

- *Relax*—Reduce your level of stress. Stress can aggravate symptoms.

Prescription and over-the-counter analgesics (such as aspirin or acetaminophen) also may provide relief. Although the cause of your burning feet may be difficult to determine, conscientious treatment of your symptoms might lessen the pain and make life more pleasant.

164

Chapter 24

Peripheral Neuropathy

Peripheral neuropathy refers to a variety of disorders that results from injury to the peripheral nerves—an intricate network of nerves that connects the central nervous system (the brain and spinal cord) to the muscles, skin and internal organs. Peripheral nerve damage, which interrupts communication between the brain and other parts of the body, can impair muscle movement, prevent normal sensation in the extremities and cause pain.

Types of Neuropathy

There are many different kinds of peripheral neuropathy with many different causes—from carpal tunnel syndrome (a common repetitive-stress injury) to Guillain-Barré syndrome (a rare, acute paralysis-related disorder).

As a group, peripheral neuropathies are common, especially among people over the age of 55 (3 percent to 4 percent of whom are affected). Neuropathies are typically classified according to the clinical syndrome, or, when known, according to the cause.

Terms used to describe the distribution of the neuropathy include mononeuropathy (in which a single nerve is affected), mononeuropathy multiplex (which involves several isolated nerves) and polyneuropathy (in which a wide range of peripheral nerves are involved symmetrically across the body). Neuropathy can affect motor nerves, sensory nerves or both. In some cases it can affect internal organs, such as the heart, blood vessels, or the bladder and intestines. Neuropathy that affects internal organs is called an autonomic neuropathy.

Development of Neuropathy

In terms of disease development, peripheral neuropathies are divided into acquired neuropathies (caused by environmental agents, diabetes, trauma, infections or other acquired illnesses); the less common hereditary neuropathy (caused by inherited genetic defects); and idiopathic neuropathy (in which no cause can be found). Cases of idiopathic neuropathy comprise as many as one-third of all neuropathies and are classified according to their signs and symptoms.

People with peripheral neuropathies may slowly lose normal use of their feet, hands and, at times, arm and leg muscles as the nerves to their extremities degenerate. Although the disorder is frequently progressive, peripheral neuropathies are rarely fatal, and symptoms can be at least partially controlled with early diagnosis and a comprehensive program of drug treatment and physical therapy.

Symptoms

Symptoms of peripheral neuropathy usually begin gradually and include:

- A tingling sensation in the toes or in the balls of the feet that eventually spreads up the legs toward the trunk. Less commonly, the sensation may begin in the hands and spread up the arms.

- Numbness in the hands and feet that spreads up the arms and legs.

- Weakness or heaviness in muscles throughout the body. This may be accompanied by cramping, especially in the feet, legs and hands.

- Sensitive skin that may be painful to the touch. Prickling, burning, tingling or sharp stabbing sensations may occur spontaneously and usually worsen at night.

- A foot-drop walking gait and/or problems with balance or coordination.

Chapter 25

Morton's Neuroma

What's the Problem?

A neuroma is a swelling or scarring of a small nerve that connects to two of your toes and provides sensation to these toes. The symptoms can come and go depending on activity, shoe style and even, weather. They consist of pain or numbness, usually affecting the third and fourth toes, counting from the big toe. Any action that shifts the body weight onto the front of the foot, such as wearing high heels, climbing stairs and running, can make a neuroma worse. Some doctors will describe a neuroma as a nerve tumor. However, don't worry because neuromas are not cancer and will not spread to other parts of your body. It is an injury to a nerve, that occurs slowly, over a long period of time.

How Does It Feel?

Neuromas frequently start as a numbness or tenderness in the ball of the foot. This is the area just behind the base of the toes. As the swelling increases, pain and strange sensations such as numbness, burning and tingling in the area can radiate out into the toes or back into the foot. The area may be hot or very swollen and, just as mysteriously, the symptoms can disappear and reappear. At first, the pain

"Morton's Neuroma—Intermetatarsal Neuroma," by Drew A. Harris, DPM, MPH, from the Podiatry Online website at http://www.footdoc.com, © 2000 Drew A. Harris; reprinted with permission.

is only present when weight bearing in tight shoes. As it gets worse, spontaneous shooting pains, often like electric shocks, can be felt even when you're off your feet.

Let's Do a Test!

Your doctor will make the diagnosis relying on your history and description of the problem and the physical examination. There is a simple test to find a neuroma. The doctor will squeeze the area between the bases of the toes to see if it is sensitive. If a neuroma is present, the doctor, and sometimes you, will feel a "click", as the soft neuroma mass squishes out between the long metatarsal bones. You may feel the pain shooting out into your toes or back into the foot. This is called a Mulder's Sign, and is the diagnostic sign of the presence of Morton's Neuroma.

Finally, the doctor will do an x-ray to see if there are any other problems present. The nerve and neuroma are soft tissue and don't show on a standard x-ray. However, the doctor can tell if the metatarsals are close together and if the toes are spread apart—both signs of a neuroma. If the diagnosis is at all unclear, a soft tissue imaging technique called an MRI (magnetic resonance imaging) may be done to actually see the neuroma mass.

How Did This Happen?

To understand why neuromas develop, it is important to know how the nerves connect to the toes. The nerve that carries sensation signals back from the toes starts in the midfoot between the metatarsals. The nerve passes beneath a strong ligament, or soft-tissue band, that holds the metatarsal heads together. Just after it passes this band, it splits in half forming a Y. Each half then connects to the adjacent sides of the two toes.

The neuroma usually develops just under or beyond the tight ligament. Why? Well, imagine that the nerve is the bow of a violin and the tight ligament is the string. The constant pulling of nerve over the ligament irritates the nerve and causes the nerve to thicken and scar. The nerve also can get pinched between the two metatarsal bones that it passes between. A scarred nerve doesn't carry signals well and may send back strange signals to the brain such as burning, pain and tingling. So, instead of beautiful music, we get terrible noise.

Anything that stretches and pulls the nerve will aggravate the condition. For instance, wearing high heels aggravates neuromas in three ways. First, the higher heel will push the toes up from the rest of the foot and cause the nerve to tighten and pull harder against the tight ligament. Second, the tight toebox squeezes the front of the foot together leaving less space between the metatarsal bones for the nerve to rest. Finally, the body weight is put more on the ball of the foot increasing the pressure on the nerve. All three are bad news for you and your neuroma.

What Can I Do for It?

The most significant help that you can give yourself to lessen the pain and allow the injured nerve to heal is to avoid tight, short or pointed shoes. If the metatarsal bones are allowed to splay or spread out naturally, as when you're barefoot, many neuromas will get better on their own. An oral anti-inflammatory medicine like ibuprofen, naproxin sodium or aspirin can help. The application of moist heat can help.

What Will My Doctor Do for It?

If the home remedies do not relieve your pain or if you have suffered several episodes, see your doctor for care. After the diagnosis is made, the doctor may apply special padding to the foot to take the pressure off the area. An injection of an anti-inflammatory medicine (cortisone) mixed with numbing medicine (xylocaine) may be put into the area surrounding the nerve to calm it down. The doctor may also prescribe a prescription anti-inflammatory medication or begin physical therapy treatments, to help the injured nerve to heal.

If these treatments are not effective at calming the neuroma down, the podiatrist may dispense orthotics to help control the abnormal mechanical structure of your foot. By preventing the arch from dropping, the nerve will not be stretched as much.

Finally, if these more conservative treatments don't work, then the faulty nerve may need to be removed or destroyed. This is not as bad as it sounds. This is only a sensory nerve that doesn't control any muscles and only provides sensation to a small area between the toes. The nerve is removed through an incision in the top or bottom of the affected area. The nerve is identified and snipped just behind the swollen part and just beyond where it splits in two. Frequently, the tight ligament between the metatarsal bones is also cut to allow more room. It is a relatively minor procedure with possible complications that include infection, swelling and pain. Rarely, a portion of the remaining nerve may become tender and require additional surgery.

Another procedure involves the destruction of the sensitive nerve through the injection of caustic medications. Either way, the area between the affected toes is likely to remain numb forever. However, this is rarely more than a minor annoyance.

Can I Prevent It from Happening Again?

When the nerve is removed, the pain rarely recurs in that spot. However, it is possible to develop another neuroma between two other toes or in the other foot. This is because the underlying conditions that caused the first one to develop are still present. So, you must be careful about what kinds of shoes you are wearing and the amount of pressure you put on the ball of the foot. If your podiatrist dispensed orthotics, then be sure you are wearing them and get them replaced regularly. Finally, if a new neuroma is developing, seek attention sooner rather than later. Early treatment may help you avoid future surgery.

Chapter 26

Tarsal Tunnel Syndrome

Introduction

Tarsal tunnel syndrome is a condition that occurs from abnormal pressure on the posterior tibial nerve (Figure 26.1). The condition is similar to carpal tunnel syndrome in the wrist. The condition is somewhat uncommon, and can be difficult to diagnose.

Anatomy

The posterior tibial nerve runs into the foot behind the medial malleolus, the bump on the inside of the ankle. As it enters the foot it runs under a band of fibrous tissue called

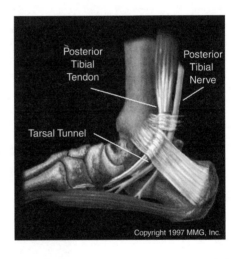

Posterior Tibial Tendon

Posterior Tibial Nerve

Tarsal Tunnel

Copyright 1997 MMG, Inc.

Figure 26.1. Posterior tibial nerve.

the flexor retinaculum (Figure 26.2.). The flexor retinaculum is a dense band of fibrous tissue that forms a sort of tunnel, or tube. Through this tunnel the tendons, the nerve, the artery and the veins that travel to the bottom of the foot are all held together. This tunnel is called the tarsal tunnel. The tarsal tunnel is made up of the bone of the ankle on one side and the thick band of the flexor retinaculum on the other side.

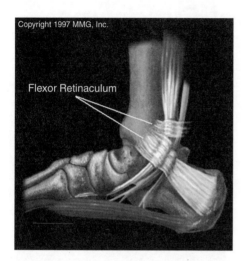

Figure 26. 2. Flexor retinaculum.

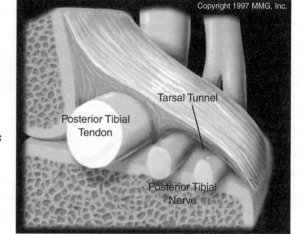

Figure 26.3. Nerve is squeezed.

Causes

Anything which takes up space in the tarsal tunnel will increase the pressure in the area, because the flexor retinaculum cannot stretch very much. As the pressure increases in the tarsal tunnel, the nerve is the most sensitive to the pressure and is squeezed against the flexor retinaculum (Figure 26.3.). This causes dysfunction of the nerve leading to the symptoms of tarsal tunnel syndrome. The term dysfunction means that something isn't working right. In the case of a nerve, this usually means that there is numbness in the area of skin that the nerve would normally supply sensation to. There may also be weakness in the muscles supplied by the nerve, and pain near the area where the nerve is being pinched.

Symptoms

Tarsal tunnel syndrome usually causes a vague pain in the sole of the foot, that most patients describe as a burning or tingling type pain. The symptoms are typically made worse by activity, and are reduced by rest. There may be pain to touch along the course of the nerve as well (Figure 26.4.). If the condition becomes worse, numbness and weakness may occur in the foot.

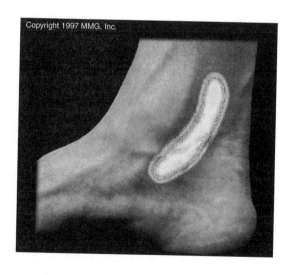

Copyright 1997 MMG, Inc.

Figure 26.4. Course of the nerve.

Diagnosis

The diagnosis of tarsal tunnel syndrome begins with a complete history and physical examination. A Tinel's sign may be present. This is a tingling sensation that shoots electric shocks into the foot when the skin above the nerve is tapped with a finger at the level of the irritation.

If more information is needed to make the diagnosis a nerve conduction velocity (NCV) may be suggested by your doctor. This test measures how fast the nerve impulses travel along a nerve. If the test shows that the impulses are traveling slowly across the ankle, this may confirm a diagnosis of tarsal tunnel syndrome.

Treatment

Treatment for this condition is varied—depending on what may be contributing to the pressure on the nerve. Anti-inflammatory medications and rest may be suggested to control the symptoms initially. If the condition is being aggravated by abnormal position of the foot, then orthotics may be suggested to relieve the stretching of the nerve. A cortisone injection may give temporary relief of symptoms.

If the symptoms fail to respond to conservative treatments, surgery to relieve the pressure on the posterior tibial nerve may be suggested.

Surgery is usually done by making a small incision in the skin behind the medial malleolus, (the small bump on the inside of the ankle), The incision is made along the course of the posterior tibial nerve. The nerve is located and released by cutting the flexor retinaculum. The surgeon will then surgically follow the nerve into the foot, making sure the nerve is free of pressure throughout its course.

This surgery can usually be done as an outpatient. The surgery can be done using a general anesthetic (where you are put to sleep) or some type of regional anesthetic. A regional anesthetic is a type of anesthesia where the nerves going to only a portion of the body are blocked. Injection of medications similar to novacaine are used to block the nerves for several hours. This type of anesthesia could be a spinal block (where the lower half of the body is asleep) or a foot block (where only the foot is asleep).

Following surgery, the skin is repaired with sutures. You will need to keep the incision clean and dry for several days. You will also need to use crutches for several days while the incision heals.

Chapter 27

Clubfoot

Clubfoot or talipes equinovarus is a complex deformity characterized by three distinct manifestations. The foot is in an equinus position; the forefoot and heel are in varus; and the entire foot is
supinated. While the exact etiology of this problem remains unknown,
many advancements have been made in the treatment of clubfeet. The
surgical procedure is progressive and tailored according the severity
of the deformity. Pain management, thorough neurovascular assessments, and education of the family are essential to caring for these
patients.

The purpose of this chapter is to increase knowledge and understanding of congenital idiopathic clubfoot. This educational activity
is designed for nurses and other health care professionals caring for
patients with congenital idiopathic clubfoot and their families.

The history of the clubfoot disorder dates back to the ancient time
of Hippocrates, who was the first to describe the affliction. Since that
time, great strides have been made in the surgical correction of this
deformity. Despite these advances, however, its precise etiology continues to elude even contemporary investigators. This chapter will
discuss what has been traditionally known about clubfoot and the
many theories that have evolved surrounding its etiology. It will also
provide insight into current management and surgical interventions
as well as nursing care guidelines for clubfoot patients.

Reprinted with permission of the publisher, the National Association of Orthopaedic Nurses, Alexander, M., Ackman, J.D., Kuo, K.N. (1999). "Congenital
Idiopathic Clubfoot," *Orthopaedic Nursing* 18(4) 47–59.

Talipes equinovarus, the Latin name for the deformity, became commonly known as clubfoot because the ankle and heel often give the foot a "club-like" appearance. Using a more anatomic description, the disorder is also known as a subluxation of the talocalcaneonavicular joint. The clubfoot is characterized by three separate and distinct deformities required for diagnosis:

- The forefoot and heel are in varus (the forefoot and heel turn inward).
- The foot is in equinus (the foot points downward).
- The entire foot is supinated (the foot is rotated upwards).

In many cases, the foot also has a cavus deformity (high arch). One foot or both feet may be affected. Figure 27.1. shows the typical appearance of clubfeet.

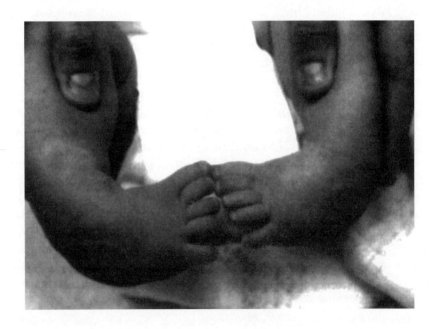

Figure 27.1. Typical appearance of clubfeet.

The incidence of clubfoot in the United States is approximately 1.2 in 1,000 live births. (The incidence varies according to geographic location with the highest incidence being in Polynesia, 6.81 per 1,000 births.)

The incidence of this deformity among offspring of first-degree relatives is 2%, for second-degree relatives 0.61%, and for third-degree relatives 0.2%. The male-to-female ratio is approximately two to one.

In twin studies, if one monozygotic twin has a clubfoot, the second twin has 32.5% chance of having it. If a male child is affected, a subsequent male has a one-in-40 chance; a lesser chance exists if the child is a female.

If a female is born with a clubfoot, a subsequent male has a one-in-16 chance and a subsequent female a one-in-40 chance. This difference between male and female inheritance is due to more of the gene/genes being required for a female to express the deformity than for a male.

If both parents and one child are affected, subsequent siblings have a one-in-four chance. Thus, clubfoot can be inherited on a genetic basis, with the inheritance pattern most likely multifactorial.

The exact etiology of clubfeet is unknown. However, many different theories have arisen regarding causality. Although no agreement exists among investigators, the diversity of these theories provides substantial insight into the development and structural and biochemical components of the clubfoot (see Table 27.1).

Assessment

The assessment of the clubfoot patient begins with a thorough history. Data should be obtained regarding the child's birth, overall health, and development. While most clubfeet are found in otherwise normal children, the condition is known to be associated with many congenital disorders. The history and physical exam should focus not solely on the diagnosis of clubfoot, but also in ruling out any other associated or incidental problems. The clubfoot deformity is often seen in children afflicted with neuromuscular diseases, genetic disorders, arthrogryposis, osteochondrodystrophies, and many syndromes, such as Larsen's syndrome. Once this information is obtained, a complete musculoskeletal exam should follow.

Foot deformities can occur as a result of spinal dysraphism. The spine and reflexes should be examined and tested. Skin pigmentation should be noted along with any masses or lesions on the trunk or along the spine. The child should spontaneously move all four extremities.

Table 27.1. Theories: Causes of Clubfoot; continued on next three pages.

Theory	Source	Description
Mechanical	Hippocrates	Mechanical/environmental factors *in utero* force the foot into equinovarus. Subsequently, as the skeleton grows, the soft tissues contract, forcing the tarsal bones (especially the talus) into malalignment.
	Parker & Shattuck[1] (1884); Nutt[1] (1925)	This theory has been largely disputed because there is not an increased incidence in multiple births, oligohydramnois or other instances where crowding occurs in utero.[2] Also, the deformity exists at a time the embryo is too small to be affected by exogenous factors.[3]
Chromosome	As cited in Simons[4] (1994)	Suggests that the deformity is a result of a genetic defect in the germ cell prior to fertilization.
Developmental Arrest	Hüter[1] (1863); Heneke & Reyher[1] (1874); Schomburg[1] (1900); Bardeen & Lewis[1] (1901); Bohm[5] (1929)	These investigators noted that during embryonic development there are three physiologic positions of the normally developing foot which resemble the clubfoot. They theorized that at one of these points developmental arrest occurred in the affected foot. This theory has been disputed by Gardner[1] (1959), Carroll[1] (1978), and Mau[1] (1927) because the embryonic foot does not have a distortion of the tarsal bones—as does the clubfoot.
Muscle Development	White[1] (1929)	Pressure in utero causes a lesion in the peroneal nerve and creates the deformity.
	Middleton[1] (1934)	Deformity is due to dysplasia of the striated muscle.
	Berchtol & Mossman[1] (1950)	During embryonic development, skeletal growth exceed muscle growth. This results in degeneration of muscle fibers. They shorten and result in deformity.
	Flinchem[1] (1953)	Skeletal changes are due to a muscle imbalance between the strong anterior tibials and the peroneals (which fail to develop).

178

Table 27.1. Theories: Causes of Clubfoot; continued from previous page; continued on next page.

Theory	Source	Description
Primary Germ Plasm	Irani & Sherman[6] (1963)	The germ cell is normal but undergoes a defect at a given point between conception and 12 weeks gestation. This produces a defect in the cartilaginous anlage of the tarsal bones.
Tendon Aberrations	Stewart[7] (1951)	The deformity is caused by abnormal development of the tendons at or near sites of attachment.
	Fried[8] (1959)	The deformity is caused primarily by a tibialis posterior which is thickened and contains fibrotic tissue. It attachments are hypertrophic.
Biochemical Defect	Isaacs, Handelsman & Badenhorst[9] (1977)	These investigators did histological and electron microscope studies of the muscles in clubfeet. Their investigation revealed a loss of microfilaments, abnormal mitochondria, severe loss of filament direction, and almost complete loss of fiber structure. They also noted that there were few sections with increased collagen fibers and suggested that fibrosis is not the primary reason for a clubfoot deformity.
Neuromuscular Defect	Ippolito & Ponseti[10] (1980)	A retraction of the muscle tendon units and soft tissue units creates the deformity. This is believed to be genetically induced.
	Gray & Katz[11] (1981); Handelsman & Badalamente[12] (1981)	The atrophy of the calf suggests a neuromuscular defect. The shortening of the posterior-medial muscles may result from fibrosis. This occurs as a result of faulty innervation, which in turn causes the muscles to degenerate. Their research revealed clubfeet to have a preponderance of type I muscle fibers. (Type I fibers are fast twitch O_2 consuming fibers). Normally the foot has a 1:1 or 2:1 ratio of type I and type II fibers. (Type II are glycogen-consuming, slow-twitch fibers). In the clubfoot the distribution of type I fibers is as high as 86-90%. They conclude clubfoot patients have a type II fiber deficiency. (Fiber type is determined by nerve innervation.)

179

Table 27.1. Theories: Causes of Clubfoot; continued from previous page; continued on next page.

Theory	Source	Description
Biochemical Defect	Zimny, Willig & Roberts[13](1985)	Examined the fascia from the medial aspect and lateral aspects of the clubfoot. They noted the medial aspect contained three cell types:
		• fibroblasts: give rise to collagen
		• myofibroblast-like cells: fibroblasts that have developed some structure and functional characteristics of smooth muscle cells.
		• mast cells: initiate an immune response by the secretion of histamine, which in turn induces contraction of the myofibroblasts in the clubfoot.
Vascular Defect	Hootnick, Packard, Levinsohn, & Wladis[14] (1994)	On the lateral aspect, fibroblast cells produce collagen as a compensatory fibrosis to maintain tissue density.
		Loss of the anterior tibial and dorsalis pedis arteries can sometimes be noted in the clubfoot. This puts the developing foot at risk for deformity as it decreases the routes for developing a collateral circulation. A teratogenic event then may further diminish blood flow and precipitate tissue damage, which in turn interferes with normal development of the foot.

Notes to Table 27.1

1. As cited in Tachdjian, M. (1985). *The child's foot.* Philadelphia: Saunders.

2. Wynne-Davies, R. (1973). *Heritable disorders in orthopaedic practice.* Oxford: Blackwell Scientific Publications.

3. Handelsman, 1963, as cited in Handelsman, J., & Glasser, R. (1994). Muscle pathology in clubfoot and lower motor neuron lesions. In G. Simons (Ed.) *The clubfoot* (pp. 21-31). New York: Springer-Verlag.

Table 27.1. Theories: Causes of Clubfoot; continued from previous three pages.

Notes to Table 27.1, continued.

4. Simons, G. (1994). Etiological theories of C.T.E.V. In G. Simons (Ed.) *The clubfoot* (p. 2). New York: Springer-Verlag.

5. Bohm, M. (1929). The embryologic origin of clubfoot. *The Journal of Bone Surgery*, 11-A, 229.

6. Irani, RN., & Sherman, M.S. (1963). The pathological anatomy of club foot. *The Journal of Bone and Joint Surgery*, 45-A(1), 45-52.

7. Stewart, S. (1951). Clubfoot: Its incidence, cause, and treatment. Anatomical-physiological study. *The Journal of Bone and Joint Surgery*, 33-A, 577.

8. Fried, A. (1959). Recurrent congenital clubfoot. The role of the m. tibialis posterior in etiology and treatment. *The Journal of Bone and Joint Surgery*, 41-A, 243.

9. Isaacs, H., Handelsman, J.E., & Badenhorst, M., et al. (1977). The muscles in clubfoot—A histological, histochemical and electron microscope study. *The Journal of Bone and Joint Surgery*, 59-B, 465.

10. Ippolito, E., & Ponseti, I.V. (1980). Congenital clubfoot in the human fetus: Histological study. *The Journal of Bone and Joint Surgery*, 45-A(1), 45-52.

11. Gray, D.H., & Katz, J.M. (1981). A histochemical study of muscle in clubfoot. *The Journal of Bone and Joint Surgery*, 63-A, 417.

12. Handelsman, J.E., & Badalamente, M.A. (1981). Neuromuscular studies in club foot. *Journal of Pediatric Orthopaedics,* 1, 23.

13. Zimny, M.L., Willig, S.J., Roberts, J.M., et al. (1985). An electron microscopic study of the fascia from the medial and lateral sides of clubfoot. *Journal of Pediatric Orthopaedics*, 5-A, 577.

14. Hootnick, D., Packard, D., Levinsohn, E., & Wladis, A. (1994). A vascular hypothesis for the etiology of clubfoot. In G. Simons (Ed.) *The clubfoot* (pp. 48-59). New York: Springer-Verlag.

The upper extremities should also be examined for complete joint range of motion, any deformity of the hands, or the presence of congenital constriction bands.

A thorough hip exam should be done on every child with a clubfoot. There is an increased incidence of hip dysplasia associated with clubfoot deformities. It is suggested that every child diagnosed with a clubfoot undergo a diagnostic study of both hips by the age of three months.

An ultrasound is the method of choice for infants under three months of age. Radiographs should be done on both hips when the child is three months of age or older. Children with pelvic obliquity, laxity in the hip joint, or any other suspicious findings should be closely watched during the first year of life.

The entire lower extremity should be assessed. Twenty-degree flexion contractures in the knee are normal findings in neonates. Knee range of motion should otherwise be full. Leg lengths should be measured since the affected leg may be congenitally shorter.

Attention can now be focused on the foot deformity. There are two types of clubfoot deformities: postural clubfoot and the true congenital clubfoot. The first task for the examiner is to discern the difference and decide which problem exists.

The postural deformity results from intrauterine positioning. Upon first observation, this foot has the equinovarus deformity; however the deformity is flexible and the foot can be easily manipulated to a straight position. The heel of the foot has normal size and appearance, skin creases are normal, and calf and leg atrophy is minimal or nonexistent. This flexible deformity is easily corrected with serial casting and generally does not require surgery.

The true clubfoot, which will be the focus of this discussion, is a rigid deformity that initially cannot be manually realigned to a normal position. The foot should be examined for the severity of its components: fixed equinus, varus of the ankle, and varus and supination of the forefoot. Also to be noted is whether a cavus deformity exists. The heel of the clubfoot is smaller and drawn upwards. In general, the smaller the heel, the more severe the deformity. Ankle range of motion is limited. The lateral malleolus is tethered to the calcaneus. This prevents rotation of the heel and restricts motion of the ankle.

The skin on the lateral side of the foot appears thin. A deep skin crease lies at the posterior aspect of the ankle joint, and a deep furrow along the foot's medial plantar border. The clubfoot is always smaller than the unaffected foot.

Muscle function can be stimulated by tickling the infant's foot. The clinician should observe for active function of the anterior and posterior tibialis, peroneal muscle, and toe extensors and flexors. The anterior and posterior tibial muscles are contracted but should exhibit active movement. The peroneal muscles, on the other hand, are generally weak, and often motor function is nonexistent.

As mentioned previously, the involved foot and leg are always smaller. Calf atrophy is one trademark of individuals with a clubfoot, as it remains this way throughout life. This atrophy is due to a decrease in muscle fiber size, not to a decrease in the number of fibers. The gastrocsoleus, posterior tibialis, flexor hallucis longus, and flexor digitorum longus are all contracted.

Pathology of the Deformity

To understand the pathoanatomy of the clubfoot requires a knowledge of the bones of the foot and their normal relationships (see Figures 27.2., 27.3., and 27.4.). The deformities noted in the clubfoot are the sequelae of changes in the talocalcaneonavicular joint. In a clubfoot, the joint is displaced in a medial and plantar direction and internally rotated.

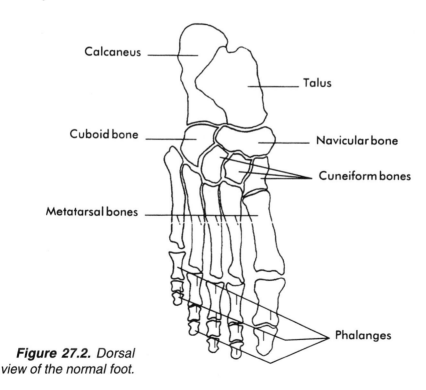

Figure 27.2. Dorsal view of the normal foot.

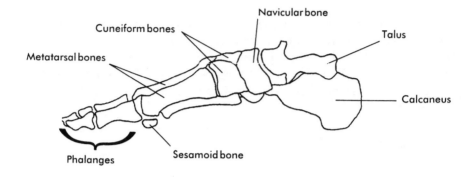

Figure 27.3. *Medial view of the normal foot.*

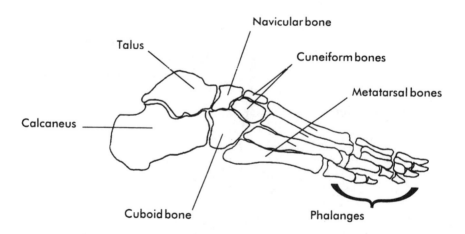

Figure 27.4. *Lateral view of the normal foot.*

A significant aspect of the deformity lies within the talus. As part of the hindfoot, it normally rests on the calcaneus and joins in front with the navicular. It articulates with both medial and lateral malleoli and supports the tibia. The talus consists of three parts: the body, head, and neck. In the clubfoot, the talus assumes an equinus position with its body externally rotated in the ankle mortise (see Figure 27.5).

The head and neck of the talus, however, angulate plantarly and medially. The talus is smaller in size, and its center of ossification may be delayed in appearing.

The calcaneus, also part of the hindfoot, is deformed to a lesser degree than the talus. The calcaneus is the strongest and largest of the tarsal bones and constitutes the heel of the foot. Normally, its long axis is directed forward and outward. In the clubfoot, the calcaneus, also, rests in an equinus position. Its posterior aspect rotates laterally and upward and is tethered to the lateral malleolus. The anterior portion should be lateral to the head of the talus; instead, it rotates medially and downward and lies beneath the talus. The entire hindfoot is then in equinus and varus.

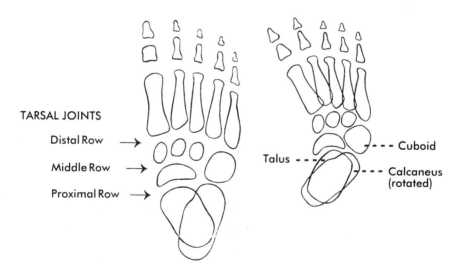

Figure 27.5. Left: *the normal foot.* Right: *A clubfoot. Note the forefoot adduction, displacement of the talanovicular and calcaneocuboid joints and external rotation of the body of the talus.*

The navicular bone is displaced medially on the head of the talus. In the normal foot, the navicular articulates with the head of the talus. In the clubfoot, it is shifted to the medial aspect of the foot; and often the displacement is so extreme that it lies next to the medial malleolus (see Figure 27.5.). While maintaining a normal shape, the navicular in the clubfoot is usually smaller than normal in size.

Changes in the soft tissue are apparent as well. Shortening of the soft tissue occurs at the medial and posterior portions of the foot and ankle. The tendon sheaths encompassing the posterior tibialis and toe flexor tendons are thickened. The capsules of the posterior ankle, subtalar and talonavicular and peroneal tendons are contracted. The talofibular, calcanofibular, deltoid, long and short plantar ligaments, and the bifurcate ligament are all contracted. The cavus deformity is due to tight plantar fascia, abductor hallucis, and flexor digitorum brevis.

Treatment

When the history and physical exam are complete, a thorough explanation of the deformity and its severity should be provided to the infant's parents. The focus can turn to the treatment plan.

The initial treatment for all clubfeet is serial manipulation and casting. Since the bones of the newborn's foot consist mainly of cartilage, and the soft tissues are quite moldable, this procedure should begin a day or two after birth. Manipulation is a gentle and gradual method of elongating the contracted soft tissues.

A long-leg plaster cast is applied during the procedure from the toes up to the midthigh. The toes are left open for neurovascular checks. The clubfoot is gradually corrected by passive stretching while the cast maintains the new position. The casts are removed every one to two weeks, the foot is further manipulated to achieve greater correction, and then the casts are reapplied.

Much time should be spent teaching the family the importance of follow-up visits for the cast to be changed. They will also require detailed information on cast care and neurovascular checks. Each time the casts are changed, the skin should be assessed for any signs of erythema or breakdown.

Manipulation and casting should continue as long as progress is observed up to a three-month period. At that point, there are no longer any gains from continuing this process. At the three-month period, a decision is made as to whether surgery is required and when it will be done.

Criteria for surgery are based not only on clinical assessment but on radiographic findings as well. Abnormal bony alignment indicates the need for surgical intervention. Stress views should be taken when evaluating the clubfoot.

Ordinarily, on the lateral view, lines drawn through the long axis of the talus and the calcaneus should intersect and form a 30-40° angle. The lines should not be parallel. Parallelism of the talus and calcaneus indicates a deformity persists, and surgery is indicated. Likewise, on the anterior/posterior view, the talus and calcaneus should form a divergent angle distally. An overlapping of these two bones indicates abnormal alignment.

The timing of the surgery depends on the child's age and weight, the severity of the deformity, and the surgeon's preference. In general, the accepted time for performing surgery ranges from three months to one year of age. If manipulation and casting are completed and the surgeon chooses to do surgery at a later time, the infant can be placed in an ankle-foot orthosis to maintain correction until surgery is performed.

Soft tissue releases are the only procedures done on the infant's foot. Reduction is accomplished by releasing or elongating the contracted soft tissues at the posterior, medial, lateral, and plantar aspects of the foot. The calcaneofibular ligament and posterior capsule of the ankle joint is released along with the tendon sheaths. The surgery is done sequentially and is a progressive procedure. The surgeon does as many releases as necessary to properly reduce the bones, bringing them into normal alignment without overcorrecting the foot. Table 27.2. outlines the specific anatomic structures that are contracted and may be released during the surgical procedure.

To hold the foot in the corrected position, smooth pins are placed through the talonavicular and sometimes through the talocalcaneal or calcaneocuboid joint. The pins remain in the entire length of time the child is in the cast. One end of the pin remains outside of the foot, facilitating easy removal when the cast is discontinued.

A question commonly asked by the infant's parents is about the location of the surgical incision. The type of incision used is based on the surgeon's preference. Several methods are currently used. These include the Turco incision (along the medial aspect of the foot from the base of the first metatarsal to the Achilles tendon and curved proximally) and the Carroll incision (actually two incisions: the first extends along the medial aspect of the foot, and the second is a longitudinal lateral incision along the Achilles tendon).

Probably the most widely used incision is the Cincinnati incision. This is a transverse incision that extends across the posterior aspect of the foot. It offers several advantages: improved visualization of the anatomic structures, better healing, and minimum scar formation. In addition, the location of the scar is cosmetically appealing.

In the immediate postoperative period, the child is placed in a plaster long-leg cast for approximately six weeks. (The exact length of time for casting may vary.) To prevent wound healing problems, the foot is initially casted in a slight degree of equinus in order to place less stress on the newly stretched skin. A week or two after surgery, the cast is changed and the foot repositioned to neutral. The new cast remains on until it is removed for the final time.

Table 27.2. Structures That Are Contracted and Released during the Surgical Procedure

Releases	Muscles/Fascia	Joint Capsules	Ligaments
Posterior	Achilles tendon	Ankle joint, Subtalar joint	Posterior talofibular ligament, Posterior portion of superficial deltoid ligament
Medial	Posterior tibial tendons, Toe flexors, Abductor hallucis, Knot of Henry	Tibionavacular junction, Medial capsule of subtalar joint	Bifurcate ligament, Spring ligament
Plantar	Plantar fascia, Short toe flexors	Medial calcaneo-cuboid joint	Calcaneonavacular and calcaneocuboidal ligaments
Lateral		Lateral calcaneocuboid joint	Calcaneofibular ligament, Talofibular ligament

188

Complications

The earliest complication of the clubfoot surgery is vascular compromise. It has been reported that a deficiency of the anterior tibial and dorsalis pedis arteries occurs in approximately 90% of clubfeet. These arteries are responsible for the major portion of the blood flow to the dorsum and medial aspect of the foot. Obviously, the clubfoot is then at greater risk for necrosis after surgery should any further disruptions compromise the vascularity of the foot.

Every precaution should be taken to avoid the undue swelling that can put the infant at risk for this serious problem. After surgery, the child's leg should be immediately elevated on a pillow with the child lying on his/her back with the head flat. Often, the infant's legs are taped onto the pillow to help the child maintain elevation. The child's foot/feet should remain elevated for 48 hours when the greatest risk for swelling and neurovascular compromise is over. The patient's neurovascular status should be closely monitored and documented during this period.

Other complications can include excessive bleeding and infection. Parents should also be informed prior to the procedure that additional complications might include wound dehiscence, over-correction of the clubfoot, injury to the neurovascular bundle, loss of reduction, and reoccurrence of the deformity.

Nursing Care

Pain is readily controlled for the first 24 to 48 hours with parenteral morphine. After this period, the child can be switched to an oral narcotic such as acetaminophen with codeine. If irritability persists, one should take into account that the cast(s) and immobilization may be a major portion of the child's discomfort. Infants, however, easily adapt and pain resolves over a few short days. Thus, if irritability is persistent, further investigation is warranted.

Many children have an elevated temperature for the first 48 hours after surgery. Rarely does this require a work-up. After the third day a fever of 101°F or higher may be indicative of a problem. One should keep in mind, however, that infants often have other problems which may be concurrent such as teething, ear or upper respiratory infections, or gastrointestinal problems. These should be ruled out before cutting the cast to examine the incision.

When the child is discharged, parents should be given instructions on cast care, neurovascular assessment, and the signs and symptoms of infection (see Table 27.3.). Parents are often advised not to let the child's legs hang in a dependent position for one week following surgery to prevent further swelling after discharge.

When the final cast and pins are removed, the child is placed in an ankle-foot orthosis for six months to maintain the corrected position. The brace is usually worn over a sock and under a shoe. Parents often inquire what type of shoe the child is required to wear after

Table 27.3. Discharge Instructions for Parents

Potential Problem	Assessment	Intervention
Neurovacsular compromise	Assess toes for color, movement, and capillary refill. • Toes should be pink and warm, and the child should move them while in the cast. • Capillary refill should be less than 2 seconds.	Call doctor or nurse immediately if parents suspect neurovascular compromise. Be sure all 5 toes are visible and not obscured by cast.
Infection	Assess for fever, irritability, listlessness, restlessness, difficulty in sleeping, poor feeding, and foul odor from cast.	Call doctor or nurse if fever is greater than 101°F or other problems persist.
Swelling	Assess for increased swelling of toes.	Keep legs horizontal for 12 weeks following surgery. (Patient does not have to have legs elevated beyond the first 48 hours, but legs should not hang in a vertical position.)
Skin irritation	Assess skin around edges of cast. Also assess skin on back for signs of breakdown.	Moleskin should be applied to cast borders. Sharp edges should be trimmed. Remind parents to assess skin.
Other		Keep cast dry at all times.

clubfoot surgery. There are no special shoes required, and the parents may put the child in any type of shoe they prefer.

Clubfoot surgery should not delay the child's normal growth and development. The foot will continue to grow while casted, and the child will meet the normal developmental milestones at the appropriate time.

Many believe that if the clubfoot is untreated, the child will be unable to walk. Development, however, is controlled by the brain, and when the child is ready to walk, he or she will ambulate regardless of the foot deformity. The child will, unfortunately, walk on the lateral aspect of the foot if not corrected and place pressure on the lateral malleolus. The gait is awkward, painful callus develops, and shoe wear is difficult. Over time, the deformity progressively becomes more rigid, and growth in the foot is hindered.

Parents should be encouraged to promote normal growth and development while the child is in the cast(s). The child can sit up as well as crawl while wearing the cast(s). Parents are encouraged to take the child places and provide the same sensorimotor stimulation as they would normally.

Parents of clubfoot patients are always concerned about the long-term outcome and future implications on the child's lifestyle. They should be informed that the clubfoot and calf will always remain smaller than the normal foot. Lateral skin creases will remain as well. The child, however, will have a straight, plantigrade, functional foot that will allow the child to participate in sports and other physical activities.

Parents should be made aware that there is always a chance that future procedures may be required and the child will require yearly follow-up visits until growth is complete. If the peroneal tendon fails to recover function after the initial surgery, the child may develop a recurrent varus deformity and supinate or toe-in when he/she begins to walk. In this situation, a tendon transfer is required when the child is a few years older.

Other bony procedures may also be necessary for any persistent deformities when the child reaches adolescence. It is important to emphasize to parents that each child's case is different, and the treatment plan and surgical intervention is individualized to meet their child's specific needs.

Working with clubfoot patients and families requires a knowledgeable and skilled team of clinicians that can address both the short-term and long-term physiologic and developmental needs of the child as well as the educational and psychosocial needs of the parents.

Chapter 28

Intoeing (Pigeon Toes)

Many babies are born with feet that turn in. This is called intoeing and is a part of growing up for many toddlers. Intoeing is often the result of the child's position in the uterus. This is usually not a serious problem and corrects itself with time. Some children intoe because there is a temporary twist to the bone in one of the following areas:

The Foot: When the twist is in the foot, it is called metatarsus adductus [met-ah-tar'-sus ah-duk'-tus]. Most cases are mild and correct without treatment in the first several years of life. This condition is most obvious when the child first stands up and bears weight and then starts to walk. A few children require corrective cast treatment. Treatment can also include stretching exercises or wearing a shoe on the wrong foot.

The Shin: When the twist is below the knee, it is called internal tibial torsion [in-ter'-nal tib'-e-al tor'-shun]. The tibia is the shin bone. This is easy to see when the child sleeps face down with the feet turned in.

Both of these conditions (metatarsus adductus and internal tibial torsion) usually improve and often resolve before children start school. Bracing and night splints were used for many years to treat this.

Many of today's adults were treated with a Denis Browne splint when they were young. Braces and splints are uncommon today. Growth and development produce similar results. Correction occurs despite what is sometimes a striking appearance when the child is young. Falling and tripping are normal at this age.

The Thigh: Some children toe in because there is a twist in the thigh, between the hip and the knee. This is called femoral anteversion [fem'-or-al an-te-ver -zhun] or internal femoral torsion [in-ter'-nal fem'-or-al tor'-shun]. Children with this condition find it very easy to sit in the "W" position. We encourage children to avoid this position as it may delay or prevent the normal correction that occurs with growth and development. Sitting with the legs crossed is encouraged, but can be more difficult for these children.

For 50 years, children were placed in braces, splints, twister cables, special shoes and given exercises in an attempt to overcome femoral anteversion. Several excellent research studies have shown that this equipment makes no difference. Such treatment is no longer recommended. Most children show a tendency to improve until the age of eight to 12 years. For the rare case that does not improve, there remains the possibility of correction by an operation. In practice, this is rarely necessary. Surgical correction is not even considered at a young age since most children show complete correction on their own.

In summary: Children with intoeing rarely require orthopedic treatment. Once your child has been evaluated to be certain that no serious condition exists, you can expect improvement with time.

Chapter 29

Helping Children with Genetic Foot Disorders

For the scores of mainstream children that enter your practice, inevitably you'll encounter a young patient with muscular dystrophy, spina bifida or another severe abnormality. While their overall disabling affects have been well documented, many genetic disorders also leave deforming, distressing and often painful foot problems in their wake.

Foot deformities can be inherited by either simple Mendelian genetics, chromosomal abnormalities or, most commonly, polygenetic (multifactorial) inheritance (Table 29.1). Management of pediatric foot deformities focuses on proper shoe gear and orthotic therapy for the milder deformities, and on intensive physical therapy, bracing and surgical correction for the more severe disorders.

Above all, early detection and diagnosis are crucial to effectively managing genetic foot disorders. Podiatrists can play a crucial role either in steering the child toward a normal life, or in reducing the physically challenged child's distress.

The Language of Genetic Disorders

Let's review some basic terminology pertaining to genetic foot disorders. In a genetic disease, the chromosomes or genes figure prominently

"Helping Children with Genetic Foot Disorders—Detection and Management Strategies for Treating Pediatric Patients with Muscular Dystrophy, Spina Bifida or Other Serious Genetic Conditions," in *Podiatry Today,* September 1998, by Ellen Sobel, DPM, PhD, and Renato Giorgini, DPM. © HMP Communications, LLC; reprinted with permission.

195

in its etiology. A genetic disorder often can be passed on to succeeding generations, but this is not always the case. In fact, the more severe the trait or disease, the more likely it will be transmitted by a fresh mutation rather than inherited from the parents.

For example, while achondroplastic dwarfism occurs as an autosomal dominant trait, 80 percent of all cases arise from a fresh mutation with no family history.

Congenital means present at birth. Clubfoot, calcaneovalgus, and metatarsus adductus all are congenital foot deformities. Each abnormality is transmitted by multifactorial inheritance and, therefore, is both congenital and inherited.

A disorder can be congenital and not inherited, however, Phocomelia, a congenital absence or severe shortening of limbs, can be caused by the drug Thalidomide, for example. Also, congenital rubella is caused by a virus passed from the mother to the embryo during gestation. Foot deformities can be classified as malformations or deformations. Although the two terms often are used interchangeably, each has a precise meaning.

A malformation or anomaly is a primary structural abnormality arising from an error in morphogenesis, or a "defect in manufacturing." The genetics of a congenital malformation are determined at fertilization. Malformations caused by chromosomal disorders usually are determined during meiosis of the gametes.

Because malformations usually involve multiple tissues and organs, the podiatrist must look beyond the foot for evidence of disease when either Mendelian genetics or chromosomal aberration causes the etiology. Marfan's syndrome, an autosomal dominant disorder,

Table 29.1. Genetics of Foot Deformities

Autosomal Dominant Mendelian Inheritance	Multi-factorial Inheritance
Polydactyly	Clubfoot
Syndactyly	Metatarsus adductus
Clinodactyly	Calcaneovalgus
Brachydactyly	Hallux valgus
Ectrodactyly	Pes planus
Calcaneonavicular coalition	
Vertical talus	
Idiopathic toe walking	

manifests as a flatfoot secondary to ligamentous laxity, but the disorder also strikes the cardiovascular and skeletal systems and the eyes. An abnormality in the protein fibrillin, which is distributed throughout all affected tissues, causes the disease to affect multiple systems.

A deformation is an alteration in a previously formed structure's shape, a "defect in packaging." Most genetic foot disorders meet this criteria and are transmitted by multifactorial inheritance (Table 29.1). Deformations occur in utero and usually affect a single structure, resulting in localized foot deformities. Common examples include clubfoot, metatarsus adductus and calcaneovalgus.

Fetal constraint inside the womb usually causes congenital deformations that tend to correct spontaneously after birth. This often is the case with calcaneovalgus and metatarsus adductus, both multifactorial genetic positional deformities. Congenital deformities with multifactorial inheritance that do not correct spontaneously after birth—such as clubfoot and congenital dislocated hip—require immediate treatment.

Chromosomal Disorders

The incidence of serious chromosomal anomalies is five per 1,000 births, or .05 percent. The risk to a subsequent child after an older sibling is affected is about one in 400, or .25 percent (Table 29.2). Few chromosome disorders are inherited even though they are genetic in nature, so family history always is negative and the risk of recurrence is minuscule for subsequently born children after a first child is affected.

About 20 recognized chromosomal disorders exist. Down Syndrome, the trisomy of chromosome 21, is the most-common and well-recognized congenital anomaly, occurring once every 700 births. The incidence rises sharply with maternal age. One in 2,500 babies is born with Down Syndrome to women younger than 30. The risk increases to one in 50 for mothers older than 45. After one child in a family is born with Down Syndrome, the risk of recurrence in a second child is about one percent.

Down Syndrome usually is apparent at birth. The pronounced muscle hypotonia and the characteristic facies are the first signs of mental retardation. The disorder's young victims are profoundly retarded, with IQs ranging between 25 and 50. Independent ambulation is delayed by about 1½ years. Children with Down Syndrome become disabled because they cannot wear shoes. The severe hypotonia with ligamentous laxity results in a widely splayed, hyperpronated flat-foot, often with pronounced hallux abductovalgus, making it hard for the child to fit into shoes.

Pes planovalgus is the most common orthopedic problem among children with Down Syndrome. The foot tends to be flexible and asymptomatic during the first two decades of life, and becomes more rigid and painful when the patient reaches his or her 20s.

A wide-soled running sneaker is excellent for the child with this condition. The sneaker should have a removable sock liner so that an additional scaphoid pad can be applied without excessively bulking the shoe. Custom or prefabricated orthoses can be added and are well tolerated by children who still have foot flexibility.

Surgery is indicated for painful bunion deformity when conservative treatment fails.

Table 29.2. Risk to Subsequent Child after First Child Is Affected

Inheritance Pattern	Risk to Second Born
Simple Mendelian inheritance	25%-50%
Multifactorial inheritance	5%
Chromosomal disorders	.25%

Mendelian Inheritance

Classic Mendelian genetics consists of traits inherited in an autosomal dominant, recessive, or sex-linked manner. About one-half of all known single-gene defects are autosomal dominant traits. An autosomal dominant inheritance pattern occurs in idiopathic toe walking, for example. Most musculoskeletal structural anomalies—including polydactyly, syndactyly, ectrodactyly, brachydactyly and other digital deformities—also fall under this category (Table 29.3).

Polydactyly occurs as an isolated autosomal dominant trait. It sometimes is associated with syndactyly and other digital deformities, and can also be a component of several genetic afflictions, including Apert's syndrome, Ellis van Creveld syndrome, and tuberous sclerosis.

The severity of polydactyly varies greatly and is characteristic of dominant genes; this is referred to as expressivity. For example, polydactyly ranges from a rudimentary duplicated digit to total duplication involving the entire metatarsal. This also means that a parent with a relatively minor expression of the trait risks having a child in whom the gene produces a far more severe effect.

Some individuals with polydactyly report that the trait "skips a generation" in their families, or that the condition exists only in "distant cousins." This actually reflects a lack of gene penetrance, another characteristic of autosomal dominant inheritance. This means that the trait is present, but it's barely noticeable in physical appearance.

A certain percentage of individuals who genetically possess a trait will not clinically show it. About two-thirds of those with polydactyly report no family history, indicating a fresh mutation rather than autosomal inheritance.

Digit duplication can become an impediment because in most cases the child cannot wear shoes. If the duplicated digit is fleshy and devoid of bone, it can be tied off in the nursery. The accessory digit should be removed between ages six months to one year, before the child begins to walk.

Amputation of the medial-most toe generally is performed when the first toe is duplicated; the lateral-most toe is amputated in small-toe duplication cases.

Other digital deformities occurring as autosomal dominant traits include:

- Clinodactyly, or curly toes, which is characterized by overlapping toes; the fifth toe frequently is curled over the fourth.

  Treatment consists of passively stretching the involved toes several times per day for children younger than age six. Taping the involved toe to the adjacent digit with nonallergenic tape at bedtime may produce gradual stretching. Six months of conservative therapy is attempted before surgical treatment.

- Ectrodactyly, sometimes called "lobster foot" because of the large cleft between the toes. This rare deformity occurs about once every 90,000 births.

  Although ectrodactyly is a cosmetic heartache, it rarely interferes with function and responds well to surgical foot narrowing.

- Brachydactyly, or short fingers and toes, which results from a localized vascular growth plate disturbance. Treatment generally is unnecessary.

Table 29.3. Genetic Etiologies of Musculoskeletal Disease

Genetic Etiology	Manifestations in the Foot
Autosomal Dominant Mendelian Inheritance	
Acrocephalosyndactyly (Apert's syndrome)	Syndactyly
Achondroplastic dwarfism	Varus ankle deformity
Charcot Marie Tooth disease	Cavus and drop foot
Idiopathic toe walking	Ankle equinus
Marfan's syndrome	Flatfoot
Multiple epiphyseal dysplasia	Varus foot deformities
	Valgus ankle deformity
	Brachydactyly
Multiple hereditary exostosis	Valgus ankle
Myotonic dystrophy	Drop foot
Osteogenesis imperfecta	Pathological fractures
Autosomal Recessive Mendelian Inheritance	
Diastrophic dwarfism	Clubfoot
Friedrich's ataxia	Cavus foot/poor balance
Limb girdle muscular dystrophy	Cavus foot/poor balance
Most inborn errors of metabolism that do not affect musculoskeletal system	None
Sex-Linked Mendelian Inheritance	
Duchenne's muscular dystrophy	Equinus/toe walking
Vitamin D-resistant rickets	None
Chromosomal Anomalies	
Down syndrome—trisomy 21	Flatfoot
Edward's syndrome—trisomy 18	Vertical talus
Patau's syndrome—trisomy 13	Polydactyly
Multifactorial Inheritance	
Congenital dislocated hip adductus	Associated with metatarsus
Excessive femoral anteversion	Associated with intoe gait
Meningomyelocele	Clubfoot, vertical talus, equinus, valgus

- Syndactyly, or fused digits. This problem also is solely cosmetic, and surgical treatment usually is not indicated unless another deformity is present.

- Macrodactyly, or local toe gigantism. This often is associated with neurofibromatosis, which is inherited as an autosomal dominant trait. Treatment involves multiple surgical debulking so that the child can fit into shoes.

Managing Muscular Dystrophy

Duchenne's muscular dystrophy is the most-common genetic sex-linked musculoskeletal system disorder among children, affecting one in 3,500 newborn males. A mutation in a single gene (called the dystrophin gene) found on the short arm of the X chromosome causes the disorder. The dystrophin gene codes for the dystrophin muscle protein normally found in the muscle fiber membrane. The absence or abnormality of the dystrophin muscle protein in human muscle cells results in sex-linked muscular dystrophy.

A positive family history is present in only 65 percent of Duchenne's muscular dystrophy cases; the other 35 percent occurs by a new mutation. The child is born healthy and initially presents with static foot deformities, toe walking and waddling gait. The parents complain that the child falls frequently and has trouble keeping up with other children his age.

All progressive neuromuscular disorders clinically manifest with weakness, atrophy, contracture and deformity. In Duchenne's muscular dystrophy cases, the proximal muscle groups (hip extensors and quadriceps) weaken first. Pseudohypertrophy of the calves then develops as fibrosis and fat replace muscle mass. Foot and ankle instability makes it progressively harder for the youth to stand and walk. Inevitably the child becomes wheelchair bound, usually between ages eight and 12.

Management of related foot problems should begin while the child still can walk, and should be directed toward minimizing contractures. Physical therapy should be performed daily (often with the family's help) to maintain the foot's full range of motion. Use of night splints can help maintain the ankle at 90 degrees to the tibia with the forefoot in neutral rotation. Night splints also minimize progression of equinus contractures and discourage younger patients from placing their feet in the equinus and varus positions, as children typically do while asleep.

201

Braces, which often are indicated for youths with neuromuscular disease, should combine strength and lightness. A vacuum-molded plastic brace with a molded foot plate lined with plastazote is most commonly utilized. If the equinus contractures become significant, serial plaster casting should be attempted to return the foot to a neutral position. Running shoes are excellent to wear with a brace because of their lightness and rubber soles. Younger patients confined to a wheelchair should be fitted for shoes that are soft, non-confining and porous.

Multifactorial Inheritance Defects

Disorders inherited by multi-factorial inheritance are caused by a combination of genes and intrauterine environment. Multi-factorial inheritance accounts for 60 percent of congenital malformation cases. More than 500 multi-factorial genetic disorders, including most common foot defects, are recognized.

Clubfoot deformity ranges from the so-called postural clubfoot to a severe rigid teratologic malformation. The incidence, range of clinical severity and risks of clubfoot recurrence are characteristic of foot deformities inherited by multi-factorial genetics. Congenital clubfoot is among the most-common birth defects, with an incidence of about one in 1,000 live births. The risk of recurrence increases to one in 20 for a second child.

Treatment should begin at birth. The most common non-operative strategy involves gently manipulating or realigning the foot, then applying a series of corrective plaster casts. Serial casting is continued for about six months. If casting does not provide adequate correction, surgery should be performed between ages six months and two years. Bracing and night splints often are necessary for several years to maintain the surgical correction.

Spina bifida is a relatively common yet severe multi-factorial inheritance defect, occurring once every 700 live births. The odds of recurrence in a second child are one in 40. The disorder, which is caused by the neural tube's failure to close, occurs during the fourth week of pregnancy. Spina bifida clinically manifests with lower-extremity paralysis, loss of sensation, and bowel and bladder paralysis. The amount of paralysis depends on the level of the spinal cord lesion.

Most children need braces to substitute for weak, paralyzed muscles. Eighty-five percent of children with spina bifida also suffer with paralytic foot deformities caused by muscle imbalances. Clubfoot and congenital vertical talus are most common among children with spina bifida and casting for these deformities should begin in the nursery. Because clubfoot secondary to spina bifida usually is more severe than isolated clubfoot deformity, serial plaster casting should be started as early as possible. Surgical intervention for either clubfoot or congenital vertical talus is delayed until the child is 12 months to 18 months old.

Equinus deformity is seen primarily in completely paralyzed children. Surgery often is needed to obtain a plantigrade foot—just so that the young patient can sit comfortably in a wheelchair without buildup of pressure areas.

Young spina bifida patients also are prone to lower-extremity sensory deficits and are at increased risk of ulceration and amputation, in much the same way that neuropathy threatens adult diabetic patients. The insensitive foot secondary to spina bifida should be managed in the same way, with periodic sensory testing and use of a protective shoe.

When treating a severely handicapped child, though, medical expertise is only part of the equation. The podiatrist's ability to advise and comfort the young patient's parents is just as important as treating the foot problem. Make it a point to thoroughly explain to Mom and Dad your treatment strategy, and to reassure them at each visit.

Podiatrists can greatly improve the quality of life for a young patient with a genetic disorder—either by correcting a foot deformity and allowing the child to walk away from his or her pain, or by providing comfort to a boy or girl who faces a lifetime of physical challenge. By effectively treating a severely deformed or handicapped child, the podiatrist can perform an invaluable service both to the young patient and to his or her family.

Chapter 30

Structural Deformities of the Foot

The two most prevalent foot deformities encountered in office practice are the flatfoot (pes planus) and the foot with an excessively high arch (pes cavus).

Pes Planus

The flatfoot is difficult to classify; there is no real standard as to how flat is flat. The integrity of the medial plantar ligament (spring ligament) seems to be a primary determining factor in the shape of the longitudinal arch. In 10-20% of the population, this ligament does not tighten and varying degrees of flatfoot develop. Approximately one in 1,000 affected persons will have pain. The asymptomatic flexible flatfoot requires no treatment—except possibly in children, where some controversy still remains. You may need time, however, to convince a demanding patient of this.

At the age of 12-14 months, all children have flat feet. At 24 months, the arch starts to develop, and by five-to-seven years in girls and eight-to-ten years in boys the ligaments are starting to tighten significantly. The appearance of the parents' feet, although often similar, is not a statistically proven determinant of what the child's feet will look like and should not influence management.

Excerpted from "Effective Approaches to Common Foot Complaints," *Patient Care*, March 15, 1997, Vol. 31, No. 5, Pg. 158(16), by Stephen J. Dale, Daniel J. David, and Ted F. Sykes. © 1997 Medical Economics; reprinted with permission of *Patient Care*.

Even older children with pes planus rarely have foot pain. If they do, it is usually in the legs and at night. The pain most often is coming from spasm in the posterior tibial muscle, which has been stretched during daytime play. Parents may be suffering sleepless nights, prompting them to show up in your office for answers.

Massage and warm soaks to the calves help, but if the child is older than four and the symptoms persist, scaphoid pads, inner heel wedges, or soft orthoses lessen or relieve the painful spasms. Some clinicians use this treatment protocol in asymptomatic flatfoot with severe deformity or in obese children. Rigid orthoses should be avoided unless the deformity is neurologic in origin.

Symptomatic flatfoot in a child older than four should be carefully evaluated and treated. Two congenital conditions frequently cause a painful flatfoot in an otherwise healthy child: the peroneal spastic flatfoot that is secondary to a coalition or bony bar between the calcaneus and navicular (sometimes the calcaneus and talus); and the prehallux (accessory navicular) that manifests as a painful prominence over the medial navicular bone.

- **Peroneal spastic flatfoot.** In any painful flatfoot, the heel position, examined with the patient bearing weight and then on tiptoe, is the key to diagnosis and treatment. In the weight-bearing position, normal heel eversion is 5 degrees. On tiptoe, the peroneal spastic flatfoot will show heel eversion greater than 10 degrees that is rigid. In contrast, when the patient has symptomatic flexible flatfoot, the heel will revert to normal inversion on toe standing. Peroneal spastic flatfoot plus a finding of decreased or absent subtalar motion are clues for further work-up. This should include oblique x-rays and possibly tomograms or a CT scan looking for a bony bar.

  When the diagnosis is made, initial treatment should be conservative, with casting for six weeks, followed by an ankle-foot orthosis. This approach affords relief in about 50% of patients, and, more often than not, surgery is not required.

- **Accessory navicular.** In an adolescent with a tender medial bump over the navicular and increasing foot pain, consider the diagnosis of accessory navicular. The pull of the posterior tibial tendon on the abnormal navicular attachment, plus increased rubbing of the shoe on the bump, causes the pain. A bursa over the prominence occasionally contributes to the pain pattern.

Treatment includes early casting and oral NSAIDs. If symptoms do not improve after about three weeks, referral for further treatment, which may include surgery, is indicated.

On occasion, an adult with a previously asymptomatic flexible flatfoot will become symptomatic. The history often includes prolonged weight bearing, changes in work environment, some type of minor trauma, or a sudden weight gain. A dull, achy, diffuse pain develops after two-to-three hours of standing that is relieved by sitting down. With the patient sitting, the arch appears normal, but it flattens on weight bearing and the heel deviates into valgus. With the patient on the toes, the heel reverts to normal varus and examination of the subtalar joint shows normal flexibility. Further examination usually demonstrates a tight heel cord.

Treatment should be conservative, starting with a spacious, comfortable shoe with an adequate arch support and a trial of medial heel wedges to tilt the calcaneus into varus. This alone, or in combination with heel cord stretching exercises if necessary, may be sufficient treatment for most patients. Any modifications inside the shoe should be made gradually, allowing the foot to adapt to change. If symptoms persist, the foot is placed into a University of California Biomechanics Laboratory type insert. Surgical evaluation is a last resort.

Pes Cavus

The cavus foot, because of its multitude of possible deformities, is much more difficult to treat than the flatfoot. Pes cavus varies widely in severity, from a mild, flexible high arch to a rigid, extremely deformed neurologic foot. Symptoms increase with severity but appear early and are resistant to treatment.

More than 65% of patients with a diagnosis of cavus foot have a neurologic lesion. The most common are Charcot-Marie-Tooth disease, followed by myelodysplasia and polio. In idiopathic pes cavus, half of patients have a positive family history and one third have abnormal electromyographic and nerve conduction studies. Most remaining patients have sustained trauma and a postcompartment syndrome, crush injury, or fracture malunion. The clinician's first duty is to establish the classification, which may require referral to a neurologist.

Whatever the cause, the basic problem is muscle imbalance. A dorsal tilt of the calcaneus of more than 30 degrees is seen on a lateral x-ray, and the plantar fascia is extremely thick and prominent. The foot cannot absorb the impact of running without severe pain, which limits repetitive activities such as sports. The foot tires easily and readily forms huge calluses; the patient is susceptible to lateral ankle sprains.

Treatment aims to provide pain relief by maintaining as much of a plantigrade foot as possible to even out pressure distribution. If the foot has potential flexibility, a stretching program is essential. A spacious shoe with a well-molded, flexible fiberglass orthosis is recommended. Custom shoes may be necessary. If a plantigrade foot cannot be maintained and the foot starts collapsing, referral for surgical correction is appropriate.

Part Three

Diseases that Affect the Foot

Chapter 31

The Diabetic Foot: Ulcers and Amputations

Incidence and Prevalence of Ulceration

Ulceration with infection is one of the leading causes of hospitalization for patients with diabetes mellitus. Approximately 15% of all patients with diabetes will develop a foot or leg ulceration at some time during the course of their disease. However, solid data pertaining to the true incidence and prevalence of diabetic foot lesions are still lacking. Some of the information concerning such pathology is based on National Hospital Discharge Survey (NHDS) data, which does not capture the majority of ulcerations treated in the outpatient setting. Population-based and cross-sectional studies provide a general picture of the frequency and distribution of diabetic foot lesions, while case-control (retrospective) and prospective cohort studies are helpful in determining the associated risk factors for these disorders.

The recent comprehensive epidemiologic review by Reiber et. al. indicates that chronic ulcers were present in 2.7% of all diabetes-related hospitalizations and 46% of all hospitalizations listing any ulcer condition. This NHDS data also indicates that the highest rates were found in individuals ages 45 to 64 years, with males having a higher ulcer rate than females. The average length of stay (LOS) for

Used with permission from Frykberg, Robert G., "Epidemiology of the Diabetic Foot: Ulcerations and Amputations," in *Advances in Wound Care: The Journal for Prevention and Healing,* April 1999, Vol. 12. Issue 13, p. 139(1). © Springhouse Corporation.

diabetes discharges with ulcerations was 59% longer than for discharges without ulceration, approximately 14 and 8 days, respectively.

Several population-based studies report an annual incidence of diabetic foot ulceration in the range of 2% to 3% in patients with either Type 1 or Type 2 diabetes, while the prevalence varies between 4% and 10%. A three-year prospective study of diabetic outpatients found an annual foot ulcer incidence of 5.6%, while the prevalence of prior foot lesions was 28%.

Numerous putative risk factors for diabetic foot ulceration have been ascertained. Aside from the major factors of neuropathy, ischemia, pressure (trauma), and infection, multiple other contributory factors interact to produce foot lesions. Intrinsic risk factors include metabolic or biologic characteristics that may or may not be causally related to diabetes but do contribute to the etiology of ulceration. Such factors include duration of diabetes, glycosylated hemoglobin level, peripheral neuropathy, peripheral vascular disease, limited joint mobility, structural deformity, nephropathy, obesity, and impaired visual acuity. Extrinsic risk factors are the result of the patient's interaction with the environment, and they include trauma, abnormal stress, occupational hazards, social considerations, and cigarette smoking.

Amputation Incidence and Risk Factors

Approximately 50% of all non-traumatic lower extremity amputations (LEAs) in the United States occur in people with diabetes. In 1994, there were 67,000 diabetes-related LEA discharges, accounting for 98,400 days of hospital stay, with an average LOS of 14.7 days. This is nearly a two-fold increase in the number of LEAs in 1980, which was reported as 36,000. Between 1990 and 1994, the NHDS rate of diabetes-related LEAs averaged 56,000 per year. Depending on the study, the annual incidence of LEA can range from 37 to 137 per 10,000 people with diabetes, a rate 15 to 40 times higher than that found in individuals without diabetes. The 1994 age-adjusted rate based on hospital discharge data was 82 per 10,000 diabetic persons. Lower level amputations (toe, foot, and ankle) are more common in this population as compared with above-knee amputations, which are more frequent in non-diabetic individuals. Below-knee amputations, comprising 23% of all LEAs, seem to occur with similar frequencies in both populations. LEA rates increased with age, were 1.6 times higher in males than in females, and were 1.2 times higher among African Americans than among Caucasians in 1990. Native Americans have even higher rates of LEAs, reported as three- to four-times higher than in Caucasians. A study of California discharge data from

1991 indicates similar rate distributions between African Americans and Caucasians, but the incidence of diabetes-related LEAs in Latinos was approximately 20% lower than that found in Caucasians. However, diabetes accounted for 83% of all LEAs within the Latino population.

Risk factors for diabetic LEA, based on several types of analytic studies, are quite similar to those for foot ulceration. In fact, foot ulceration itself seems to be a major predisposing risk factor for LEA, preceding approximately 85% of amputations. Most studies indicate that duration of diabetes, level of glucose control, and various measures of neuropathy are independent predictors for amputation, as are blood pressure, retinopathy, nephropathy, and peripheral vascular disease or low TcPO2. Cigarette smoking is an inconsistent risk factor across a variety of study designs.

In their landmark paper, Pecoraro et. al. determined the causal pathways responsible for LEAs in a series of consecutive male diabetic patients. Using the model established by Rothman, the causal sequence was defined by both component and sufficient causes. Component causes are risk factors that are insufficient by themselves to cause the outcome of interest (LEA or ulceration) but are required components of a complete causal pathway that is sufficient to produce the outcome. A sufficient cause, therefore, is a constellation or grouping of the minimal number of specific component causes that, in concert with each other, inevitably produce disease. There can be a number of sufficient causes with various combinations of component causes that produce the same outcome. However, removal of any component cause will block the completed pathway to the sufficient cause and thereby prevent disease through this specific pathway.

Pecoraro found that the particular triad of minor trauma, cutaneous ulceration, and wound healing failure preceded 72% of amputations, often in combination with gangrene and infection. Eighty-four percent of the amputations could in part be attributed to cutaneous ulceration, 81% to faulty wound healing, 81% to initial minor trauma, 46% to ischemia, 55% to gangrene, 59% to infection, and 61% to neuropathy. A pivotal triggering event was identifiable in 86% of the cases that led to the sequence of events completing the causal chain to amputation. Most of the pivotal events were minor trauma that caused ulceration, and most could have been prevented.

Preventing Amputations

Prevention takes on immediate significance when one evaluates the survival data after LEA in diabetic patients. The three- and five-year survival rates are about 50% and 40%, respectively, with the major cause of death being from cardiovascular disease. Following one LEA, there is a 50% incidence of serious contralateral foot lesion within two years and a 50% incidence of contralateral amputation in two to five years. A Swedish study reported only a 27% five-year survival rate after LEA, with a four-fold excess risk of mortality when compared with an age- and sex-matched Swedish population. These authors also found a three-year cumulative additional amputation rate of 48% after an initial diabetic LEA. As all studies suggest, the majority of these amputations could be prevented through programs that are designed to prevent and treat foot ulcers and that recognize the essential role of patient education pertaining to diabetic foot care.

The U.S. Public Health Service estimates that up to 50% of diabetic LEAs can be prevented through aggressive treatment and education programs. The American Diabetes Association (ADA) projects that given an annual incidence of 80 per 10,000 people, 15,000 amputations per year can be prevented should this target be achieved. Aside from morbidity, mortality and disability associated with LEA, the cost savings attendant with prevention programs are quite significant. The total cost of an amputation is estimated to be between $24,000 and $40,000, with approximately $600 million spent on the 54,000 LEAs performed in 1990. If just 15,000 cases per year can be prevented as predicted by the ADA, a cost savings of $360 million could be realized annually. This amounts to 60% of the direct costs for amputations performed in 1990.

Clearly, this tragic outcome of diabetic foot lesions must be adequately addressed and controlled if quality of life is to be improved for the 16 million people in the United States with diabetes. Recognizing both the necessity and morbidity attendant with diabetic LEAs, the United States Department of Health and Human Services has set a goal to reduce the incidence of such procedures by 40% by the year 2000.

— by Robert G. Frykberg, DPM, MPH

Robert G. Frykberg, DPM, MPH, is Clinical Instructor in Surgery, Harvard Medical School and Beth Israel Deaconess Medical Center, Boston, MA. This text is based on his lecture at the 13th Annual Clinical Symposium on Wound Care, in Atlanta, GA.

Chapter 32

Charcot Joints

Charcot arthropathy, or neuropathic arthropathy, is a condition that affects some diabetic patients with peripheral neuropathy (loss of sensation) after eight to 10 years. Jean Martin Charcot was a French physician who in 1868 described neuropathic arthropathy primarily in patients with advanced syphilis. At that time, people with diabetes did not live very long because insulin was unavailable to treat diabetes. Once insulin was available and diabetes treatable, it was in the 1930s that neuropathic arthropathy was recognized in diabetics. It may also occur with several other diseases that affect the sensory nervous system (alcoholism, leprosy, syphilis, Charcot-Marie-Tooth Disease to name a few). In the United States, diabetes is the number-one cause.

So what do all these terms mean?

Neuropathy is a term used to describe problems with the nervous system. In diabetics this is called peripheral neuropathy and affects the sensory nervous system to the peripheral, or farther, points of the body (i.e., feet and hands) causing loss of feeling or numbness. Diabetic neuropathy also involves the autonomic (involuntary) nervous system, which controls regulation of blood vessels and may result in

"Charcot Joints or Neuropathic Arthropathy," excerpted from the American Orthopaedic Foot and Ankle Society (AOFAS) website at http://www.aofas.org. © 1999 AOFAS. Reprinted with permission of the American Orthopedic Foot and Ankle Society.

increased blood flow to the limb, contributing to swelling and osteoporosis of the bones as the Charcot process occurs. Arthropathy is a term used to describe a problem with a joint. Therefore, neuropathic arthropathy is used to describe problems with joints related to lack of nerve system input. It is believed that as the peripheral neuropathy progresses in long-standing diabetes, the joints are unable to recognize the forces put across them and the relative positions of the various joints, sustaining microtrauma or microfractures because the body does not adjust to these forces and positions. It would therefore be reasonable to assume that most cases of neuropathic arthropathy would occur in the lower extremities, with their weight-bearing function. This is indeed the case, although on occasion other joints can be involved.

When does neuropathic arthropathy occur?

Most patients who develop neuropathic arthropathy have peripheral neuropathy after being diabetic about 10 years or longer. So a patient with juvenile-onset diabetes (as a child) may develop this in his 20s or 30s. However, most patients with Charcot arthropathy are in their 40s or older, as more patients have adult-onset diabetes.

What are the signs and symptoms of Charcot arthropathy or neuropathic arthropathy?

There are three stages to Charcot arthropathy. The first stage is a fragmentation or destruction stage. During this stage, as the process begins, the joint and surrounding bone is destroyed. The bone fragments, the joint becomes unstable and in some cases the bone is completely reabsorbed. This stage is clinically identified by significant swelling (often with little pain to the patient) erythema (redness), and warmth or heat to the area. It is easy to see why this is often confused with an infection, especially as there is often no history of injury or trauma. As the bones and joint are affected, fractures and instability develop and the joints can dislocate or shift the bones in relationship to each other. This can lead to severe deformity of the foot and ankle. Often the midfoot joints are affected and the result is a very flat foot which is wide where the normal foot narrows in the arch. Bony prominences often develop on the plantar (bottom) surface of the foot. Diagnosis and early treatment at this stage is important to try to minimize the bone destruction and deformity. This process may last as long as six to 12 months.

The second stage is termed coalescence. During this stage the acute destructive process slows down and the body begins to try and heal itself. The swelling and heat begin to disappear. Once the acute process is resolved and the healing on-going, the third stage begins. This is a consolidation or reconstruction phase during which the bones and joints heal. Unfortunately, the foot is often deformed, and if there has been enough destruction, there may be residual instability. Fitting shoes may be very difficult, and prescription footwear and diabetic orthotics (shoe inserts) are important to help prevent ulcer formation over deformed areas.

How is Charcot arthropathy treated?

Once the diagnosis is made (for most patients in the first stage) there are several important treatment goals. The first is to get the heat and swelling under control. The second is to support or stabilize the foot to minimize deformity. A total-contact cast is applied by trained personnel. This cast has more padding than a standard cast and is often applied with the toes completely covered to prevent foreign objects (gravel, stones, etc.) from getting in the cast. The cast will need to be changed frequently initially as it will get loose very quickly as the swelling is controlled. Once the initial swelling is controlled and the patient is tolerating the casts without skin problems, the cast change interval may be lengthened to two to four weeks.

Another alternative is fabrication of a custom walking boot for diabetics. The foot must be supported until all heat and swelling has resolved. This may occur in several months but more commonly requires six to 12 months. Minimizing weight bearing on the affected foot/ankle is also important. Realistically this is extremely difficult for the patient with diabetic neuropathy and should be encouraged. Assistive aides such as a walker or cast are recommended. During this period the patient will be seen frequently in the office. Continued education about diabetic foot care and Charcot arthropathy is necessary. Also, support of the various stages of anger and denial concerning this rather profound change is necessary. After the first stage is completed, molds for appropriate diabetic footwear, orthotics and braces (if needed) are made. During treatment it is important to check the noninvolved foot and protect it, as that foot is doing much more work.

For patients who develop deformities that are unshoeable or bracable, or who develop unbracable instability, surgery may be considered. The timing for this surgery is important. Surgery done

217

during stage one has a high complication rate, often with fragmentation of any grating done. Sometimes, however, surgery must be done during this stage due to joint instability. Another option for severe deformity/instability is amputation and prosthetic fitting. Patients often have multiple medical problems that must be taken into account in consideration for any surgery.

Long-term management of patients with Charcot arthropathy is important. Once the patient is stable, periodic checkups (six to 12 month intervals) with a qualified foot and ankle specialist is important to identify early complications, address footwear, orthotic and brace issues, and continue patient education regarding the care of diabetic feet and the special needs of the patient with Charcot arthropathy. Patients should be counseled to seek medical care if they develop any redness, selling, or heat in their feet, as this could be the start of another Charcot process.

Chapter 33

Questions and Answers about Gout

This chapter contains general information about gout. It describes what gout is and how it develops. It also explains how gout is diagnosed and treated. At the end is a list of key words to help you understand the terms used. If you have further questions after reading this text, you may wish to discuss them with your doctor.

What is gout?

Gout is one of the most painful rheumatic diseases. It results from deposits of needle-like crystals of uric acid in the connective tissue, joint spaces, or both. These deposits lead to inflammatory arthritis, which causes swelling, redness, heat, pain, and stiffness in the joints. Arthritis is a term that is often used to refer to the more than 100 different rheumatic diseases that affect the joints, muscles, and bones, and may also affect other connective tissues. Gout accounts for about 5 percent of all cases of arthritis. Pseudogout, also a crystal-induced arthritis, is a condition with similar symptoms that results from deposits of calcium pyrophosphate dihydrate crystals in the joints. It is sometimes called calcium pyrophosphate deposition disease, crystal deposition disease, or chondrocalcinosis.

"Questions and Answers about Gout," National Institute of Arthritis and Musculoskeletal and Skin Diseases (NIAMS), January 1999. **Note:** Brand names included in this article are provided as examples only, and their inclusion does not mean that these products are endorsed by the National Institutes of Health or any government agency. Also, if a particular brand name is not mentioned, this does not mean that the product is unsatisfactory.

Uric acid is a substance that results from the breakdown of purines or waste products in the body. Normally, uric acid is dissolved in the blood and passes through the kidneys into the urine, where it is eliminated. If the body increases its production of uric acid or if the kidneys do not eliminate enough uric acid from the body, levels build up (a condition called hyperuricemia). Hyperuricemia may also result when a person eats too many high-purine foods, such as liver, dried beans and peas, anchovies, and gravies. Hyperuricemia is not a disease and by itself is not dangerous. However, if excess uric acid crystals form as a result of hyperuricemia, gout can develop. The excess crystals build up in the joint spaces, causing inflammation. Deposits of uric acid, called tophi, can appear as lumps under the skin around the joints and at the rim of the ear. In addition, uric acid crystals can also collect in the kidneys and cause kidney stones.

For many people, gout initially affects the joints in the big toe, a condition called podagra. Sometime during the course of the disease, gout will affect the big toe in about 75 percent of patients. Gout can also affect the instep, ankles, heels, knees, wrists, fingers, and elbows. The disease can progress through four stages:

- **Asymptomatic (without symptoms) hyperuricemia**—In this stage, a person has elevated levels of uric acid in the blood but no other symptoms. The tendency to develop gout, however, is present. A person in this stage does not usually require treatment.

- **Acute gout, or acute gouty arthritis**—In this stage, hyperuricemia has caused the deposit of uric acid crystals in joint spaces. This leads to a sudden onset of intense pain and swelling in the joints, which may also be warm and very tender. An acute attack commonly occurs at night and can be triggered by stressful events, alcohol or drugs, or another acute illness. Early attacks usually subside within three to 10 days, even without treatment, and the next attack may not occur for months or even years. Over time, however, attacks can last longer and occur more frequently.

- **Interval or intercritical gout**—This is the period between acute attacks. In this stage, a person does not have any symptoms and has normal joint function.

- **Chronic tophaceous gout**—This is the most disabling stage of gout and usually develops over a long period, such as 10 years. In this stage, the disease has caused permanent damage to the affected joints and sometimes to the kidneys. With proper treatment, most people with gout do not progress to this advanced stage.

What causes gout?

A number of risk factors are related to the development of hyperuricemia and gout:

- Genetics may play a role in determining a person's risk, since six to 18 percent of people with gout have a family history of the disease.

- Being overweight increases the risk of developing hyperuricemia and gout because excessive food intake increases the body's production of uric acid.

- Excessive use of alcohol can lead to hyperuricemia because it interferes with the removal of uric acid from the body.

- Eating too many foods that are rich in purines can cause or aggravate gout.

- An enzyme defect that interferes with the way the body breaks down purines causes gout in a small number of people.

- Exposure to lead in the environment can cause gout.

Some people are at risk for high levels of uric acid in body fluids because of certain medicines they take or other conditions they may have. For example, the following types of medicines can lead to hyperuricemia because they reduce the body's ability to remove uric acid:

- Diuretics, which decrease the amount of uric acid passed in the urine. Many people take diuretics for hypertension, edema, or cardiovascular disease.

- Salicylates, or medicines made from salicylic acid, such as aspirin.

- The vitamin niacin, also called nicotinic acid.

- Cyclosporine, a medicine used to control the body's rejection of transplanted organs.

- Levodopa, a medicine used to treat Parkinson's disease.

Who is likely to develop gout?

Gout occurs in approximately 275 out of every 100,000 people. Men are more likely to develop gout than women, and men aged 40 to 50 are most commonly affected. Women rarely develop gout before menopause. The disease affects men and women differently: Men tend to develop gout at an earlier age than women, and alcohol is more often associated with the development of the disease in men. Gout is rare in children and young adults.

What are the signs and symptoms of gout?

- Hyperuricemia
- Presence of uric acid crystals in joint fluid
- More than one attack of acute arthritis
- Arthritis that develops in one day
- Attack of arthritis in only one joint, usually the toe, ankle, or knee
- A painful joint that is swollen, red, and warm

How is gout diagnosed?

Gout may be difficult for doctors to diagnose because the symptoms may be vague and often mimic other conditions. Although most people with gout have hyperuricemia at some time during the course of their disease, it may not be present during an acute attack. In addition, hyperuricemia alone does not mean that a person has gout. In fact, most people with hyperuricemia do not develop the disease.

To confirm a diagnosis of gout, doctors typically test the fluid in the joint, called synovial fluid, by using a needle to draw a sample of fluid from a person's inflamed joint. The doctor places some of the fluid on a slide and looks for monosodium urate crystals under a microscope. If the person has gout, the doctor will almost always see crystals. Their absence, however, does not completely rule out the diagnosis. Doctors may also find it helpful to examine joint or tophi deposits to diagnose gout. A doctor who suspects a joint infection may check for the presence of bacteria.

How is gout treated?

With proper treatment, most people with gout are able to control their symptoms and live normal lives. Gout can be treated with one or a combination of therapies. Treatment goals are to ease the pain associated with acute attacks, prevent future attacks, and avoid the formation of new tophi and kidney stones.

The most common treatments for an acute attack of gout are high doses of nonsteroidal anti-inflammatory drugs (NSAIDs) and injections of corticosteroid drugs into the affected joint. NSAIDs reduce the inflammation caused by deposits of uric acid crystals. The NSAIDs most commonly prescribed for gout are indomethacin (Indocin[1]) and naproxen (Anaprox, Naprosyn[1]), which are taken by mouth (orally) every day. Patients usually begin to improve within a few hours of treatment, and the attack goes away completely within a few days.

When NSAIDs do not control symptoms, the doctor may consider using colchicine. This drug is most effective when taken within the first 12 hours of an acute attack. Doctors can give colchicine by mouth (usually every hour until symptoms go away), or they can inject it directly into a vein (intravenously). When taken by mouth, colchicine frequently causes diarrhea.

For some people, the doctor may prescribe either NSAIDs or oral colchicine in small daily doses to prevent future attacks. If attacks continue and tophi develop, however, the doctor may prescribe medicine to treat hyperuricemia, most commonly allopurinol (Zyloprim) and probenecid (Benemid).

What can people with gout do to stay healthy?

* To help prevent future attacks, take the medicines your doctor prescribes. Carefully follow instructions about how much medicine to take and when to take it. Acute gout is best treated when symptoms first occur.

* Tell your doctor about all the medicines and vitamins you take. He or she can tell you if any of them increase your risk of hyperuricemia.

* Plan follow-up visits with your doctor to evaluate your progress.

* Maintain a healthy, balanced diet; avoid foods that are high in purines; and drink plenty of fluids, especially water. Fluids help remove uric acid from the body.

* Exercise regularly and maintain a healthy body weight. Lose weight if you are overweight.

What research is being conducted to help people with gout?

Scientists are studying whether other NSAIDs are effective in treating gout and are analyzing new compounds to develop safe, effective medicines to treat gout and other rheumatic diseases. For example, researchers are testing to determine whether fish oil supplements reduce the risk of gout. They are also studying the structure of the enzymes that break down purines in the body, in hopes of achieving a better understanding of the enzyme defects that can cause gout.

Where can people find more information about gout?

Arthritis Foundation

1330 West Peachtree Street
Atlanta, GA 30309
Telephone: 404-872-7100
Toll Free: 800-283-7800
Fax: 404-872-0457
or call your local chapter (listed in the telephone directory)
Website: http://www.arthritis.org

This is the main voluntary organization devoted to arthritis. The foundation publishes free pamphlets on many types of arthritis and a monthly magazine for members that provides up-to-date information on arthritis. The foundation also provides physician and clinic referrals.

National Arthritis and Musculoskeletal and Skin Diseases Information Clearinghouse (NAMSIC)

National Institutes of Health
1 AMS Circle
Bethesda, MD 20892-3675
Toll Free: 877-22-NIAMS
Telephone: 301-495-4484
TTY: 301-565-2966
Fax: 301-718-6366
Website: http://www.nih.gov/niams
E-Mail: niamsinfo@mail.nih.gov

This clearinghouse, a public service sponsored by the National Institute of Arthritis and Musculoskeletal and Skin Diseases (NIAMS), provides information about various forms of arthritis and rheumatic diseases. The clearinghouse distributes patient and professional education materials and also refers people to other sources of information.

Acknowledgments

The NIAMS gratefully acknowledges the assistance of John H. Klippel, M.D., NIAMS; N. Lawrence Edwards, M.D., of the University of Florida in Gainesville; and Lawrence Ryan, M.D., of the Medical College of Wisconsin, in the preparation and review of this fact sheet.

Key Words

Arthritis: Literally means joint inflammation. It is a general term for more than 100 conditions known as rheumatic diseases. These diseases affect not only the joints, but also other parts of the body, including important supporting structures, such as muscles, tendons, and ligaments, as well as some internal organs.

Cartilage: A tough, resilient tissue that covers and cushions the ends of the bones and absorbs shock.

Colchicine: A medicine used to treat gout. It may be given by mouth (orally) or injected directly into a vein (intravenously).

Connective tissue: The supporting framework of the body and its internal organs.

Corticosteroids: Potent anti-inflammatory hormones that are made naturally in the body or synthetically for use as drugs. The most commonly prescribed corticosteroid is prednisone.

Crystal-induced arthritis: An accumulation of crystalline material in various parts of the body, especially the joints. Gout and pseudogout are examples of crystal-induced arthritis.

Gout: A type of arthritis caused by the body's reaction to needle-like crystals that accumulate in joint spaces. This reaction causes inflammation and extreme pain in the affected joint, most commonly the big toe. The crystals are formed from uric acid. Gout is caused by either increased production of uric acid or failure of the body to eliminate uric acid.

Hyperuricemia: Increased amount of uric acid in the blood.

Inflammation: A characteristic reaction of tissues to injury or disease. It is marked by four signs: swelling, redness, heat, and pain.

Joint: A junction where two bones meet. Most joints are composed of cartilage, joint space, fibrous capsule, synovium, and ligaments.

Joint space: The volume enclosed within the fibrous capsule.

Ligaments: Bands of cord-like tissue that connect bone to bone.

Nonsteroidal anti-inflammatory drugs (NSAIDs): A group of drugs, such as aspirin and aspirin-like drugs, used to reduce the inflammation that causes joint pain, stiffness, and swelling.

Pseudogout: Similar to gout; however, the crystals in the synovial fluid are composed of calcium pyrophosphate dihydrate and not uric acid. As in gout, the crystals in the joint space cause an intense inflammatory reaction in the joint.

Purines: Components of all human tissue that break down to form uric acid. Purines are also found in many foods in varying amounts.

Rheumatic diseases: A general term that refers to more than 100 conditions that affect joints, muscles, bones, and other connective tissues.

Synovial fluid: A substance found around the joints that nourishes and lubricates them.

Tendons: Fibrous cords of tissue that connect muscle to bone.

Tophus (plural tophi): A hard deposit of crystalline uric acid that may appear as a lump just under the skin, particularly around the joints and at the rim of the ear.

Uric acid: An organic substance that results from the breakdown of purines or waste products in the body. It is dissolved in the blood and passes through the kidneys into the urine, where it is eliminated. Most patients with gout have high levels of uric acid in their blood. If the concentration of uric acid in the tissues rises above normal levels, crystals can form in the joints and cause inflammation.

Uric acid crystals: Caused by high concentrations of uric acid. When uric acid crystals form in the blood, they can collect in connective tissue, joints, and kidneys. Some kidney stones are made of uric acid.

Notes

Brand names included in this fact sheet are provided as examples only, and their inclusion does not mean that these products are endorsed by the National Institutes of Health or any other Government agency. Also, if a particular brand name is not mentioned, this does not mean that the product is unsatisfactory.

The National Institute of Arthritis and Musculoskeletal and Skin Diseases (NIAMS), a part of the National Institutes of Health (NIH), leads the Federal medical research effort in arthritis and musculoskeletal and skin diseases. The NIAMS supports research and research training throughout the United States, as well as on the NIH campus in Bethesda, MD, and disseminates health and research information. The National Arthritis and Musculoskeletal and Skin Diseases Information Clearinghouse (NAMSIC) is a public service sponsored by the NIAMS that provides health information and information sources. Additional information can be found on the NIAMS website at http://www.nih.gov/niams.

Chapter 34

Getting in Step with Arthritis

Arthritis of the Foot and Ankle

The pain and stiffness you feel in your foot and ankle as you grow older could be arthritis. If left untreated, this nagging pain can grow worse, eventually becoming so excruciating that you can no longer walk even short distances. Severe arthritis can restrict your mobility and limit your quality of life, but with proper treatment, you can slow the development of arthritis and lead a more productive life.

This article answers basic questions about the arthritic foot and offers information on treatment of this condition. For more information, you should speak with your orthopedic surgeon.

What Is Arthritis?

Arthritis is a broad term for a number of conditions that destroy the workings of a normal joint.

Arthritis may occur in your back, neck hips, knees, shoulders or hands, but it also occurs in your feet and ankles. Almost half of people in their 60s and 70s have arthritis of the foot and/or ankle. There are many different types of arthritis.

"Getting in Step With Arthritis," excerpted from the American Orthopaedic Foot and Ankle Society (AOFAS) website at http://www.aofas.org. © 1999 AOFAS. Reprinted with permission of the American Orthopedic Foot and Ankle Society.

The most common type, osteoarthritis (OSS-tee-oh-ar-THRIE-tiss), results from the "wear and tear" damage to joint cartilage (the soft tissue between joint bones) that comes with age The result is inflammation, redness, swelling and pain in the joint.

Also, a sudden and traumatic injury such as a broken bone, torn ligament, or moderate ankle sprain can cause the injured joint to become arthritic in the future. Sometimes a traumatic injury will result in arthritis in the injured joint even though the joint received proper medical care at the time of injury.

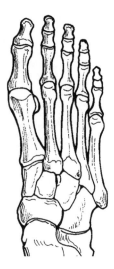

Figure 34.1. Right foot—normal.

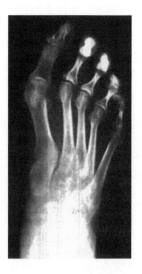

Figure 34.2. Right foot—rheumatoid arthritis.

Another common type, rheumatoid arthritis, is an inflammatory condition caused by an irritation of the joint lining (the synovium). People with rheumatoid arthritis for at least 10 years almost always develop arthritis in some part of the foot or ankle.

Other types of inflammatory arthritis include gout, lupus, ankylosing spondylitis, and psoriatic arthritis.

Foot Anatomy

The foot has 28 bones and over 30 joints. Tough bands of tissue called ligaments hold these together. The muscles, tendons, and ligaments work together with the many joints of the foot to control motion. This smooth motion makes it possible for a person to walk well. When you get arthritis in the foot, you develop pain and limited motion and can't walk as well.

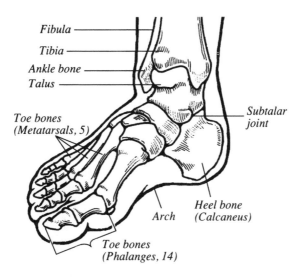

Figure 34.3. Anatomy of the foot.

Treatment of Arthritis of the Foot and Ankle

Proper treatment of foot and ankle arthritis addresses both pain and joint deformity. Pain develops when the joint is injured. Injury to the joint may result from swelling caused by inflammatory arthritis or from the loss of joint surface (cartilage), often caused by trauma. If left untreated, the foot and ankle may eventually become deformed.

231

If your doctor suspects you have arthritis of the foot and ankle, he/ she will ask you to have a complete medical history and physical examination. X-rays and laboratory tests often can confirm the type and extent of the arthritis. Other tests such as a bone scan, computed tomography (CT) scan, or magnetic resonance imaging (MRI) may be used to evaluate your condition.

Once your doctor confirms you have arthritis, he/she will recommend a treatment regimen, which may include medications by mouth (anti-inflammatories), injections (steroids), physical therapy, occupational therapy, or orthotics such as pads in your shoes, shoe inserts, additions to the insoles or heels of your shoes, or custom-made braces. Surgery may be necessary. This may mean cleaning the arthritic joint, eliminating the painful motion of the joint, replacing the joint with an artificial joint or a combination of all these.

After surgery, you will require a period of rehabilitation when your foot might have to be in a cast and you might have to wear special shoes or braces for a while.

Who Will Care for You?

Orthopaedic surgeons, medical doctors who specialize in the non-surgical and surgical care of foot and ankle problems, can diagnose and treat your arthritis. In addition to your orthopedic surgeon, other health care professionals may care for you, including a rheumatologist (medical arthritis specialist), physiatrist (rehabilitation specialist), pedorthist (footwear specialist), physical therapist, orthotist (brace specialist), occupational therapist, nurse, and clinical social worker.

Community resources also are available to people with arthritis. The local chapter of the National Arthritis Foundation offers exercise programs, educational information and support groups. Look under "Arthritis Foundation" in your local telephone directory to find the number you can call for information.

You Are an Important Part of the Treatment

You are often told you must live with arthritis, but that does not mean that you have to stop living. You should take an active part in your treatment; seek treatment for arthritis as early as possible to help control pain and reduce damage to the joint; take medications as directed, exercise, control your weight, and participate in all aspects of your care.

Remember, if you have questions about the need for a test, or the risks or benefits of your treatment, ask your doctor.

Even with the best of treatment, arthritis of the foot and ankle may continue to cause you pain or changes in your activities. However, proper diagnosis and treatment will help to minimize these limitations and allow you to lead a more productive, active lifestyle.

The American Orthopaedic Foot and Ankle Society

The American Orthopaedic Foot and Ankle Society (AOFAS) is a group of orthopedic surgeons who have special interest and training in the foot and ankle. Its members are medical doctors who, after completing medical school, have taken at least five years of additional training to become specialists in the care of diseases and deformities of the foot and the ankle and its surgical treatment. Remember, AOFAS members are the MDs who specialize in foot care. For further information, contact:

The American Orthopaedic Foot and Ankle Society
2517 East Lake Avenue, East
Suite 200
Seattle, WA 98102
Tel: 206-223-1120
Fax: 206-223-1178
Website: http://www.aofas.org
E-Mail: aofas@aofas.org

Chapter 35

Parkinson's Disease: Treating Foot Cramps

Drugs mentioned:

- levodopa/carbidopa (Sinemet/Dupont-MSD)
- selegiline (Eldepryl/Somerset)
- pergolide (Permax/Lilly)
- bromocriptine (Parlodel/Sandoz)
- trihexyphenidyl (Artane/Lederle)
- cyclobenzaprine (Flexeril/Merck)
- baclofen (Lioresal/Geigy)
- clonazepam (Klonopin/Roche)
- botulinum toxin (Botox/Allergan).

Aching and cramping of the feet are common complaints, often occurring after injury (strains and sprains) or excessive exercise, or in association with arthritis or poor circulation in the legs. In Parkinson's disease (PD), cramping of the feet is also very common, but the cause is central rather than peripheral. Foot cramping is just one of several focal dystonias—abnormal, sustained tightening of muscles—that appear to be due to neurochemical abnormalities in the basal ganglia, that part of the brain involved in PD. Patients show a particular type of cramping characterized by downward clenching of the toes or inward turning of the foot. Cramping can occur throughout the day

"Parkinson's Disease: Treating Foot Cramps," from *Medical Sciences Bulletin* at http://www.pharminfo.com/ © 2000 Pharmaceutical Information Associates, Ltd.; reprinted with permission.

or night, and can be especially annoying when it interferes with sleep. Foot cramping is more common among those individuals whose PD affects just one side of the body.

Dystonias are often mistaken for other causes of cramping or painful muscles. Some individuals with orthopedic foot problems, such as hammer toes, are actually suffering from Parkinsonian dystonia. Patients with dystonias may be entirely unaware of any Parkinsonism; indeed, muscle cramping can precede the onset of Parkinsonian symptoms by years. There are no laboratory tests that distinguish dystonia from other causes of cramping, although a thorough neurologic examination and specialized tests should pinpoint the cause. Some dystonic features—such as blepharospasm (involuntary closing of the eyelids) or torticollis (involuntary turning of the neck)—are common in the general population.

In the PD patient receiving levodopa/carbidopa (Sinemet/DuPont Pharmaceuticals), focal dystonias may be caused by either too much of the drug or too little. Patients may experience dystonia when peak drug levels are attained one to two hours after administration, or hours later when drug effects wear off. Changing the dose or dosage schedule of Sinemet, or using the sustained-release product (Sinemet CR) may help. The monoamine-oxidase B inhibitor selegiline (Eldepryl/Somerset) may also help. A bedtime dose of Sinemet CR, pergolide (Permax/Lilly), or bromocriptine (Parlodel/Sandoz) may prevent foot dystonia during early morning hours. Some patients respond to anticholinergics such as trihexyphenidyl (Artane/Lederle), muscle relaxants such as cyclobenzaprine (Flexeril/Merck) and baclofen (Lioresal/Geigy), and the anticonvulsant clonazepam (Klonopin/Roche). Another treatment giving excellent relief is botulinum toxin (Botox/Allergan). Injected into the dystonic or cramping muscle, botulinum toxin reduces the intensity of the spasms; the effects may last months after injection. The toxin is also used for Parkinsonian tremors, benign essential tremor, and a number of dystonias not always associated with PD. These include blepharospasm, torticollis, dysphonia (cramping of the vocal cords), strabismus (wandering eye), stuttering, and large-muscle spasms associated with conditions such as stroke, head trauma, and multiple sclerosis.

A careful evaluation of the temporal relationship between foot cramping and the levodopa dosage schedule should help the physician decide how best to treat this uncomfortable manifestation of PD. Modifying the levodopa regimen or adding other anti-PD agents can alter signals from the brain that trigger the contractions, or the muscle itself can be "paralyzed" with botulinum toxin. (LeWitt PA. UPF Newsl. 1993; #3: 3-4).

Chapter 36

AIDS and Your Feet

Definition

There are thousands of people who become infected with HIV each day. HIV stands for the Human Immunodeficiency Virus. This virus weakens the body's immune system making it unable to do its job effectively. During the late stage of the HIV infection, AIDS (Acquired Immunodeficiency Syndrome) develops. People who are infected with HIV may not develop AIDS for many years. This means that people with HIV can appear to be healthy and normal but their health will eventually decline. It is important for people to understand that they can pass the virus to other people even though they have not developed AIDS at that point of time.

Different illnesses that effect AIDS patients include severe diarrhea, pneumonia, tuberculosis, skin cancer, fever and skin infections. Due to the body's weakened immune system, people infected with the AIDS virus are unable to fight off infections. In addition to these illnesses, people with AIDS often develop peripheral neuropathy. Peripheral neuropathy is a disease that effects the nerves located outside the central nervous system. Neuropathy leads to insensitivity, stiffness, and numbness in the feet. These problems can also lead to foot deformities such as bunions, hammer toes, metatarsalgia, and many others. These complications should be taken care of immediately to prevent more serious problems such as the development of ulcers and possibly even amputation.

Cause

AIDS develops from the virus HIV. Scientists have traced the origin of the HIV virus to an African primate, specifically to a subspecies of the chimpanzee.

The HIV virus is found in fluids such as: blood, vaginal secretion, semen, and breast milk. Therefore, the virus can be passed on by the following:

• Sex with an infected person

• Passed from a mother to her unborn child

• Blood transfusions with infected blood

• Injections with unsterilized equipment

One of the highest growing age groups infected with the HIV virus are young adults under the age of 25. They account for about half of all new HIV infections in the United States alone. AIDS is the second leading cause of death among people between the ages of 25 and 44.

Peripheral Neuropathy

Approximately 30 percent of those infected with AIDS develop a condition called peripheral neuropathy. Peripheral neuropathy is a disease of the nerves. These nerves are located outside the central nervous system. Neuropathy can cause insensitivity or a loss of ability to feel pain, heat, and cold. People suffering from neuropathy can develop minor cuts, scrapes, blisters, or pressure sores that they may not be aware of due to their inability to sense pain. If these minor injuries are left untreated, complications may result and lead to ulceration and possibly even amputation. Neuropathy can also cause foot deformities such as bunions, hammertoes, metatarsalgia, and Charcot feet.

It is very important for people with AIDS to take the necessary precautions to prevent all foot-related injuries. Due to the consequences of neuropathy, daily observation of the feet is critical. By following the necessary preventative foot care measures you can reduce the risk of developing serious foot conditions.

Treatment and Prevention

There is no vaccine or cure for the HIV virus that causes AIDS. HIV is most frequently transmitted sexually. Because of this, the key to prevention is education. The best way for people to prevent the disease from spreading among the population is to know how to protect themselves from becoming infected.

People with AIDS are at high risk for developing neuropathy and other serious foot complications. Because of this fact, special attention must be focused on foot health management. Footwear and orthotics play an important role in footcare. Orthotics designed with Plastazote foam are recommended to protect the insensitive, neuropathic AIDS foot. Plastazote is a material designed to accommodate pressure "hot spots" by conforming to heat and pressure. By customizing to the foot, Plastazote provides superior comfort and protection for feet. For these reasons, footwear constructed with Plastazote is highly recommended for the people who have AIDS.

Footwear for people with AIDS should also provide the following protective benefits:

- High, wide toe box (high and wide space in the toe area).

- Removable insoles for fitting flexibility and the option to insert orthotics if necessary.

- Rocker soles. These soles are designed to reduce pressure in the areas of the foot most susceptible to pain, most notably the ball of the foot.

- Firm heel counters for support and stability.

If you have AIDS and are experiencing a foot problem, immediately consult with your foot doctor.

Part Four

Foot Injuries

Chapter 37

Heel Pain

That first step out of bed in the morning really catches your attention—it feels just like someone poked you in the heel with a knife. But after walking for a few minutes, the pain slowly disappears.

Heel pain is very irritating, but rarely serious. Although it can result from a pinched nerve or a chronic condition, such as arthritis or bursitis, the most common cause is plantar fasciitis (PLAN-tur fase-I-tis). Plantar fasciitis is an inflammation of the plantar fascia, the fibrous tissue that runs along the bottom of your foot and connects to your heel bone (calcaneus) and toes.

The plantar fascia also acts as a bowstring for the arch of your foot to keep the arch from collapsing. Treatment for plantar fasciitis involves simple steps to relieve the pain and inflammation. But don't expect a quick cure. It can take six months or longer before your heel is back to normal.

Stretching under Stress

A flattening of your arch or overuse can cause your plantar fascia to stretch and pull on your heel bone. That can result in microscopic tears in the fascia, inflammation, and a piercing pain or burning sensation. The pain usually develops gradually, but can come on suddenly

"Heel Pain," originally published in *Mayo Clinic Health Letter*, last updated July 14, 1999. ©1999 Mayo Foundation for Medical Education and Research. Reprinted with permission from Mayo Foundation for Medical Education and Research, Rochester, MN 55905.

243

and severely. It tends to be worse in the morning, when the fascia is stiff. Although both feet can be affected, it usually occurs in only one foot. The pain generally goes away once your foot limbers up. But it can recur if you stand or sit for a long time. Climbing stairs or standing on your tiptoes can also produce pain.

In severe cases, your foot may hurt whenever you put pressure on it, making walking difficult. You may also develop a bone spur that forms from tension on your heel bone. In most cases, the spur doesn't cause pain.

Common Causes

Plantar fasciitis can affect people of all ages. Factors that increase your risk include:

- *Age*: As you get older, your plantar fascia loses some of its elasticity and doesn't stretch as well. In addition, the fat pad covering your heel bone thins out and isn't able to absorb as much shock when you put weight on your foot. That places more stress on your heel bone and the tissues attached to it.

- *Weight-bearing activities*: Walking, jogging, lifting heavy objects and standing for long periods place added pressure on your feet. When performed regularly, they may stress your plantar fascia. Plantar fasciitis can also occur if you've been physically inactive and then plunge into a weight-bearing activity, such as playing golf or walking more than you're used to while vacationing.

- *Shoes*: Shoes with thin soles, poor arch support, that are too loose around your heels, lack shock absorbency, or are worn out can be harmful to your feet. In addition, regularly wearing high heels (greater than two inches) can shorten your Achilles' tendon, which attaches to your heel bone, and tighten your calf muscles. This increases the strain on your heels when you switch to a flatter shoe.

- *Weight*: Excess weight increases pressure on your feet.

- *Poor biomechanics*: A flat foot, high-arched foot, or abnormalities in your gait may prevent your weight from being evenly distributed when you walk or run. This stresses your plantar fascia.

Treatment Steps

The goal of treatment is to heal the tears and decrease inflammation, as well as prevent the condition from recurring. Although you may find the slow course of healing frustrating, patience is important.

There are several steps you can take to relieve plantar fasciitis. But if these aren't effective, or you believe your condition is due to a foot abnormality, see your doctor. Treatment options include:

- *Custom orthotic devices*: If you have a foot deformity, a custom shoe insert from an orthopedist or podiatrist can compensate for the deformity and distribute pressure to your foot more evenly.

- *Night splints*: While you sleep, your plantar fascia relaxes and starts to heal in that position. When you bear weight on the foot, you can stretch and tear your fascia all over again. Splints worn at night keep tension on the tissue so it heals in a stretched position.

- *Ultrasound*: Deep heat may increase blood flow and promote healing.

- *Corticosteroids*: An injection in your heel can often help relieve the inflammation when other steps aren't successful. But multiple injections aren't recommended because they can weaken and rupture your plantar fascia, as well as shrink the fat pad covering your heel bone.

- *Surgery*: Doctors can detach your plantar fascia from your heel bone, but this is only recommended when all other treatments have failed. Side effects can include continued pain and weakening of your arch.

Additional options may be available in the future. Mayo Clinic and other medical centers are investigating a number of alternative therapies, including low-intensity laser treatments.

Stepping Away from the Pain

Heel pain can be frustrating, but it doesn't have to keep you from your daily routine or favorite exercise program. Most people are able to relieve the pain by following simple treatment recommendations and gradually working back into normal activities. Maintaining a stretching program and continued attention to proper footwear may help prevent the condition from returning.

Chapter 38

Overuse Injury in Adolescents: Sever's Disease

Sever's Disease (calcaneal apophysitis) is an inflammation in the area between the sections of bone that make up the heel. This problem occurs in young people whose bones have not yet fused and fully matured. The back of your heel may hurt, forcing you to limp or walk on your toes.

What is Sever's Disease?

Sever's disease occurs in children when the growing part of the heel is injured. This growing part is called the growth plate. The foot is one of the first body parts to grow to full size. This usually occurs in early puberty. During this time, bones often grow faster than muscles and tendons. As a result, muscles and tendons become "tight." The heel area is less flexible. During weight-bearing activity (activity performed while standing), the tight heel tendons may put too much pressure at the back of the heel (where the Achilles tendon attaches). This may injure the heel.

When is my child most at risk for Sever's Disease?

Your child is most at risk for this condition when he or she is in the early part of the growth spurt in early puberty. Sever's disease is most common in physically active girls eight to 10 years old and in physically active boys 10 to 12 years old. Soccer players and gymnasts often get Sever's disease, but children who do any running or jumping activity may be affected. Sever's disease rarely occurs in older teenagers, because the back of the heel has finished growing by the age of 15.

How do I know if my child's heel pain is caused by Sever's Disease?

In Sever's disease, heel pain can be in one or both heels. It usually starts after a child begins a new sports season or a new sport. Your child may walk with a limp. The pain may increase when he or she stands on tiptoe. Your child's heel may hurt if you squeeze both sides toward the very back. This is called the squeeze test. Your doctor may also find that your child's heel tendons have become tight.

How is Sever's Disease treated?

First, your child should cut down or stop any activity that causes heel pain. Apply ice to the injured heel for 25 minutes three times a day. If your child has a high arch, flat feet or bowed legs, your doctor may recommend orthotics, or heel cups. Your child should never go barefoot. Physical therapy consisting of hydrotherapy (whirlpool) and electrical stimulation will help stimulate circulation to the painful heel and thereby help to reduce the inflammatory process. The athlete must still continue to ice and stretch at home.

If your child has severe heel pain, medicines such as acetaminophen (Tylenol) or ibuprofen (Advil) may help. It is important that your child performs exercises to stretch the hamstring and calf muscles, and the tendons on the back of the leg. The child should do these stretches five times each, two or three times a day. Each stretch should be held for 20 seconds.

Your child also needs to do exercises to strengthen the muscles on the front of the shin. To do this, your child should sit on the floor, keeping his or her hurt leg straight. One end of a bungee cord or piece of rubber tubing is hooked around a table leg. The other end is hitched around the child's toes. The child then scoots back just far enough to stretch the cord. Next, the child slowly bends the foot toward his or her body. When the child cannot bend the foot any closer, he or she slowly points the foot in the opposite direction (toward the table). This exercise (15 repetitions of "foot curling") should be done three times. The child should do this exercise routine twice daily.

When can my child play sports again?

With proper care, your child should feel better within two weeks to two months. Your child can start playing sports again only when the heel pain is gone. Your doctor will let you know when physical activity is safe.

Are there any problems linked with Sever's Disease?

No long-term problems have been linked with Sever's disease. However, call your doctor if your child's heel pain does not get better or if it gets worse, or if you notice changes in skin color or swelling.

Can Sever's Disease be prevented?

Sever's disease may be prevented by maintaining good flexibility while your child is growing. Your child should avoid excessive running on hard surfaces.

If your child has already recovered from Sever's disease, stretching and putting ice on the heel after activity will help keep your child from getting this condition again.

Chapter 39

Foot Injuries and the Weekend Warrior

Most sports involve running and jumping, both of which sharply increase strains on the legs and feet. Of all sports-related injuries, between 55% and 90% occur between the hip and the toe,[1] and 15% affect the foot alone.[2] No wonder, then, that foot problems are common among running, jumping, and kicking weekend warriors.

During running, for example, the loads absorbed by the foot are two to three times the body weight. Since runners may take more than 5,000 steps per hour with each leg, it is easy to understand why so many of them have overload problems.

Of foot injuries suffered in typical weekend sports, 9% are associated with tennis, 11% to 26% with running, 4% to 8% with basketball, 8% to 14% with cycling, and 6% with volleyball.[3] In this article, we will discuss the most frequent overuse injuries to the foot among amateur athletes: an explanation of how they occur, predisposing factors, and practical advice on their evaluation and management.

Factors Affecting Injury

The main risk factors for development of foot problems can be summed up as "too much, too often, too soon." A basic principle of exercise is that training leads to specific adaptation to the loads used.

"Foot Injuries: Office Management for the Woes of Weekend Warriors," by Lars Engebretsen and Roald Bahr, in *Consultant*, February 1996, Vol. 36, No. 2, p. 209(8). Copyright 1996 by Cliggott Publishing Co. Reprinted with permission.

If a training load exceeds the adaptive ability of any given tissue, injury results.

In a study of sedentary prison inmates, 30-minute aerobic training sessions (jogging, stationary biking, and walking) three times a week for 12 weeks caused injuries in 12% of the subjects; an increase in training frequency to five times a week led to injuries in 39%.[4] About 10% of these injuries were to the foot and ankle. When the sessions were increased to 45 minutes, more than half the subjects were injured.

Table 39.1—Factors that may influence exercise injury

Intrinsic	Extrinsic
Physical characteristics	Type of sports activity
Age	Knowledge and skill of coaches
Sex	Practice or training methods
Genotype	Level of competition
Somatotype	Environmental conditions
Strength	Playing surfaces
Speed	Equipment
Agility	
Coordination	
Physical fitness	
Joint flexibility or laxity	
Malalignment	
Physical maturity level	
Growth rate	
Muscle composition	
Anatomic variation	
Previous injuries	
Personality traits	
Conscientiousness	
Self-confidence	
Tough-mindedness	
Responsiveness to coaching	
Discipline	
Determination	

In a similar study of army trainees, 12 weeks of training caused injuries in 20% of those already accustomed to running four or more times weekly. The same program led to injuries in 44% of the sedentary subjects.[5]

Treatment and prevention of any injury require recognition of the responsible conditions. In addition to obtaining the patient's training history, you must be aware of the intrinsic and extrinsic factors that may contribute to injury (Table 39.1). Foot injuries incurred during running are caused by factors that influence the distribution of load: anatomic features, body weight, shoes, running surface, training program, and technique. Knowledge of the normal biomechanics of running helps in preventing these injuries. Often, it is not difficult to analyze the cause of problems.

Biomechanics of Running

During running, the foot is slightly supinated just before the heel strikes. The outside of the heel touches the surface first; this is followed by loading of the arch, which then flattens. The foot then pronates; together with contraction of the calf muscles, this dissipates the generated forces throughout the entire foot and leg. The longitudinal arch continues to flatten until the arch ligament (plantar aponeurosis) is tightened.

During takeoff, the forefoot supinates to stabilize the foot until the great toe leaves the ground. Depending on the runner's speed, the foot is in pronation during 40% to 70% of the supporting phase.

Injury Analysis

Take a history centering on the intrinsic and extrinsic variables listed in Table 39.1. Palpate the feet, and examine their alignment, flexibility, range of motion, and stability. This should give sufficient information to suggest differential diagnoses. In a "worst-case" (if not typical) example of the weekend athlete with foot problems, a runner is overweight and flat-footed; has a training program involving too much, too often, too soon; wears old shoes; and runs on a hard surface.

Running shoes. The longevity of a shoe's shock absorbency is related to the distance that has been run; this usually ranges between 500 and 1,000 miles, after which the shoe offers little or no protection.[6] The hindfoot stability of a jogging shoe is critical in managing overuse problems attributed to excess pronation. Evidence corroborating the effect of controlling pronation is provided by the results of treating injured runners with orthotic devices: the condition improved in 70% to 90% of the runners, and they were able to resume training.[7]

Surface. Hard surfaces are associated with a higher incidence of injury in any sports activity. Impact forces and excess load (e.g., produced by overweight runners on a hard surface) have been emphasized as causes of many conditions, ranging from osteoarthritis to shin splints to stress fractures.

Differential Diagnosis of Overuse Injuries

Insufficiency of the Longitudinal Arch (Flat Foot)

When the foot is under load (as during sports activity on a hard surface) and is overloaded because of tendon or ligament injury, excess body weight, or prolonged standing, the arch may collapse. The result is a flat foot.

Initial workup. The patient may complain of pain and fatigue in the foot, leg, knees, and/or groin. You will often find calluses on the sole of the foot. The soles of training shoes show a typical pattern: greater wear on the medial edge of the shoe than on the lateral edge. The patient's metatarsal bones and toes are often externally rotated.

Additional testing. When a runner complains of long-standing foot pain, an x-ray study or even, occasionally, a bone scan is necessary to rule out a stress fracture.

Management. Prescribe arch supports, and have the patient change the training program from running to another activity. Biking or swimming is a good substitute.

Insufficiency of the Anterior Transverse Arch

If the ligaments between the metatarsal bones slacken, the arch loses its load-absorbing capacity. The foot widens, a hallux valgus and/or hammertoes may develop, and calluses are typically seen under the forefoot.

Initial workup. Assess the alignment while the patient walks, runs, and stands.

Management. Prescribe orthotic shoes with a pad for the anterior transverse arch. A patient with prominent hallux valgus or hammertoes may require surgery.

Pes Cavus

An unusually high longitudinal arch and relative inflexibility of the foot characterize pes cavus. In most cases, the patient also has a tight Achilles tendon and plantar fascia. Pain follows long-distance running.

Initial workup. Calluses are often seen on the big toe, and patients have a tendency toward hammertoes.

Additional testing. A radiograph may detect a metatarsal stress fracture, a possible result of running with a cavus foot.

Management. Advise the patient to stretch before and after athletic activities. Prescribe arch supports that also have good shock-absorbing properties. Change the training pattern away from running and toward cycling, Nordic track, or swimming.

Painful Heel Cushion

The heel cushion is divided into small compartments containing fat and surrounded by connective tissue fasciae, which can become ruptured by repeated jumping. When the heel makes contact with the ground, fat is squeezed out—thus decreasing the cushioning effect of the fat pad. In some cases, there is an inflammatory response.

Initial evaluation. The patient generally gives a history of repeated jumps on a hard surface or one faulty, hard landing on the heel. The area is painful on palpation. A radiograph may show cysts in the calcaneus—signs of irritation.

Management. The athlete can use a plastic heel insert that fits snugly around the heel and has shock-absorbing flanges. Nevertheless, this problem can be difficult to treat. The patient may need to reduce or curtail jumping and running activities for as long as three months to allow the fat pad to heal.

Haglund's Heel

Also known as "pump bumps," this pain and swelling in the posterior superior portion of the calcaneus may be associated with retrocalcaneal bursitis, enlargement of the superior bursal prominence of the calcaneus, and Achilles tendinitis. This is most often a complaint of runners and those who play basketball and tennis.

Initial evaluation. Palpation of the swelling between the Achilles tendon and the calcaneus elicits pain.

Additional testing. A lateral standing film of the calcaneus demonstrates the bony deformity on the posterior margin of the posterior facet.

Additional test. We usually obtain a lateral view of the calcaneus with the patient standing to evaluate the posterior margin of the posterior facet.

Management. Most patients can be successfully treated nonsurgically with the following regimen:

* Reducing (or discontinuing) the usual mileage run weekly

* Temporarily terminating interval training and workouts on hills

* Changing to a softer running surface

* Adding a 1/4- to 1/2-inch lift inside the shoe until the symptoms cease (for at least three months)

* Starting an exercise program that stretches and strengthens the gastrocnemius-soleus complex, to be continued as long as the patient runs.[8]

In addition, anti-inflammatory medication and padding of the painful area may be useful. If the condition does not respond to these modalities after three to six months, consider referral for surgery (usually excision of the retrocalcaneal bursa and calcaneal exostosis). About 70% of affected patients are able to return to their previous activity level following this procedure.[6]

Plantar Fasciitis

Pain that radiates distally from the volar aspect of the calcaneus—plantar fasciitis—is a frequent complaint of middle-aged runners.

Particularly at risk for this problem are those with excessive prona-tion, which places increased strain on the plantar fascia, or aponeuro-sis. Repetitive trauma produces microruptures in the fascia near its insertion on the calcaneus and leads to chronic inflammation. Plan-tar fasciitis may be associated with subcalcaneal plantar bone spurs; these are found in only 15% of adults with asymptomatic feet but in nearly half of those with plantar pain.[9]

Initial evaluation. Pain is felt in the heel (at the origin of the aponeurosis) when patients put weight on the foot. Morning stiffness in the foot is typical; it decreases with activity, but prolonged activ-ity may produce pain. Weight-bearing on the heel becomes impossible, and patients typically walk on the forefoot.

Additional testing. An x-ray study reveals a spur in approxi-mately 40% to 50% of patients with plantar fasciitis. It may also show signs of a stress fracture, in which case further work-up with a bone scan or MRI is indicated. Nerve entrapment syndromes can be ex-cluded by carrying out sequential nerve blocks or nerve conduction studies. Rule out stress fractures with a technetium 99m bone scan.

Management. During the acute phase, prescribe rest, icing, and anti-inflammatory medication. After three to five days of this treat-ment (and also for a chronic complaint), arch supports or heel cups plus stretching and physical therapy may give relief.

Up to 10% of patients do not respond to conservative treatment.[10] For those who have had six to 12 months of pain that prevents them from continuing their desired activity, consider surgical intervention. This consists of releasing the central slip of the plantar fascia at its origin and excising a bone spur, if present. Up to 90% of patients are able to return to their former activity levels after surgery.

Nerve Entrapment

In several areas of the foot, nerves pass through rigid compart-ments, through fibrous or fibro-osseous canals, or over bony promi-nences. Table 39.2 lists the most frequently involved areas.

Initial evaluation. Look for signs and symptoms as listed in Table 39.2.

Additional testing. An x-ray study and, occasionally, a bone scan will be necessary to rule out stress fracture.

Management. Conservative treatment may be beneficial: wider shoes, padding, and corticosteroid injections around the nerve. We have found that surgery is frequently necessary, although the results are not invariably successful. Tarsal tunnel syndromes are relieved by surgery in only 70% to 90% of cases and interdigital neuromas in 80%.[11]

Table 39.2—Nerve entrapment problems

Area of involvement	Signs and symptoms	Diagnostic aids
Posterior tibial nerve or plantar nerves (tarsal tunnel syndrome)	Burning, tingling, numbness of sole	Excessive pronation is risk factor; nerve conduction studies helpful
Medial calcaneal nerve	Pain on medial side of heel	Clinical diagnosis
Motor branch to abductor digiti quinti muscle	Vague burning pain in heel pad	Nerve conduction studies usually not helpful
Sural nerve	Pain and numbness extend to lateral border of foot	Clinical diagnosis
Superficial peroneal nerve	Pain, numbness on dorsum of foot except for first web space	Usual entrapment is high on the leg; rule out L-5 radiculopathy; nerve conduction studies helpful
Deep peroneal nerve	Vague pain over dorsomedial surface of foot, numbness in first web space	Nerve conduction studies helpful
Interdigital nerves (Morton's neuroma)	Pain usually in third web space; predominantly in women	Clinical diagnosis based on pain pattern

Turf Toe

The use of lightweight, flexible shoes on artificial turf predisposes the forefoot to injury.[10] Metatarsophalangeal (MTP) joint injuries frequently occur in athletes who compete on wooden or synthetic surfaces (e.g., playing football, basketball, squash, and racketball). The first MTP joint will normally undergo an average of 60 degrees of dorsiflexion.[10] As the phalanx approaches this limit, the usual joint sliding action is replaced by axial compression onto the cartilage surfaces of the joint. This may cause an exaggerated hyperextension, resulting in a sprain and varying degrees of soft-tissue capsular injury. Turf toe syndrome is classified as first-, second-, and third-degree, depending on the severity of swelling, tenderness, reduction in range of motion, and extent of ecchymosis.[12]

Initial evaluation. Periarticular swelling and ecchymosis are usually apparent. The patient's gait is antalgic in an effort to protect the joint from dorsiflexion.

Additional testing. Although AP, lateral, and oblique x-ray views may detect small bone chips, they are otherwise of no help.

Management. In the acute phase, rest, icing, and elevation are combined with anti-inflammatory medication. The discomfort may be decreased by taping the toe to decrease dorsiflexion. When the athlete returns to sport, a shoe with a less flexible sole will help prevent relapse.

Subungual Exostosis

This reactive bony prominence commonly develops on the dorsomedial aspect of the terminal phalanx of the great toe. Typically, it is found in basketball players whose toes have repeatedly been stepped on.

Initial evaluation. The athlete may recall an episode of trauma followed by pain under the nail of the great toe. Direct pressure over the toenail may be very painful. The exostosis is frequently misdiagnosed as a toenail deformity, onychomycosis, or chronic ingrown toenail.

Additional testing. The key to correct diagnosis is radiographic demonstration of an exostosis on a lateral or oblique view.

Management. Treatment of exostosis is usually surgical excision of the toenail and the exostosis.

Sesamoid Dysfunction

The two sesamoid bones, located under the MTP joint, play a significant role in the function of the great toe. They protect the tendon of the flexor hallucis brevis, absorb the majority of weight-bearing on the medial side of the forefoot, and increase the mechanical advantage of the intrinsic musculature of the hallux.

Initial evaluation. Suspect sesamoiditis if a young athlete has tenderness on palpation over the sesamoids, pain while playing sports, restricted range of motion in the first MTP joint, and diminished strength on plantar and dorsal flexion of the toes.

Additional testing. Oblique and axial x-ray views demonstrate fractured or bipartite sesamoids. The latter condition (more often the medial bone) occurs normally in up to 30% of the general population.[13] A bone CT scan is necessary to show a stress fracture.

Management. The diagnosis of a fractured sesamoid is often delayed because of confusion with the frequent finding of bipartite sesamoids. Fracture is managed by immobilization (taping or casting) for six weeks. For those with chronic sesamoiditis, orthotic treatment (molded shoe inserts with a metatarsal relief bar to unload the sesamoids) may give relief. The orthoses must be worn constantly for at least six months, and their use should be resumed if symptoms recur.[14] Surgical excision of the bones is occasionally necessary if there is prolonged pain.[15]

Freiberg's Infarction

This is an avascular necrosis of subchondral cancellous bone of the metatarsal head, followed by a repair process. It most commonly develops in young athletes who perform on their toes, as in sprinting or jumping activities.

Initial evaluation. The athlete complains of pain and occasional swelling, usually in the second or third metatarsal head. An x-ray film showing osteosclerosis (early in the course) or osteolysis (after one or two months) confirms the diagnosis.

Management. Metatarsal arch pads generally bring relief; patients should refrain from running and jumping activities for six to 12 weeks. In refractory cases, surgery may be carried out in adolescence or early adulthood.

Stress Fractures

At least 30% of all stress fractures occur in the foot and ankle—about 50% in the metatarsals and up to 30% in the lateral malleolus.[16] This injury is usually caused by a combination of intrinsic and extrinsic factors that include malalignment, overweight, over-training, old shoes, and hard surface.

Initial evaluation. History is particularly important when you suspect stress fracture. There is a well-known correlation between this injury and eating disorders, menstrual dysfunction, and osteoporosis. Women who run a great deal often suffer from menstrual problems, reduced estrogen levels, increased incidence of osteoporosis and, subsequently, risk of stress fracture. Suspect this diagnosis if patients experience pain on deep palpation; verify it with an x-ray study, CT bone scans, or MRI.

Management. Although this depends on the fracture site, it always includes decreasing loading activities. Patients may, however, be able to exercise in water. If eating or menstrual disorders exist, appropriate management is necessary.

Two more commonly injured areas warrant special comments. The well-known tarsal navicular stress fracture requires immobilization for six to eight weeks; initially, only touch-down weight-bearing is allowed.[17] Nonunion of this fracture is not infrequent.

Stress fracture of the proximal diaphysis of the fifth metatarsal bones can be treated with three to four weeks of relative rest. If this does not lessen the symptoms, however, patients require either casting with complete immobilization for six weeks or insertion of an intramedullary screw with possible bone graft.[18] We prefer early surgical intervention for active athletes to expedite their return to activity.

References

1. Garrick JG. Characterization of the patient population in a sports medicine facility. *Physician Sportsmed.* 1985; 13:73-76.

2. Garrick JG, Requa RK. The epidemiology of foot and ankle injuries in sport. *Clin Sports Med.* 1988; 7:29-36.

3. Clanton TO. Etiology of injury to the foot and ankle. In: DeLee JC, Drez D Jr, eds. *Orthopaedic Sports Medicine.* Philadelphia: WB Saunders Company; 1994:1642-1704.

4. Pollock MI, Gettman LR, Milesis CA, et al. Effects of frequency and duration of training on attrition and incidence of injury. *Med Sci Sports Exerc.* 1977;9:31-36.

5. Jones BH, Cowan DN, Tomlinson JP, et al. Epidemiology of injuries associated with physical training among young men in the army. *Med Sci Sports Exerc.* 1993;25:197-203.

6. Cook SD, Kester MA, Brunet ME. Shock absorption characteristics of running shoes. *Am J Sports Med.* 1985; 13:248-253.

7. Donatelli R, Hurlbert C, Conaway D, St Pierre R. Biomechanical foot orthosis: a retrospective study. *J Orthop Sports Phys Ther.* 1988; 10:205-212.

8. Schepsis AA, Leach RE. Surgical management of Achilles tendinitis. *Am J Sports Med.* 1987; 15:308-315.

9. Mann RA. *Surgery of the Foot.* 5th ed. St Louis: CV Mosby Co; 1986:244-247.

10. Lutter LD. Surgical decisions in athletes' subcalcaneal pain. *Am J Sports Med.* 1986; 14:481-485.

11. Mann RA. Entrapment neuropathies of the foot. In: DeLee JC, Drez D Jr, eds. *Orthopaedic Sports Medicine.* Philadelphia: WB Saunders Company; 1994:1831-1841.

12. Clanton TO, Butler JE, Eggert A. Injuries to the metatarsophalangeal joints in athletes. *Foot Ankle.* 1986; 7:162-176.

13. Bloomfield J, Fricker PA, Fitch KD, eds. *Textbook of Science and Medicine in Sport.* Champaign, Ill: Human Kinetics Books; 1992:417.

14. Axe MJ, Ray RL. Orthotic treatment of sesamoid pain. *Am J Sports Med.* 1989; 16:411-416.

15. Richardson EG. Injuries to the hallucal sesamoids in the athlete. *Foot Ankle.* 1987;7:229-244.

16. McBryde A. Stress fractures of the foot and ankle. In: DeLee JC, Drez D Jr, eds. *Orthopaedic Sports Medicine*. Philadelphia: WB Saunders Company; 1994:1970-1981.

17. Hullko A, Orava S, Pellinen P. Stress fracture of the navicular bone. Nine cases in athletes. *Acta Orthop Scand*. 1985; 56:503-505.

18. Lehman RC. Fractures of the base of the fifth metatarsal distal to the tuberosity: a review. *Foot Ankle*. 1987;7:245-252.

— by Lars Engebretsen and Roald Bahr

Dr. Engebretsen is associate professor of orthopedic surgery at the University of Minnesota Medical School, Minneapolis. Dr. Bahr is associate professor of sports medicine at the Norwegian University of Sport and Physical Education, Oslo.

Chapter 40

Detecting and Treating Common Foot and Ankle Fractures

Part 1: Ankle and Hindfoot Fractures

In Brief

Some of the most common and potentially serious ankle and hindfoot fractures seen in a primary care sports medicine practice are fractures of the tibial plafond, malleolus, calcaneus, and talus (including osteochondral lesions). Making a careful physical exam to detect for sites of tenderness and ordering the appropriate diagnostic images—usually plain films—are important in pinpointing the diagnosis, but some injuries, like Maisonneuve fractures, can be difficult to detect. Certain injuries, like many fractures of the lateral process of the talus, can be managed conservatively with casting, but severe or displaced fractures usually require surgery. Rehabilitation typically focuses on rest and proper strengthening and stretching exercises.

Fractures of the foot and ankle immediately impair a recreational or elite athlete's ability to perform competitively in virtually any sporting activity. Fractures of the ankle and hindfoot usually occur acutely in a traumatic episode; chronic injuries like stress fractures are more likely in the midfoot and forefoot. Some of the more common fractures

"Detecting and Treating Common Foot and Ankle Fractures: Part 1: The Ankle and Hindfoot, and Part 2: The Midfoot and Forefoot," by David B. Thordarson, MD in *The Physician and Sportsmedicine*, Vol. 24, No. 9, September 1996, and Vol. 24, No. 10, October 1996. ©1996 The McGraw-Hill Companies. Reproduced with permission of McGraw-Hill, Inc.

heal well with nonoperative care and some require surgical treatment, so an accurate diagnosis is essential.

Ankle Fractures

Ankle fractures have been classified in various ways. An important initial distinction is whether a fracture is of a malleolus, or is a much more severe tibial plafond (pilon) intra-articular impaction fracture.

Tibial plafond: Tibial plafond fractures generally result from a high-energy axial load, as can occur in a fall from a height or a motor vehicle accident. Patients experience immediate pain and cannot walk. On exam, they generally have significant swelling with or without deformity.

These fractures—in contrast to malleolus fractures—involve the weight-bearing surface of the plafond and generally require open reduction and internal fixation. Results are frequently poor despite operative intervention.[1] Fortunately, tibial plafond fractures are uncommon in athletes.

Malleolus: Fractures involving the malleolus are a much more common type of ankle fracture. They can involve the lateral or medial malleolus, or both, and they usually result from an external rotation injury to the ankle. Ligament damage is typical, generally of the deltoid ligament and of the anterior and posterior tibiofibular ligaments. Patients feel immediate pain and have difficulty walking or cannot walk. Moderate-to-severe swelling and bony tenderness exist over the fracture site(s), with or without a visible deformity.

Malleolus fractures are typically classified by one of two systems. The Lauge-Hansen fracture classification relies on the position of the foot at the time of injury and includes four types:

1. supination-lateral rotation
2. supination-adduction
3. pronation-abduction, and
4. pronation-lateral rotation.[2]

The Danis-Weber system is based on the level of the fibular fracture relative to the ankle joint.[3] It includes type A, fracture below the ankle joint; type B, fracture at the level of the joint, in which the tibiofibular ligaments are most likely intact; and type C, which occurs above the joint and disrupts the syndesmotic ligaments. In both the Lauge-Hansen and Danis-Weber classifications, a fracture higher on the fibula indicates more instability and, therefore, a greater likelihood of surgical intervention.

The initial treatment for all displaced malleolus fractures is closed reduction and casting followed by ice and elevation. If an anatomic reduction is obtained, these fractures can be managed with a cast. However, postreduction radiographs must show that the joint space is symmetric on a mortise view because even 1 to 2 mm of displacement of the talus within the mortise can cause dramatic changes in the contact area and pressures within the ankle. One study[4] demonstrated a 40% decrease in contact area with a 1-mm lateral shift of the talus.

Because of this potential for change in the contact area and pressure in the ankle with an intra-articular fracture, surgeons recommend open reduction and internal fixation of persistently displaced malleolus fractures to guarantee an anatomic reduction. An added benefit of operative treatment in an athlete is a more aggressive, early rehabilitation. Range-of-motion exercises can be started after wound healing, but compliance with non-weight bearing must be emphasized.

Most patients with a malleolus fracture require six weeks of immobilization. Patients with a displaced ankle fracture that has undergone successful closed reduction will typically require two to four weeks in a long-leg cast and then an additional two to four weeks in a short-leg non-walking cast. Patients with an initially non-displaced fracture or who were treated surgically will generally require four weeks of non-weight bearing in a short-leg cast or removable walking boot, followed by two weeks in a walking cast or boot. The removable boot will allow for earlier range-of-motion exercises.

In patients treated non-operatively, follow-up radiographs must be obtained weekly for the first two to three weeks following injury to rule out fracture displacement. Following fracture healing, patients can begin physical therapy for range-of-motion and strengthening exercises. Most patients who sustain a malleolus fracture will miss at least three months from most sports, and frequently six months or more from cutting-type sports.

Maisonneuve: A Maisonneuve fracture—an external rotation injury of the ankle with an associated fracture of the proximal third of the fibula—is a serious injury that can have deceptively minor radiographic findings. Although less common than other types of ankle fractures, it is often misdiagnosed and can result in long-term disability.

The typical mechanism and presentation are external rotation of the foot and medial ankle pain. On examination, the patient will have tenderness over the deltoid ligament and over the fracture site on the proximal fibula. Any patient who has proximal fibular tenderness after a twisting injury to the ankle should have radiographs taken of both the ankle and the tibia and fibula.

Radiographs of the ankle generally reveal no fracture or only a small avulsion injury of the medial malleolus with variable widening of the space between the tibia and fibula. A radiograph of the whole tibia and fibula, however, will demonstrate a high fibula fracture. These patients require open reduction and internal fixation with one or two screws placed between the distal fibula and tibia to maintain the bones' normal relationship while ligament healing occurs. The screws are generally removed eight to 12 weeks after surgery.

Calcaneus Fractures

Like tibial plafond fractures, calcaneus fractures occur most commonly after high-energy axial loads. They can also stem from an avulsion of the Achilles tendon. Approximately 75% of calcaneus fractures extend into the subtalar joint.[5] Both high-energy fractures and avulsion are relatively uncommon in athletes because of the mechanism of injury, but either can result in permanent disability. Following a fracture, patients have severe heel pain and cannot walk. They have moderate-to-severe hindfoot swelling and tenderness on exam.

Intra-articular fractures that result from an axial load need to be carefully assessed for displacement on lateral and axial radiographs any displacement warrants a computed tomography (CT) scan. Initial treatment for displaced and non-displaced intra-articular fractures includes immobilization in a bulky dressing and splint, with ice and elevation to control edema. Most displaced fractures are managed operatively, but these patients typically experience residual stiffness of their subtalar joint that will adversely affect future athletic performance. For non-displaced extra-articular calcaneus fractures, patients wear a short-leg cast or walking boot for about six weeks.

Avulsion fractures occur during a violent contraction of the gastrocnemius and soleus. If not displaced or if minimally displaced, they can be managed in a plantar-flexed short-leg cast for six weeks followed by physical therapy involving stretching. Most of these fractures, however, are significantly displaced and frequently require immediate surgery to repair the fracture and relieve the pressure on the skin overlying the bony fragment.

Talus Fractures

Talus fractures typically involve either the talar neck or lateral process, or an osteochondral fracture of the talar dome.

Talar neck: Although talar neck fractures are relatively uncommon and represent high-energy injuries involving hyperdorsiflexion of the ankle, they deserve mention because of the potential devastating complication of avascular necrosis of the talus. A typical mechanism of injury is a motor vehicle accident in which the ankle is hyperdorsiflexed by the brake pedal. Patients experience severe hindfoot pain and moderate-to-severe edema, tenderness, and ecchymosis. The body of the talus may be palpable in the posteromedial ankle area.

Displaced talar neck fractures are true surgical emergencies. The fracture must be reduced immediately to minimize the risk of avascular necrosis or skin slough. The talus has limited vascularization; most of its blood supply enters the neck via an anastomotic sling and flows posteriorly. A fracture, therefore, disrupts the intraosseous portion of the blood supply, and the greater the displacement, the greater the disruption of the blood supply and likelihood of necrosis. Avascular necrosis may lead to collapse of the body of the talus, resulting in arthritic changes that necessitate ankle fusion. Even without avascular necrosis, many patients develop a significant degree of subtalar arthrosis or arthritis, which leads to residual hindfoot stiffness and pain. Treatment for patients who have a non-displaced talar neck fracture typically involves a short-leg non-walking cast for six to eight weeks followed by range-of-motion exercises.

Lateral process: Although fractures of the lateral process of the talus are relatively uncommon, they can be a source of chronic lateral ankle pain following an inversion injury. The typical mechanism of injury is acute hyperdorsiflexion with inversion.[5] The patient will experience lateral ankle pain and have edema and tenderness in this area. Radiographs reveal a variable-sized fragment of the lateral process along the inferior aspect of the talus. This defect is most easily identified on a lateral radiograph.

Non-displaced fractures require six weeks in a short-leg cast. Large displaced fragments (generally greater than 1 cm in diameter) should be treated with open reduction and internal fixation. Small displaced fragments can be treated symptomatically and can be excised if symptoms persist.

Osteochondral injury: A more common talus injury in sports is an osteochondral fracture of the dome of the talus that results from an inversion injury. A related, chronic condition probably caused by repetitive trauma is osteochondritis dissecans (OCD). A typical post-traumatic osteochondral fracture or an OCD lesion occurs in the anterolateral aspect of the talar dome. It is postulated that the corner of the talus fractures as the dome rotates laterally through the mortise.[5]

Patients who sustain an acute osteochondral fracture have pain with weight bearing. If the fragment displaces, they will experience locking or clicking. On exam, they have tenderness over the lateral aspect of the talar dome. Radiographs typically show a small flake of bone off the lateral dome of the talus. Occasionally, plain radiographs will be negative, and magnetic resonance imaging can establish the diagnosis and define the extent of the lesion.

An OCD lesion may appear as a cyst or loose piece of bone in either the anterolateral or posteromedial dome of the talus. Patients report a gradual onset of pain that is generally activity related and, if the fragment displaces, mechanical symptoms such as locking. If the fragment is non-displaced and follows an acute injury, the patient can be treated with a short-leg non-walking cast for six weeks followed by range-of-motion exercises. In more chronic cases, or if the fragment is displaced, the fragment can be removed arthroscopically and the bony defect can be drilled to encourage fibrocartilage formation. These patients should avoid weight bearing for six weeks while fibrocartilage is forming, but they can do range-of-motion exercises at this time.

Dual Strategies

Although fractures of the foot and ankle can be a source of significant disability and require surgery, many ankle and hindfoot fractures sustained in athletic activities are amenable to non-operative treatment. Primary care sports medicine physicians, therefore, must not only make astute diagnoses, they must be well-versed in rehabilitation strategies for both conservative and postoperative treatment.

Part 1 References

1. Chapman MW: Fracture and fracture-dislocations of the ankle, in Mann RA, Coughlin MJ (eds): *Surgery of the Foot and Ankle*, ed 6. St Louis, CV Mosby Co, 1993, pp 1439-1464.

2. Lauge-Hansen N: Fractures of the ankle: combined experimental-surgical and experimental-roentgenologic investigations. *Arch Surg* 1950;60(5):957-985.

3. Muller ME, Allgower M, Schneider R, et al (eds): Manual of Internal Fixation: Techniques Recommended by the AO-Group, ed 2. New York City, *Springer-Verlag*, 1979, pp 282-299.

4. Ramsey PL, Hamilton W: Changes in tibiotalar area of contact caused by lateral talar shift. *J Bone Joint Surg (Am)* 1976;58(3):356-357.

5. De Lee JC: Fractures and dislocations of the foot, in Mann RA, Coughlin MJ (eds): *Surgery of the Foot and Ankle*, ed 6. St Louis, CV Mosby Co, 1993, pp 1465-1703.

Part 2: Fractures of the Midfoot and Forefoot

In Brief

Midfoot and forefoot fractures commonly seen in a primary care practice include navicular and metatarsal stress fracture, tarsometatarsal fracture-dislocation, and acute fracture of the metatarsals, sesamoid, great toe, or lesser toes. A careful history to determine the mechanism of injury and a methodical physical exam to detect sites of tenderness are essential. X-rays are usually required, but stress fractures may warrant bone scans. Compared with ankle and hindfoot fractures, sports-related midfoot and forefoot fractures are more often treated conservatively with casting or wooden shoes. Tarsometatarsal disruption and Jones fractures are more likely to require surgery.

When a person sustains a foot or ankle fracture, his or her ability to perform virtually any athletic activity is immediately impaired. Several types of sports-related ankle and foot fractures occur in the midfoot and forefoot. These injuries are often acute, but stress fractures, which are frequently due to improper technique, commonly occur in this region as well. Exact diagnosis based on physical exam findings and diagnostic images will determine treatment, whether conservative or surgical.

Navicular Stress Fracture

Traumatic fractures of the navicular require high energy and are thus uncommon in sports. The navicular, however, is one of the more

271

common locations of stress fractures in the foot and ankle. These fractures are frequently due to the repetitive trauma of running, and patients will typically describe chronic activity-related pain localized to the region of the navicular along the midmedial arch.

Radiographs are often negative, but in patients who have persistent tenderness in the navicular region, a technetium bone scan will reveal increased activity at the site of the fracture. Computed tomography or tomograms can then help to definitively diagnose the fracture.

Patients who sustain a navicular stress fracture should wear a short leg non-walking cast for six to eight weeks. An alternative is a short leg brace for the same period of non-weight-bearing to allow for mobilization. A highly competitive athlete, however, may not comply with the period of non-weight-bearing if placed in a removable brace. If immobilization does not lead to healing, these patients can be treated surgically.

Lisfranc (Tarsometatarsal) Fracture-Dislocation

A Lisfranc injury, which involves disruption of the tarsometatarsal joint with or without associated fracture, can be a source of prolonged disability for an athlete. Most Lisfranc injuries involve the first three metatarsals, but the intercuneiform or naviculocuneiform joints may also be affected.

Although typically a high-energy injury, a Lisfranc fracture-dislocation can occur during athletic activities. The typical mechanisms of injury include twisting of the forefoot, axial load on the forefoot, and a crush injury.[1] A twisting injury can occur, for example, when a person falls from a horse and gets a foot caught in a stirrup, or when a person is thrown from a sailboard while his or her feet are secured in the straps. A classic sports-related Lisfranc injury occurs when a football player falls onto the heel of another player's plantar-flexed foot, causing an axial load along the metatarsals.

A high index of suspicion is necessary to diagnose this injury. The patient will report severe midfoot pain, and examination will reveal moderate-to-severe swelling along the midfoot region with variable flattening of the arch or abduction of the forefoot. Severe tenderness will be present along the midfoot. Passive plantar flexion and dorsiflexion of the toes should be assessed to rule out a compartment syndrome of the foot.

Radiographic evaluation includes anteroposterior (AP), lateral, and oblique views of the foot. A normal AP or oblique radiograph should reveal that the medial and lateral aspects of the first three metatarsals align with the medial and lateral aspects of the cuneiforms with which they articulate, and the medial aspect of the fourth metatarsal aligns with the medial aspect of the cuboid on the oblique view. Any alteration of these normal relationships demonstrates the site or sites of displacement. Other radiographic signs include diastasis or a fleck fracture between the base of the first and second metatarsals on an AP radiograph or dorsal displacement of the metatarsals on lateral view.

A non-displaced Lisfranc injury can be treated conservatively in a short leg non-walking cast for six weeks followed by six weeks in a short leg walking cast. Most of these injuries, however, will have some degree of displacement and require open reduction and internal fixation.

Metatarsal Fractures

With the exception of stress fractures and injuries of the fifth metatarsal, metatarsal fractures typically result from a direct blow to the foot. Fractures are generally classified according to their anatomic location as neck, shaft, or base fractures, and AP and lateral radiographs are generally sufficient for assessment.

Acute fracture: A single, traumatic fracture of a metatarsal is usually minimally displaced because of the restraining forces of the intermetatarsal ligaments. Patients describe pain with weight bearing. On examination, they will have swelling and tenderness localized to the fracture site. These fractures can generally be treated conservatively in a cast or wooden shoe for six weeks with weight bearing as tolerated until the patient's pain and tenderness subside.

Stress fracture: Metatarsal stress fractures generally involve a single metatarsal, usually the second or third. They typically result from training errors such as too rapid an increase in mileage in a runner. Patients will report activity-related pain that gradually increases. They will generally have tenderness over the fracture site with minimal edema. Poor shoes can also contribute. These fractures can be treated with a stiff-soled shoe or wooden shoe, and the patient should cross-train in low-impact activities such as swimming or stationary cycling until tenderness resolves.

Multiple fracture: Multiple fractures frequently require open reduction and internal fixation because of significant displacement.

273

Residual displacement of a metatarsal fracture can predispose a patient to develop a callus. This is because a displaced metatarsal, whether plantar or dorsally displaced, alters the pressure pattern in the forefoot, and a callus forms in the area of increased pressure. The callus, or intractable plantar keratosis, will cause persistent pain with weight bearing and will require an orthosis or possibly even surgical correction of the underlying bony deformity.

Fifth-metatarsal fracture: The most common injury of the fifth metatarsal is an avulsion fracture at the insertion of the peroneus brevis tendon, which occurs with an inversion injury to the hindfoot. Patients will say that they sprained their ankle, but the tenderness will be localized over the base of the fifth metatarsal. These fractures heal reliably and can be treated with a wooden shoe, tennis shoe for support, or other symptomatic treatment, provided that no displacement of the intra-articular base of the metatarsal exists.

A much more serious fracture of the fifth metatarsal is the Jones fracture. This fracture occurs at the diaphyseal-metaphyseal junction of the base of the fifth metatarsal. A watershed area of the blood supply of the fifth metatarsal exists in this region, thus predisposing this area to delayed healing, nonunion, or stress fracture. Patients who sustain a Jones fracture may experience a sudden onset of pain with trivial trauma, or they may develop a gradual onset of pain in the midlateral border of the foot.

Traumatic or stress fractures in this area must be treated with six weeks in a non-walking cast. Despite this aggressive non-operative treatment, a significant proportion of these patients will develop a nonunion.[1] Primary open reduction and internal fixation of this fracture may be preferred in competitive athletes to compress the fracture site to facilitate healing and thus minimize the period of disability.

Sesamoid Fracture

Fractures of the sesamoid bones can occur acutely as a result of direct trauma or indirectly from hyperdorsiflexion of the hallux metatarsophalangeal joint, such as in a football player. Because of their poor blood supply, the sesamoids are also prone to stress fractures.

With either an acute or a stress fracture, patients typically will have pain over the plantar aspect of the first metatarsal head and localized tenderness over the affected sesamoid. The medial sesamoid is usually involved—probably because it is located more directly beneath the first metatarsal.[1] These fractures can be very recalcitrant, and patients must be warned that symptoms will frequently persist for four to six months. Radiographic evaluation includes AP and lateral views of the foot and a sesamoid x-ray—a tangential view of the plantar aspect of the first metatarsal with the toe extended.

For an acute fracture, most authors advocate a short leg walking cast for three to six weeks followed by a stiff-soled shoe with a metatarsal pad to elevate the metatarsal head until symptoms resolve. Stress fractures are more difficult to treat and require six to 12 weeks in a short leg walking cast. Patients must avoid all high-impact activities until tenderness subsides. Patients with pain persisting for three to six months despite adherence to the above regimen may require partial or complete surgical excision of the sesamoid. However, sesamoid excision can be complicated by hallux valgus (with a medial sesamoid excision), hallux varus (lateral sesamoid excision) or stiffness, and thus should be avoided if possible. A few authors even advocate bone grafting.[1]

Great Toe Fracture

Fractures of the great toe generally result from a direct blow or an axial load. Pain and tenderness will be localized over the fracture. Non-displaced fractures can be treated with either a walking cast with a toe plate or a wooden shoe and crutches as needed. A fracture displaced into the metatarsophalangeal or interphalangeal joint should be surgically repaired to prevent osteoarthritis. AP and lateral radiographs will demonstrate the fracture anatomy.

Lesser Toe Fracture

Lesser toe fractures are typically caused by an axial load or direct trauma. Even displaced fractures or intra-articular fractures are generally amenable to non-operative treatment. These patients are able to walk despite the fracture but have problems with footwear. Again, AP and lateral x-rays will help pinpoint the fracture.

Patients are instructed to tape the injured toe to an adjacent uninjured toe (buddy taping) and to place a small piece of gauze between the toes to prevent maceration of the skin. A wooden shoe can be used until tenderness subsides to the point where the patient can begin using tennis shoes. Most fracture tenderness resolves in three to four weeks. Typically, follow-up radiographs are unnecessary since they will not influence subsequent treatment decisions.

Attuned to Foot Fractures

Fractures of the midfoot and forefoot are similar to those of the ankle and hindfoot in that they can often be treated non-operatively. But each fracture has its own distinguishing characteristics and treatment options, so physicians need to be attuned to both detection and management of these injuries. Misdiagnosing a Jones fracture, for example, can have serious consequences to an active patient.

Part 2 References

1. De Lee JC: Fractures and dislocations of the foot, in Mann RA, Coughlin MJ (eds): *Surgery of the Foot and Ankle*, ed 6. St Louis, Mosby, 1993, pp 1465-1703.

— by David B. Thordarson, MD

Dr. Thordarson is an assistant professor of orthopedic surgery and the chief of Foot and Ankle Trauma and Reconstructive Surgery in the Department of Orthopaedic Surgery at the University of Southern California in Los Angeles.

Chapter 41

Ankle Sprains

The most common type of ankle injury is a sprain. A sprain is stretching and tearing of ligaments (fibrous bands connecting adjacent bones in a joint.) There are many ligaments around the ankle and these can become damaged when the ankle is forced into a position not normally encountered.

The most frequently seen sprain occurs when weight is applied to a foot which is on an uneven surface, and the foot "rolls in" (inversion). Because the sole of the foot is pointing inward as force is applied, the ligaments stabilizing the lateral—or outside—part of the ankle are stressed. Many patients report hearing a "snap" or "pop" at the time of the injury. This is usually followed by pain and swelling on the lateral aspect of the ankle.

The Most Important Initial Management of a Sprain Is

- **R**—rest
- **I**—ice
- **C**—compression
- **E**—elevation

Many of the problems resulting from sprains are due to blood and edema in and around the ankle. Minimizing swelling helps the ankle heal faster. The **RICE** regimen facilitates this.

"Ankle Sprains," from the SportsMed website hosted by Rice University at http://www.rice.edu. © 1995-2000 SportsMed Web; reprinted with permission.

- **Rest**—no weight bearing for the first 24 hours after the injury possibly longer, depending upon severity.

- **Ice**—apply ice packs using a towel over a plastic bag to the area that is painful. Be careful to avoid frostbite. Ice should be intermittently applied for the first 24 hours.

- **Compression**—an ACE bandage or other soft elastic material should be applied to the ankle to help prevent the accumulation of edema.

- **Elevation**—elevating the ankle helps in removing edema. By having the foot higher than the hip (or heart), gravity is used to pull edema out of the ankle.

Avoid

In the initial 24 hours, it is very important to avoid things which might increase swelling.

1. hot showers,

2. heat rubs (methylsalicylate counterirritants such as "Ben Gay", etc.),

3. hot packs,

4. drinking alcohol,

5. aspirin—prolongs the clotting time of blood and may cause more bleeding into the ankle. (Tylenol or Ibuprofen may be taken to help with pain, but will not speed up the healing process.)

When to Seek Medical Attention

If the ankle is obviously fractured or dislocated, then medical attention should be sought immediately. If you are fairly certain that it is sprained then use the **RICE** regimen and get a professional opinion regarding diagnosis and treatment. It is always a good idea to make an appointment with a physician to assess the severity of the injury, determine if X-rays are necessary, and to receive instruction on proper rehabilitation of the injury.

In some instances a fracture of one of the bones in the leg or ankle may occur along with a sprain. Pain alone is not necessarily a reliable guide of the presence or absence of a fracture. Fractures can usually be diagnosed with an X-ray examination.

Anyone who sprains his or her ankle on a Friday night can usually follow the **RICE** regimen and see a physician on Monday or Tuesday.

Because it is not possible to predict or discuss every possible situation that might arise, it is recommended that the injured person use common sense in dealing with his or her injury.

Degree of Severity of Ankle Sprains

- Grade I—stretch and/or minor tear of the ligament without laxity (loosening).

- Grade II—tear of ligament plus some laxity.

- Grade III—complete tear of the affected ligament (very loose).

Treatment

After the initial 24 hours, the patient can begin partial weight bearing using crutches. Gradually progressing to full weight bearing over several days as tolerated. The patient should try to use a normal heel-toe gait. An ankle brace may be necessary to protect the joint from re-injury. As soon as pain allows, rehabilitation exercises should be done. **THE REHABILITATION EXERCISES ARE THE MOST IMPORTANT ASPECT OF RECOVERING FULL FUNCTION OF THE ANKLE.**

One simple exercise that can be begun early in the course of treatment is the "alphabet" exercise. This is non-weight bearing and involves trying to draw the letters of the alphabet with your toes. Your health care provider should be able to provide you with a complete list of rehabilitation exercise for your ankle.

Most sprains heal completely within a few weeks. The more severe the injury, the longer the time to heal. Often it is necessary to continue rehab exercises for a month or two following the injury. Grade III injuries are usually managed conservatively—rehabilitation exercises, etc.—but a small percentage may require surgery.

Chapter 42

Managing Injuries of the Great Toe

In Brief

Most of the common great-toe injuries that affect active people are self-limiting and easily treated if detected early. Reviewed here are the causes, symptoms, diagnosis, and treatment of hallux valgus, turf toe, hallux rigidus, sesamoid dysfunction, nail abnormalities, dislocations and fractures, calluses, and blisters. Conservative treatment will usually enable patients to return to activity relatively quickly. Continued disability may require referral to an orthopedist.

Great-toe injuries are common in people who are involved in all kinds of sports, but particularly in dancers, runners, and soccer players. Without proper care, these injuries can interrupt a person's exercise program or severely limit an athlete's performance. With proper diagnosis and conservative treatment, however, most patients can anticipate relief from symptoms and a resumption of previous activities.

Hallux Valgus

Hallux valgus is a subluxation of the first metatarsophalangeal (MTP) joint manifested by the medial deviation of the first metatarsal

"Managing Injuries of the Great Toe," by R. Sean Churchill, MD and Brian G. Donley, MD in *The Physician and Sports Medicine*, Vol. 26, No. 9, September 1998. © 1998 The McGraw-Hill Companies. Reproduced with permission of McGraw-Hill, Inc.

and lateral deviation of the proximal phalanx. ("Bunion" refers to any enlargement of the MTP joint caused by disorders such as osteoarthritis, enlarged bursa, or a ganglion cyst.) Originally described in 1870,[1] the condition has since been attributed to the wearing of high-fashion women's shoes.[2,3] Common causes include hereditary conditions, pes planus (flatfoot), and hyperelasticity disorders.

Hallux valgus in active individuals depends on a number of factors. Different sports put varied pressures on the foot. Walking generates a force in the forefoot equal to 80% of the body's weight; running increases it to 250% of body weight.[2] The severity and progression of deformity depend on the particular sport. For instance, dancers develop hallux valgus at a younger age than is seen in the general population.[4,5] A deformity may affect one patient differently from another

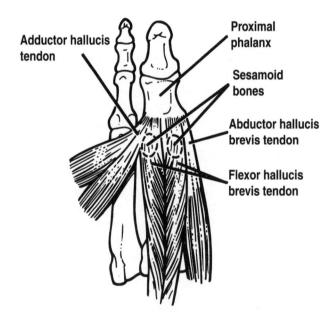

Figure 42.1. *A plantar view of the left great toe shows the metatarsophalangeal (MTP) region. The abductor hallucis tendon inserts medially and the adductor hallucis tendon inserts laterally into the proximal phalanx; their locations are more plantar then dorsal, and the forces exerted on them balance each other. The two separate heads of the flexor hallucis brevis insert into the second sesamoid bones and continue distally to join the adductor and abductor tendons. Figure 42.1: courtesy of Mary Albury-Noyes.*

because various sports make different demands on the foot. For example, sprinters require an extended range of motion in both dorsiflexion and plantar flexion of the first MTP joint, while middle- and long-distance runners do not.[6]

Anatomy: The anatomy of the first MTP joint is complex (Figure 42.1). Since no muscles insert into the head of the first metatarsal, its position is primarily influenced by the position of the proximal phalanx. With increasing lateral deformity of the proximal phalanx, the first metatarsal head is progressively deformed medially, resulting in widening between the first and second metatarsals. This widening, coupled with lateral deviation of the great toe, creates a prominent and painful bunion along the medial aspect of the first metatarsal head.

Diagnosis: The patient's primary symptom is pain over the prominent medial eminence, often caused by irritation and pressure from shoes. Repetitive athletic activities such as running can lead to the development of an inflamed bursa, skin blistering, and skin breakdown. Localized pressure can even cause compression of the dorsal medial sensory nerve to the great toe, causing neuritic pain or numbness.

As the deformity progresses, the first metatarsal can no longer support the forces across the forefoot, and increasing forces subsequently are transferred to the second metatarsal. Ultimately, this leads to the development of a painful, intractable plantar keratosis (callus) beneath the second metatarsal head.

The physical examination should begin with the patient standing. Hallux valgus deformities are often accentuated with weight bearing. Observe for other postural abnormalities, such as pes planus, or a contracted Achilles tendon, which may contribute to the deformity. Check for decreased great-toe range of motion, joint crepitus, and pain, which are often the first signs of degenerative arthritis. Local irritation may occur over the medial eminence and the plantar calluses, and either site may be tender to palpation. Finally, a thorough vascular and neurologic examination should be completed.

Radiographic evaluation should consist of weight-bearing anteroposterior (AP), lateral, oblique, and sesamoid views. The severity of the deformity can be quantified using the AP view (Figure 42.2).

Treatment: Conservative care is the cornerstone of treatment for patients who have hallux valgus. This is especially true for athletically active individuals because postoperative stiffness can occur.

283

Shoe modifications can be helpful. Stretching of shoes in constricted areas may relieve symptoms, but custom-made shoes, though expensive, may provide more relief. In any case, wearing shoes with a broad toe box to accommodate the prominent medial eminence should help. High-heeled shoes should be replaced with flatter dress shoes that do not increase the downward pressure that forces the toes into a narrow toe box.

Besides footwear modifications, bunion pads, night splints, and toe spacers can also offer relief. Orthoses can help redistribute weight away from a painful callus under the second metatarsal head. Athletes who have a tight Achilles tendon may benefit from daily stretching exercises. Conservative treatment of hallux valgus generally should continue indefinitely or until pain and discomfort force the patient to make significant changes in athletic activities.[7]

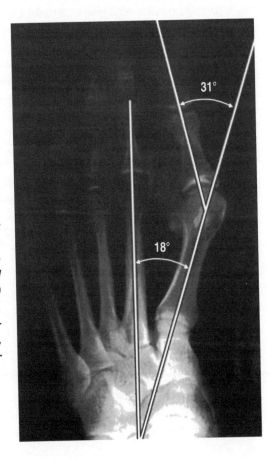

Figure 42.2. Hallux valgus is evident in this weight-bearing AP view of a 35-year-old female volleyball player's great toe. Note the medial deviation of the first metatarsal and the lateral deviation of the proximal phalanx. Lines drawn along the shafts of the first and second metatarsals and the proximal first phalanx on an AP view can be used to evaluate the severity of the deformity. The hallux valgus angle (lateral deviation of the first phalanx) in this patient is 31° (normal, less than 15°), and the intermetatarsal angle is 18° (normal, less than 9°). Figure 42.2 courtesy of Brian G. Donley, MD.

Surgery may then be considered, but the patient should first be counseled regarding options. Post-surgery stiffness can make running more difficult than the pain the athlete was trying to eliminate in the first place.[8] If a patient is willing to change activities—for example, to substitute a non-impact sport such as bicycling for running—he or she may reduce pain and further deformity and avoid surgical intervention. If a patient is unwilling to make such changes, an orthopedic surgeon should be consulted.

Turf Toe

Turf toe is simply a hyperextension injury to the great toe. The term was originally coined for football and soccer players who injured their great toes on artificial turf.[9-11] Runners and other athletes who do not compete on artificial turf can also sustain this injury.

Anatomy: The first metatarsal head articulates with the medial and lateral sesamoids on its plantar aspect (Figure 42.3). The sesamoids are contained within the flexor hallucis brevis tendon and are distally connected to the base of the proximal phalanx by the plantar plate. Medial and lateral stability of the sesamoids is imparted by the tendons of the abductor and adductor hallucis as well as by the intersesamoidal ligament. This complex stabilizes the plantar aspect of the first MTP joint.

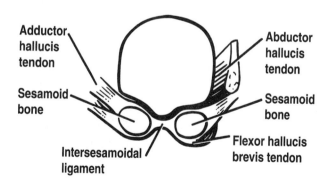

Figure 42.3. *A cross-section through the first metatarsal head shows the relationship of the sesamoid bones to the abductor and adductor hallucis tendons and intersesamoidal ligament, all of which stabilize the plantar aspect of the first MTP joint. Figure 42.3 courtesy of Mary Albury-Noyes.*

A forced hyperextension of the first MTP joint results in a capsular injury of varying severity, with associated compression injury to the dorsal articular surface in severe cases.

Diagnosis: Patients usually report a sudden onset of great-toe pain after a forced dorsiflexion, such as can occur when a football player whose crouched position has already maximally extended his MTP joint takes the weight of a falling opponent.[12]

On physical exam, the patient walks with an antalgic gait, either externally rotating the lower extremity to avoid first MTP dorsiflexion during push-off or walking on the outside of the foot to minimize pressure on the first MTP joint. Periarticular swelling and ecchymosis vary according to the severity of the injury. Passive motion at the MTP joint is painful[13] and demonstrates decreases in dorsiflexion, plantar flexion, or both. Normal active range of motion of the first MTP joint is from 80° of dorsiflexion to 25° of plantar flexion (Figure 42.4).[7] An additional 25° of dorsiflexion can be obtained passively.[14]

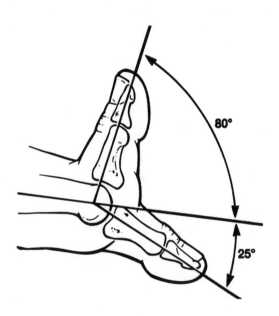

Figure 42.4. *The normal range of motion of the first MTP joint is 80° of extension and 25° of flexion. Injuries such as turf toe, caused by hyperextension of the joint, result in a reduced range of motion. Figure 42.4 courtesy of Mary Albury-Noyes.*

AP, lateral, oblique, and sesamoid radiographs often show no bony abnormalities. However, occasionally a capsular avulsion fracture on the first metatarsal head or proximal phalanx can be identified. Other radiographic findings in more severe injuries include sesamoid bone fracture or intra-articular loose bodies caused by a compression fracture.

Turf toe injuries are classified into three grades, as described in Table 42.1.[12]

Treatment: The initial treatment for all grades of turf toe is rest, ice, compression dressings, elevation, and non-steroidal anti-inflammatory drugs (NSAIDs), but other treatment measures vary with the grade.

Grade 1 injuries can usually be treated effectively with conservative measures. Patients may continue sports activity if (1) they wear stiff-soled shoes to prevent dorsiflexion beyond 30° during the push-off phase, and (2) the great toe is taped by bringing tape from the

Table 42.1. Grading of Turf Toe Injuries

Grade	Signs and Symptoms	Tissue Disruption
1	Plantar or medial tenderness, minimal swelling, no ecchymosis, negative x-rays	Stretched plantar capsuloligamentous complex
2	Diffuse tenderness, moderate swelling, ecchymosis, restriction of motion	Partially torn plantar capsuloligamentous complex without articular injury
3	Severe dorsal tenderness, plantar tenderness considerable swelling, ecchymosis, marked range-of-motion restriction	Completely torn plantar capsuloligamentous complex with compression injury to dorsal articular surface; may represent a spontaneously reduced great-toe dislocation

dorsal surface of the great toe to the plantar surface to prevent dorsiflexion beyond 30°.[15]

Patients with grade 2 injuries should refrain from athletic activities for one to two weeks and wear stiff-soled shoes; a rigid orthosis should be inserted to further prevent dorsiflexion of the first MTP joint. Grade 3 injuries require the same modalities as grade 2, but the restriction of athletic activities is three to six weeks. If these conservative measures fail for grade 3 injuries, surgery for plantar capsule repair or loose-body removal may be necessary.[9]

A patient's return to activities should progress gradually from weight bearing to walking to jogging, using discomfort as a guide. A complete return to play should be permitted only after full-speed running and cutting maneuvers are pain free.[15] With proper care, the prognosis for full recovery is excellent.

Hallux Rigidus

Hallux rigidus is the painful, progressive loss of motion of the first MTP joint. Patients report a history of trauma that can be a single episode of axial compression of the first MTP while playing football or soccer or multiple, less traumatic events that can occur in many activities, from ballet to track and field. Predisposing factors include repetitive hyperextension of the first MTP joint[16] and an abnormally long first metatarsal.[17]

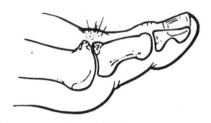

Figure 42.5. Hallux rigidus is caused by dorsal osteophytes on the first metatarsal head and first proximal phalanx that progressively impinge on each other and limit dorsiflexion. Figure 42.5: Mary Albury-Noyes.

The condition develops over months to years when a dorsal osteophyte forms on the first metatarsal head and a circumferential rim of osteophytes develops at the base of the first proximal phalanx (Figure 42.5). As these osteophytes enlarge, they eventually impinge on one another, leading to decreased range of motion and pain.

Diagnosis: The primary symptom is decreased great-toe range of motion, primarily in extension. Patients also have pain with walking and running. Pain also occurs when a patient walks without shoes and is exacerbated when he or she walks in a shoe that has an elevated heel. Intermittent swelling and pain at the base of the great toe are also common symptoms.

A physical exam reveals an enlarged, tender first MTP joint, with limited dorsiflexion. Dorsal metatarsal osteophytes, usually dorsolateral, may be palpable. Pain is produced by passive and active hyperextension and maximal plantar flexion, which tents the dorsal capsular structures over the osteophytes, resulting in increased tenderness

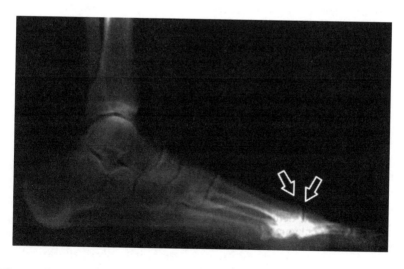

Figure 42.6. *A lateral radiograph demonstrates hallux rigidus of the foot of a 43-year-old male distance runner. The dorsal osteophytes of both the first metatarsal head and the proximal first phalanx (arrows) produced pain and limited his ability to run distances. Figure 42.6 courtesy of Brian G. Donley, MD.*

before any appreciable mechanical block. In contrast, dorsiflexion is limited but less tender, and the maneuver often seems to indicate a mechanical block, both objectively and subjectively. Pain in the chronic condition occurs only at the extremes of motion, but in the acute phase accompanied by synovitis, it occurs with any joint motion.[15]

Initial radiographs should include AP, oblique, and lateral views. Although these may be normal, they eventually show progressive osteoarthritis of the MTP joint. The lateral radiograph (Figure 42.6.) reveals dorsal osteophytes on the proximal phalanx and the first metatarsal.

Treatment: Initial treatment should include rest, ice, NSAIDs, and shoe modifications. A stiff-soled shoe to decrease dorsiflexion combined with an enlarged toe box to accommodate swelling may be adequate to relieve symptoms. A rocker-bottom shoe can be prescribed, but this may adversely affect athletic performance and thus be unacceptable.

If symptoms persist, an intra-articular corticosteroid injection[15] can provide some relief. However, injections should be used sparingly because they do cause damage to the remaining cartilage surface. Patients who have continued disability should consult an orthopedic surgeon about surgical options, which may include the removal of loose bodies from the joint, excision of osteophytes (cheilectomy), osteotomy of the proximal phalanx, or MTP joint arthrodesis.

Sesamoid Dysfunction

The primary functions of the sesamoid bones (Figures 42.1. and 42.3.) are to increase the moment arm of the flexor hallucis brevis muscle, reduce friction, and distribute the pressure of weight bearing.

Athletic injury to the sesamoids is not uncommon and can occur acutely or with repetitive stress. An acute sesamoid fracture usually follows a specific event, such as a dancer's landing from a leap[15] or a forced dorsiflexion stress in football linemen and soccer players. Sesamoiditis is a specific term that indicates inflammation and swelling of the peritendinous structures of the sesamoid complex. However, it is also used for any condition affecting the sesamoid—with or without inflammation—such as bursitis, arthritis, plantar digital nerve compression, osteochondritis, and a painful bipartite sesamoid.

Diagnosis: A physical exam typically reveals decreased range of motion of the first MTP joint and increased tenderness with dorsiflexion. Active plantar flexion is painful and thus weak. Direct palpation over the sesamoids routinely indicates whether the medial or lateral sesamoid is the source of the patient's symptoms. Ordinarily the patient who has sesamoiditis presents with pain under the head of the first metatarsal that ceases with rest and elevation.

Radiographs, including AP, lateral, oblique, and sesamoid views of the foot, should be carefully interpreted. About 19% of the population has a bipartite sesamoid, and 89% of these are the medial sesamoid.[18] The sesamoid edges are smooth and relatively sclerotic in the bipartite sesamoid (Figure 42.7), while they appear rough and irregular in an acute or stress fracture. If radiographic findings are unclear, a bone scan can help distinguish an acute fracture from a bipartite sesamoid.

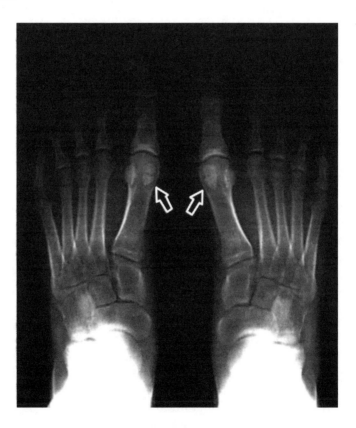

Figure 42.7. *An AP radiograph of the feet of a 25-year-old female gymnast who had no foot pain reveals bilateral sesamoids (arrows). The smooth, sclerotic edges are inconsistent with an acute or stress fracture, which has sharp, irregular edges. Figure 42.7 courtesy of Brian G. Donley, MD.*

Treatment: Treatment for sesamoid pain is conservative. Symptoms can be relieved by eliminating the use of high-heeled shoes to reduce forefoot pressure and by using a J-shaped pad or orthotic donut to decrease pressure on the affected sesamoid. NSAIDs are also prescribed to reduce inflammation. Treatment for sesamoiditis may take four to six weeks.

Sesamoid fractures are treated with three weeks of great-toe immobilization and the use of crutches. When the patient resumes bearing weight, he or she should use a stiff-soled shoe until pain subsides. Following a sesamoid fracture, dancers may gradually resume practice when symptoms resolve,[15] but complete recovery may require a full year.

If the condition fails to respond to six weeks of treatment, radiographs should be repeated. These may reveal a loss of joint space between the sesamoid and the metatarsal head, characteristic of degenerative arthritis, or fragmentation of the involved sesamoid, indicating osteonecrosis. Treatment of degenerative arthritis and osteonecrosis should be similar to that of sesamoiditis but should last four to six months. If the condition fails to improve, referral to an orthopedic surgeon for possible excision of the involved sesamoid should be considered.

Toenail Abnormalities

Ingrown nails: Ingrown toenails are ordinarily a minor nuisance, but they can disable an active person if they are not treated early. The condition occurs most commonly in athletes in their teens and early 20s and can be caused by an acute trauma, such as stubbing the toe, or repetitive stress such as occurs in long-distance running. Improper nail care is a common cause. Cutting on a curve or tearing predisposes nails to be ingrown. As the nail grows, the nail corner presses on the nail fold. If this pressure is not relieved, the nail may penetrate the nail fold and cause infection. Tight-fitting shoes can also increase pressure between the nail and nail fold, which results in ingrowth.[19]

Diagnosis: Physical examination reveals a characteristic erythematous nail fold that is edematous and tender to palpation. Care should be taken to verify that there is no fluctuance to the nail fold, indicating a purulent fluid collection that would require drainage and antibiotics. In chronic or more severe acute cases, radiographs should be obtained to rule out coexisting osteomyelitis.

Treatment: Initial treatment involves local measures. The affected border of the toenail should be gently elevated from the nail fold, and a wisp of cotton carefully inserted beneath the nail plate edge. The patient should soak the toe twice daily in a warm salt solution, carefully dry the toe, and wipe the area with alcohol.

Follow-up should occur in five to seven days, when the cotton should be changed. Cotton packing should be continued until the nail plate has grown beyond the distal nail fold edge. Patients should be instructed on proper nail cutting: trimming straight across the nail without curving the medial and lateral edges. The fit of the patient's street and athletic shoes should be checked to prevent recurrence.

Patients who have chronic or severe conditions and severe cases that do not respond to local measures are candidates for operative treatment.

Subungual Hematoma

This common condition usually occurs when someone steps forcibly on the great toe or when the toe is repeatedly jammed against the end of the toe box during activities such as soccer or tennis. In fact, the average soccer player loses two to three toenails per year of soccer playing time from subungual hematomas.[15]

If the patient presents acutely, the hematoma can easily be decompressed by penetrating the nail plate vertically with a hot paper clip, providing immediate relief. The patient should be told that the nail will eventually detach as the new nail grows. Chronic cases can result in deformed and thickened nails.

Dislocations and Fractures

Dislocations of the first MTP joint are usually the result of a violent force, as when the forefoot strikes an immovable object or a blocked ball.[15] Dorsal dislocation is more common than plantar dislocation and may be associated with intra-articular fractures.

Patients will usually present with a history of trauma, followed by spontaneous or self-reduction of the joint at the scene. The physical examination should focus on the neurovascular status of the great toe. A subungual hematoma is often present and is not diagnostic of a phalanx fracture. AP, lateral, sesamoid, and oblique views of the foot should be obtained and evaluated for fractures and small, loose bone fragments in the first MTP joint.

The foot should be immobilized in a splint and the patient referred to an orthopedic surgeon. Final treatment depends on injury severity. For a simple dislocation, treatment may include rest, ice, and a stiff-soled shoe, with return to play four weeks after injury. More complicated injuries may require operative reduction of fractures and removal of cartilage fragments from the joint. Aggressive treatment of great-toe dislocations and fractures is warranted because of the toe's importance in daily and sports activities.

Plantar Calluses

Calluses are hyperkeratotic lesions. Primarily located on the sole of the foot under the metatarsal heads, they are a protective response to imbalanced weight distribution. They are commonly seen under the first metatarsal head and on the plantar medial aspect of the great toe in soccer players[16] and may eventually become symptomatic as their size increases.

In symptomatic patients, examination reveals tenderness with deep compression of the callus. A plantar wart and a callus can be confused, but distinguishing them is quite simple: Plantar warts are painful on medial-lateral compression, but calluses are not. In addition, shaving causes pinpoint bleeding in a plantar wart but not in a callus.

Treatment involves thinning the callus by shaving it, followed by daily filing with a pumice stone after showering. Total-contact molded inserts manufactured by a local orthotist will help redistribute uneven weight-bearing forces and prevent recurrence. Patients whose calluses do not respond to this program should be referred to an orthopedist to be evaluated for possible structural foot abnormalities that may require surgical correction.

Blisters

Blisters are a common annoyance for most people, but can impair the performance of an athlete. They form as a result of friction and resulting shearing forces on the skin that cause the accumulation of fluid between the epidermal layers. A common cause of foot blisters is wearing new shoes that have not been properly broken in.

A large blister that interferes with an athlete's performance should be drained by sterile aspiration with a 27-gauge needle. The skin should be kept intact to prevent infection and should be protected with gauze and tape for the first 24 hours. A patient can continue athletic activity comfortably by placing a donut pad around the blister for protection. Preventive measures include properly fitted athletic shoes, adequate shoe break-in before hard workouts or competition, and the use of lubricants such as petroleum jelly on susceptible areas of the foot.

Excellent Prognosis

Active patients are susceptible to a wide spectrum of injuries to the great toe, from the minor annoyance of a blister to the severely disabling dislocation or fracture. With the exception of the fracture or dislocation, primary care physicians can manage most of these conditions. Early diagnosis and conservative treatment should enable most patients to recover fully and resume previous levels of activity.

References

1. Hueter C: Klinik *der Gelenkkrankheiten mit Einschluss der Orthopadie*. Leipzig, FCW Vogel, 1871.

2. Lam SF, Hodgson AR: A comparison of foot forms among the non-shoe and shoe wearing Chinese population. *J Bone Joint Surg (Am)* 1958;40:1058-1062.

3. Mann RA, Coughlin, MJ: Hallux valgus and complications of hallux valgus, in Mann RA (ed): *Surgery of the Foot*, ed 5. St Louis, *CV Mosby*, 1986, pp 65-130.

4. Sammarco GJ, Miller EH: Forefoot conditions in dancers: part 1. *Foot Ankle* 1982;3(2):85-92.

5. Sammarco GJ, Miller EH: Forefoot conditions in dancers: part 2. *Foot Ankle* 1982;3(2):93-98.

6. Lillich JS, Baxter DE: Bunionectomies and related surgery in the elite female middle-distance and marathon runner. *Am J Sports Med* 1986;14(6):491-493.

7. DeLee JC, Drez D Jr (eds): *Orthopaedic Sports Medicine, Principles and Practice*. Philadelphia, WB Saunders Co, 1994, pp 1842-1935.

8. Lutter LD: Forefoot abnormalities in runners. *Presented at the 18th Annual Meeting of the American Orthopaedic Foot and Ankle Society*, Atlanta, February 7, 1988.

9. Coker TP, Arnold JA, Weber DL: Traumatic lesions of the metatarsophalangeal joint of the great toe in athletes. *Am J Sports Med* 1978;6(6):326-334.

10. Sammarco GJ: Turf toe. *Instr Course Lect* 1993;42:207-212.

11. Rodeo SA, O'Brien S, Warren RF, et al: Turf-toe: an analysis of metatarsophalangeal joint sprains in professional football players. *Am J Sports Med* 1990;18(3):280-285.

12. Clanton TO, Butler JE, Eggert A: Injuries to the metatarsophalangeal joints in athletes. *Foot Ankle* 1986;7(3):162-176.

13. Bowers KD Jr, Martin RB: Turf toe: a shoe surface related football injury. *Med Sci Sports* 1976;8(2):81-83.

14. Joseph J: Range of movement of the great toe in men. *J Bone Joint Surg (Br)* 1954;36:450-457.

15. Nicholas JA, Hershman EB (eds): *The Lower Extremity and Spine in Sports Medicine, ed 2.* St Louis, *CV Mosby*, 1995, pp 1509-1557.

16. Jack EA: The etiology of hallux rigidus. *Br J Surg* 1940;27:492.

17. Bonney G, Mcnab I: Hallux valgus and hallux rigidus: critical survey of operative results. *(J Bone Joint Surg Br)* 1952; 34:366.

18. Dobas DC, Silvers MD: The frequency of the partite sesamoids of the first metatarsophalangeal joint. *J Am Podiatr Assoc* 1977;67(12):880-882.

19. Dockery GL: Nails: fundamental conditions and procedures, in McGlamry ED (ed): *Comprehensive Textbook of Foot Surgery.* Baltimore, Williams & Wilkins, 1987, pp 3-37.

−by R. Sean Churchill, MD and Brian G. Donley, MD

Dr. Churchill is a resident and Dr. Donley an associate staff orthopedic surgeon in the section of foot and ankle surgery in the Department of Orthopaedic Surgery at the Cleveland Clinic Foundation in Cleveland.

Chapter 43

Mid-Foot Injuries

Just as anywhere else in the body, the bulk of foot problems are overuse injuries. You try something new, or do more of your usual activity, overusing the muscles, which subsequently tighten up and pull against the tendons, which, being the most vulnerable in the chain of bone-muscle-tendon, cannot bear the strain and tear. It's an old story, repeated often. The foot, however, offers a couple of unique wrinkles.

Tendinitis

One is that you can get a kind of tendentious that you don't see anywhere else: tendentious that is the result of external pressure. Think about it. We really don't put constraining clothing around our arms, our legs, or the rest of our body. But we wedge our feet into all sorts of confining footwear, sometimes for reasons that have little to do with comfort or protection. And this footwear can actually cause tendentious in and of it self. When dealing with feet, therefore, we're in a world in which clothing can cause problems. (More on that later).

The other thing about the foot is that it enables you to identify problems quickly and accurately, more so than elsewhere in the body. There's not a lot of fat in the foot, not a lot of muscle. You can see almost all the tendons. Anything that's kind of rigid, that feels like a

"The Midfoot—Tendinitis," excerpted from "Foot Injuries" at Center for Sports Medicine website at http://www.centerforsportsmed.org. Copyright 1999 Catholic Healthcare West. Reprinted with permission.

little rope, is a tendon. When you move your feet, these little ropes move—you can't mistake them. So if one of them hurts when you move your foot, you probably have tendentious. Sometimes you'll get the same thing that's possible with Achilles Tendinitis: snowball crepitation—the tendon actually can squeak. And because there's little padding in the foot between the skin and tendons, the injured area may become red and swollen. So self-diagnosis in the foot is pretty easy.

Now, back to footwear. Because there's no padding in the foot, just lacing your shoes too tightly for a three- or four-mile run can cause so much irritation that you may be on the sidelines for three or four weeks. The tendons that run along the top of the foot are virtually on the surface. They're extremely sensitive to pressure. As you run, the tendons slide beneath the skin. Running puts the foot through a wide range of motion, and the tendons must move a long way. If there's outside pressure curtailing their ability to slide, the tendons can easily become inflamed. So, particularly when you're breaking in new shoes and haven't yet figured out how tightly or loosely to lace them, opt for loosely.

The same problem may arise in skiing. A too-tight center buckle on a ski boot is a common cause of tendinitis. Sometimes people have ill designed or ill-fitting boots and find that they can't keep their heel down inside the boot. The first thing they do is tighten the center buckle over the instep of their foot. That probably won't keep the heel down either, but it will keep the tendons down—mash them, in fact. And sometimes it can squash one of the little nerves that run along the tendons to the foot. Like the tendons, the nerves in the foot are virtually unprotected. It's not uncommon in November and December to hear people complain that two or three of their toes are numb. They'll probably stay numb through the entire ski season and into the summer, all from one day of skiing. It's not a major problem, but it can be very annoying to have a constant tingling in your foot.

What to Do about It

Treat tendinitis of the foot as you'd treat tendinitis anywhere: back off from doing what hurts. Also, you might try a shoe with a more rigid sole to block some of the motion of your foot. If there's swelling, give your foot contrast baths. Take aspirin. But the most important thing is to stop doing whatever it was that caused the problem in the first place. Then ease back slowly. Let pain be your guide. If it doesn't hurt, you're okay. If it hurts, you're doing too much. Back off for a while, and then push forward again.

Stress Fractures

One of the most common foot problems, stress fractures occur more often than not in those small bones between the toes and the top of the foot called the metatarsals. You can easily feel the metatarsals. Some people think that if you have what's called "Morton's foot"—your second toe is longer than your big toe—you may have a tendency to suffer stress fractures, but this is a controversial point of view. You don't incur a stress fracture because there is something wrong with the mechanics of your foot, but rather because there is something wrong with the mechanics of your head—you went off and ran nine miles when you're used to running two, that sort of thing. Stress fractures are almost always the result of training mistakes like that.

You can get a stress fracture at the base of the fifth metatarsal, that area marked by a bump on the outside of your foot. Dancers, and basketball players even more, are susceptible to those. And jumping sports like basketball can cause a stress fracture of the navicular, the bony ridge on the top of the foot. They are horrible to deal with—difficult to see on X-rays, long to heal, sometimes even requiring surgery. It is the injury that basketball player Bill Walton has struggled with for years. Navicular stress fractures also are quite common in gymnasts. Some nationally prominent gymnasts have suffered this injury. They are nasty injuries. You just don't ignore things like this in the middle part or outside of your foot.

Fortunately, these bones are right there under the skin, visible and easy to keep track of. You'll see and feel swelling. And, like stress fractures of the shinbone, there will be a discrete area of tenderness. You can cover it with a dime or a nickel. In contrast to tendinitis, in which the painful area is more diffused, if you put your finger on a stress fracture it will really hurt. A caution: the commonest reason to hurt on the outside of the foot is that your shoes aren't wide enough. So the first thing to do if you suffer any of these symptoms is look to your shoes. If you hurt only when you wear one particular pair of shoes and are fine the rest of the time, you're in luck. It's much easier to replace a pair of shoes than it is to replace a foot.

What to Do about It

If the symptoms persist no matter what shoes you wear, stop doing whatever it is that makes you hurt. Rest is the primary treatment for stress fractures. That and dealing with the swelling by icing and taking contrast baths. Getting into a stiff-soled shoe to reduce the movement of your foot can also help. Boots are very good in this regard. Hiking boots, cowboy boots—both can help. (The big problem with cowboy boots is getting them on and off. Once you're in them, they can solve a great many problems temporarily.)

If a few days of rest and reduced activity don't seem to be making headway, or if you stop your activity, the pain goes away, and then it comes back as soon as you begin again, it's a good idea to see a doctor. Because ... (see Fractures).

Contusions

Dropping something on your foot or having somebody step on your foot in one sport or another can cause contusions, which are very painful. Your foot is not well suited to being scrunched. We wear common shoes to protect not only the bottom of the foot but the top as well. If you bruise the top of your foot badly, it isn't going to work very well. It can be as painful, and debilitating, as barking your shin. Remember that the black and blue of a bruise is really blood under the skin, and when there's blood under the skin in the foot, there's nowhere for it to go. It simply pools on top of the bone. All the bones in the foot are just under the skin, so the tendons on the top of your foot must slide directly over the bone. If there's a big sea of blood there, the tendons won't slide very well. Tendinitis can easily result from the obstruction.

What to Do about It

Foot contusions should be treated the same way you treat contusions anywhere: apply a compression wrap as soon as possible. The more blood that pools under the skin, the longer it will take to get rid of it. Ice can help to prevent swelling; contrast baths can help to reduce it once it has formed.

Dislocations

The ultimate sprain is a dislocation, and there are some horrible dislocations that occur up in the foot. These are devastating injuries. There are so many bones in your foot, and so many things can go wrong with them. Again, if you really hurt your foot, and it swells and turns black and blue, don't even dream of not seeing somebody.

Chapter 44

Tendinitis and Bursitis

Tendinitis in the foot is difficult to treat, especially when it has become chronic. Prompt attention is imperative to prevent stretching, degeneration, and rupture of the tendon. Because of the stresses of weight bearing, inadequately treated tendinitis commonly leads to foot deformities. The tendons most frequently affected are the posterior tibial, Achilles', flexor hallucis longus, and peroneus longus and brevis.

Posterior Tibial Tendinitis

This condition is the most common cause of gradual, progressive, and chronic medial mid-foot pain, especially in women 50-70 years old. The posterior tibial muscle is a strong invertor and plantar flexor of the foot. It also supports the medial arch and keeps the foot from hyperpronating during the midstance phase of walking or running. Microtrauma to the tendon leads to inflammation, progressive degeneration, and possible rupture. The tendon acts much like a rope on a pulley around the medial malleolus and then attaches to the navicular at the apex of the medial arch. An accessory navicular bone may add to the pain picture and should be looked for.

Initially, the patient presents with medial ankle pain and swelling. There is localized tenderness over the tendon, notably in the portion

Excerpted from "Effective Approaches to Common Foot Complaints," *Patient Care*, March 15, 1997, Vol. 31, No. 5, Pg. 158(16), by Stephen J. Dale, Daniel J. David, and Ted F. Sykes. © 1997 Medical Economics; reprinted with permission of *Patient Care*.

from the medial malleolus to the navicular, and decreased inversion strength against resistance.

Conservative treatment at this stage consists of four-to-six weeks of cast immobilization holding the foot in slight inversion and plantar flexion. Oral NSAIDs are helpful as well. If immobilization is unsuccessful, you may consider a corticosteroid injection in the tendon sheath, being careful not to inject the tendon substance. Advise the patient to rest the foot for at least 10 days after any injection. No more than two injections should be given, with a two-week interval between them.

Excessive pronation must be prevented using a medial heel wedge or orthoses. When the tendon is stretched or ruptured, there is an abnormal forefoot pronation with accompanying heel valgus and abducted foot. This is best viewed from behind the standing patient and is often called the "too many toes" sign. In patients with this sign, pain may shift to the lateral ankle as a result of impingement of the lateral ligaments in the sinus tarsi. With any persistent signs of stretching or collapse of the medial foot, referral for surgical evaluation is necessary.

Achilles' Tendinitis

After plantar fasciitis, Achilles' tendinitis is the most frequent hindfoot disorder in active people. The cause is usually overuse—a sudden increase in training mileage, a switch to uneven terrain, a long hike, or a hurried run to catch a plane. Achilles' tendinitis may also occur secondary to use of fluoroquinolone antibiotics: Although an uncommon adverse effect, it should be mentioned to active people taking these drugs.

Achilles' tendinitis can present early as a peritendinitis in which the inflammation has a spongy feel. Upon movement of the foot, the pain tends to stay in one location. Tenderness is several centimeters proximal to the insertion of the tendon into the calcaneus. It's important to recognize and treat the condition at this stage, before repeated microtrauma and restricted blood flow produce inflammation and degeneration in the tendon that can lead to rupture.

Initially, treatment includes contrast soaks, ice massage, and NSAIDs. As the inflammation starts to subside, a temporary 3/8ths-inch felt heel pad is placed inside the shoe and a program of gentle stretching is begun to take the stress off the tendon. The patient should warm up the tendon before starting the stretches and work below the limits of pain with slow, controlled movements against an elastic cord. Maximum benefit is usually achieved if the patient can work up to five-to-six stretches performed three-to-four times a day.

If the injury does not respond to this regimen and range of motion is being steadily lost, the patient can be referred for a rapid infiltration of 15 mL of 1% lidocaine HCI (Xylocalne HCI) into the sheath, which produces a mechanical lysis of adhesions. Gentle stretching is then resumed. If this approach also fails, open lysis of the adhesions may be performed.

Some patients may present later in the disease process with true Achilles' tendinitis. Chronic repetitive stresses produce a fusiform swelling that is firm to palpation. Dorsiflexion of the ankle is decreased to less than 15 degrees (normal is 25 degrees). Strain causes pain within the substance of the tendon that moves with movement of the foot and increases with activity. Degenerative changes within the tendon predispose to rupture with repeated stress.

Treatment at this stage includes NSAIDs and one to two weeks in a non-weight-bearing cast, followed by ice, stretching, and assessment of the foot and leg alignment to determine if orthotic correction is needed. If symptoms persist beyond six months, referral for surgical evaluation is recommended.

Peroneal Tendinitis

This injury often occurs after an inversion injury of the ankle that produces a lateral ligament sprain. The sprain is treated successfully, but pain persists in the lateral mid-foot and ankle. You may note clicking laterally with an occasional sensation of giving way. Tenderness is well localized to the section of peroneal tendons from the lateral malleolus to the base of the fifth metatarsal. The tendon sheath is usually swollen, and resisted eversion reproduces the pain.

Treatment is aimed at reducing the stress on the tendon by using lateral or eversion wedges or orthoses. If symptoms are severe, a cast is used for two to three weeks to rest the tendon, followed by extensive rehabilitation. For resistant symptoms, corticosteroid injection within the tendon sheath can be used, followed by the usual injection precautions.

If the tendinitis is secondary to subluxating or dislocating peroneal tendons, the predominant pain and tenderness will be proximal and behind the lateral malleolus. In your examination, attempt to palpate abnormal movement of the tendons. If findings are positive, referral is indicated.

Flexor Hallucis Longus Tendinitis

This type of tendinitis is most commonly seen in persons who repeatedly execute push-off maneuvers—ballet dancers, for example.

Excessive forces along the tendon cause irritation and inflammation in the tendon and sheath. Patients complain of pain and tenderness in the posteromedial aspect of the ankle and sometimes in the medial arch. Passive extension of the great toe is limited with the foot in neutral position and normal with the foot plantar-flexed.

Taping of the foot, use of longitudinal arch supports and oral NSAIDs, and contrast soaks afford relief for most patients. Occasionally, surgical release will be necessary.

Bursitis

Retrocalcaneal bursitis or tendo-Achillis bursitis may occur in the posterior aspect of the heel. The retrocalcaneal bursa located between the Achilles' tendon attachment and the posterior angle of the calcaneus is the only consistent aharomic bursa in the foot. Together with the small, acquired subcutaneous bursa superficial to the tendon, it serves to protect the Achilles' tendon from external pressures. As a result, these bursae are themselves subject to tension from a tight heel counter. When an excessively prominent calcaneal bursal projection, or Haglund's deformity, is also present, inflamed bursae and pain localized to the Achilles' insertion can result. The Haglund's deformity is usually palpable, but a lateral x-ray of the heel demonstrates the prominence very nicely.

Retrocalcaneal bursitis produces diffuse swelling and fullness in an area directly in front of the tendon and posterior to the calcaneus. Tenderness is detected by applying pressure medially and laterally just anterior to and above the insertion of the tendon. Chronic inflammation of the tendo-Achillis bursa leads to a distinct, painful enlargement on the posterior aspect of the heel that is often called pump bump. This condition is most frequently seen in adolescent girls when they start wearing high heel shoes with restrictive heel counters. It may also develop in ice skaters, skiers, and hockey players secondary to poorly designed heel counters. Direct pressure over the enlargement will elicit pain.

Rest, ice, oral NSAIDs, and a change in footwear are the cornerstones of treatment and will control symptoms in most cases. Although corticosteroids should rarely be used near the Achilles' tendon, a well-localized injection using a short needle and excellent technique will usually cure retrocalcaneal bursitis. Local corticosteroid injection, however, is never advised in tendo-Achillis bursitis as it may produce Achilles' tendon rupture or skin and subcutaneous atrophy. Surgery may be an option in recalcitrant cases, but the results are frequently unsatisfactory.

Chapter 45

Common Ballet Injuries

Katy Keller, P. T., the Senior Physical Therapist at Westside Dance Physical Therapy, the New York City Ballet and the Juilliard School, provides an in-depth look at some issues that are of interest to all dancers.

Improving Your Turnout

Working to improve your turnout is an important part of dance training but you should never force or strain the hips in the process. By approximately age 12, the hip joints are formed and you can't change the amount of your skeletal turnout. You can do specific stretches and strengthening exercises to improve ease of turnout and technique. The muscles crossing the front, side and back of the hips should be gently and routinely stretched. The deep stomach muscles, hip rotators and abductors should be strengthened to keep the pelvis correctly placed.

Dancers often experience little pops and clicks of their joints and tendons which are usually not cause for concern. If however, the clicks are persistent and associated with pain or soreness then you must have the problem evaluated by an orthopedic doctor. The doctor may recommend stretching exercises, a modified dance schedule and physical therapy. Sometimes anti-inflammatory medication is prescribed.

"Turnout, Tendinitis and Bunions," by Katy Keller, P.T., from the Gaynor Minden, Inc. website at http://www.dancer.com. © 1996 by Katy Keller, P.T.; reprinted with permission.

Tightness of the muscles that cross the front or side of the hip can cause the tendon to snap over the hip joint and make a clicking sound. In addition to checking for tightness and weakness of hip muscles, the doctor also checks that the legs are equal length, the pelvis is level and the hip joints are healthy. It is very important that you see your doctor for correct diagnosis and guidance. Your dance teacher can help you correct technique faults that contribute to "snapping hip". Some of the technique faults to avoid include "sitting into the hip" of the standing leg, "hiking the hip" of the working leg, twisting the pelvis and forcing positions.

You may also want to find out about Functional Footprints©, our new exercise device to help train correct hip rotation and alignment for turnout. The device should be used with supervision by a physical therapist or teacher. Complete instructions, diagrams and cautions come with the device. For more information look at Dance Magazine's "What's New" feature by Marian Horosko in the March 1999 issue, check out our web site at http://www.dancemedicine.com or call the distributor at 1-800-343-5540 or 201-652-1989.

Dealing with Achilles Tendinitis

Many dancers develop Achilles tendinitis. Left untreated, this can become a chronic problem, but with prompt, proper care it can be resolved.

There are specific exercises that can help if you have Achilles tendinitis but first you must allow the tendinitis to calm down and begin healing. Stop taking class for at least a week and then gradually build up by taking partial class no more than three times a week, sitting out the jump and turn combinations. It is very important that you see your doctor for the correct diagnosis and guidance. A diagnosis of tendinitis means there is microtrauma and inflammation of the tendon. You should ice at least once or twice a day to help promote healing and decrease inflammation. A good way to ice is to rub the tendon up and down with an ice cube for about three minutes until it is slightly red and cold. If after two weeks you are not feeling a lot better then return to your doctor for further advice. If your tendinitis is chronic you will need to follow different guidelines.

Exercise

Exercises to stretch out tight calves, strengthen weak feet and legs, and loosen stiff insteps can help reverse tendinitis. To stretch out your calf, lie on your back with one leg out on the floor and the other leg raised straight up to the ceiling. Hold the ends of a belt in your hands with the middle of the belt wrapped under the ball of the raised foot. Flex your foot back to stretch the calf as you gently pull on the ends of the belt. The stretch should be felt along the back of the leg. Hold the stretch for 15 seconds and then repeat with the other leg. Relevés (heel rises) are a good way to strengthen weak feet and legs. Initially do relevés sitting down in a chair so there is very little weight on the feet. Make sure you are raising and lowering your heels slowly, smoothly and without sickling or winging. Progress to relevés in parallel on both feet and then to single leg relevés holding onto a stable support for balance. If relevés cause any discomfort then it is too soon to do them. Try just rocking back and forth from the heels to the balls of the feet. As you rock to your heels lift the toes and then as you rock to the balls of your feet lift the heels about two inches off the floor. Ten repetitions of these exercises at any one time is enough.

For more exercise ideas you can try some of the resistance band exercises described in the Dancers Dozen. Of course, do not do any exercises that cause discomfort, and be sure to work with the supervision of a teacher or physical therapist.

Technique

Technique faults also contribute to causing tendinitis. Technique faults to watch out for include rolling in and landing from jumps without articulating through the feet or putting the heels down. The Achilles tendon connects the calf muscle to the heel and normally the tendon runs straight up and down. When the feet roll in however, the Achilles is forced into a bowed position and is more likely to strain. Rolling in happens when the dancer incorrectly distributes too much weight on the inner boarders of the feet, forces plié too deeply or forces turnout incorrectly from the floor up. Work with your dance teacher to correct these technique faults.

Shoes

Pointe shoes can also cause strain on the Achilles and other tendons of the feet if they fit poorly or if they are too soft or the ribbons are tied too tight. Some dancers sew elastics into the pointe shoe ribbons at the area where the ribbons cross the Achilles tendon. This works very well to keep the ribbons snug and secure without excessive pressure on the tendons.

Be careful on hard floors and stages. If your tendons are bothering you and you are taking dance class on a hard floor, leave out the jumps especially the big jumps across the floor. Take class up until jumps then sit down and watch the rest of class. Or if your teacher permits, go to the back of the class and practice small jumps in first and second position holding the barre. Focus on articulating your feet for a quiet landing and getting your heels down. Then slowly and gently stretch out your calves and legs. Do no do any jumping or stretching exercises if you feel pain.

Dancers who are prone to tendinitis or who have to work on hard floors can try putting shock-absorbing insoles in their dance shoes. Drug stores and shoe repair stores usually carry Dr. Scholl's or Spenco brand insoles. If needed trim the edges of the insoles with a scissors so that they fit in your shoes without bunching up. Gaynor Minden pointe shoes are manufactured with shock-absorbing materials and can be very helpful in preventing tendinitis.

With any injury it is always important for you to see your doctor for proper diagnosis and guidance. Sometimes an extra bone in the back of the ankle can cause Achilles-like symptoms. An x-ray may be necessary to make the diagnosis. Tendinitis of the big toe tendon (flexor hallucis longus) is also common in dancers. In this case, the discomfort is usually felt just behind the inside ankle bone. Don't ignore your symptoms. The sooner you get help, the sooner you'll heal.

Avoiding Bunions

If one of your parents or a grandparent has bunions you are more likely to develop them since there is a hereditary factor, however you can still do a lot to prevent bunion development. In addition to avoiding "winging" also work to avoid rolling in at the feet—both can contribute to the development of bunions. Make sure your dance shoes and street shoes are fitted properly. Dancers often wear shoes that are too short, too narrow in the toe box or not supportive enough. Remember, your feet keep growing into your twenties. Even once you've stopped growing your feet may continue to widen over time especially if you are dancing many hours a week. Some dancers need to wear orthotics (custom made arch supports) in their street shoes to prevent biomechanical problems that contribute to bunion development. A podiatrist or physical therapist can help you determine if you need orthotics.

Additional Notes

"Winging" refers to a technique fault in which the feet are forced outward from the ankles toward the pinkie toes like wings of a bird. A small degree of "winging" can add to the beauty of the line of the leg. The dance student however, should focus more on healthy alignment of the leg than on the look. The center of the foot should be in line with the middle of ankle and leg. This alignment is particularly important for tendus, relevés and jumps. When the feet wing there is more pressure on the big toe joint. The joint can become inflamed and the big toe itself can gradually become angled creating a bunion.

Try the following exercise to improve the alignment and strength of you feet. Stand with your legs and feet parallel with a tennis ball placed between your ankles. Slowly rise up onto the balls of your feet and then lower back down while keeping the ball between your ankles. The ball helps you keep your ankles aligned without winging or sickling. Perform a maximum of 10 repetitions at any one time.

Chapter 46

Snowboarding Injuries

In Brief

Injury patterns in snowboarding differ from those in Alpine skiing. Snowboarders tend to have fewer knee and thumb injuries than skiers but more upper-extremity trauma, fractures in general, and ankle injuries. Of particular concern in snowboarding is fracture of the lateral process of the talus (LPT), which masquerades as an inversion ankle sprain, is often missed, and can lead to significant disability. Signs are typically similar to those of inversion sprains, but pain on palpation of the lateral process can be helpful in diagnosis. Standard radiographs often do not show the fracture, so CT or lateral tomography may be required. The most minor, non-displaced LPT injuries may heal with casting and rehab, but more severe fractures typically require surgery.

In recent years, snowboarding has developed into a mainstream winter sport, with an exponential increase in popularity. This increased participation, of course, means that more and more primary care physicians are seeing patients who snowboard at various skill levels. To aid in early injury recognition and optimal management of such patients, clinicians should be familiar with the injury patterns associated with this sport.

"Snowboarding Injuries," by Andrea J. Boon, MD; Jay Smith, MD; and Edward R. Laskowski, MD in *The Physician and Sports Medicine*, Vol. 27, No. 4, April 1999. © 1999 The McGraw-Hill Companies. Reproduced with permission of McGraw-Hill, Inc.

311

Compared with Alpine skiing, snowboarding entails a significantly higher risk of upper-extremity and ankle injuries, particularly fractures.[1-5] Fracture of the lateral process of the talus is unusually common among snowboarders, and knowledge of this injury is important because the condition masquerades as an anterolateral ankle sprain and frequently is undetected on plain radiographs. Misdiagnosis of this fracture may lead to severe degeneration of the subtalar joint and long-term morbidity.[6-8]

Overview of Snowboarding Injuries

Overall snowboarding injury rates are remarkably similar to those of Alpine skiing, at about five injuries per 1,000 visits to the slopes.[2,9-11] Significant differences in injury patterns, however, have been identified between the two sports, as well as differences in injury rate and patterns among sub-populations within each sport. For example, one study[9] found that only 4% of snowboard-related injuries required hospital admission for more than five days, as compared with 19% of skiing injuries.

The most common snowboarding injuries are simple sprains, followed by fractures and contusions.[2,9] The more serious snowboarding injuries usually result from collisions and often involve contusions to the vital organs, particularly the spleen and less often the liver.[3,10,12] Mild head injuries and coccygeal injuries can occur in backward falls and are well documented.[1,3,5] There appears to be less risk of serious chest or spinal injury in comparison to skiers.[12] Aerial maneuvers are associated with more abdominal, chest, spine, and head injuries than non-aerial maneuvers are.[3]

Relative to skiers, snowboarders have 2.4 times as many fractures (particularly of the upper limbs), fewer knee injuries, and more ankle injuries.[1,3,4,9,10,13] Knee injuries tend to be less severe in snowboarders than in Alpine skiers.[9,10] It appears, though, that as the level of snowboarding expertise increases, so does the risk of more serious knee ligament injuries such as anterior cruciate ligament rupture (Peter C. Janes, MD, personal communication, February 1999). This observation, should it prove accurate, may relate to the increased frequency of aerial maneuvers and the use of hard-shell boots.[4,5,9,14] Disruption of the ulnar collateral ligament of the thumb, which is relatively common in skiers, is virtually unheard of in snowboarders, presumably because they don't use poles.[1,5,13]

Only limited data are available on snowboarding fatalities, but rates appear comparable to those of skiers.[10] As with skiing, the major risk is from blunt trauma to the head or chest.[10] A potential cause of death among snowboarders, though, is immersion, in which a snowboarder is buried head first in the snow, usually in a tree well, can't free himself or herself, and suffocates. This danger underscores the importance of snowboarding with a partner. The risk of avalanche applies equally to both sports.

Most studies have found that beginning snowboarders are relatively more likely than beginning skiers to be injured. Several studies[1,4,9] report that in Alpine skiing, only a third of those injured are beginners, whereas about 60% of snowboarding injuries occur in novices. A recent study,[15] however, found that although injury rates for first-time snowboarders and skiers were similar, snowboarders sustained a higher percentage (53%) of upper-extremity injuries, while skiers had a higher percentage (63%) of lower-extremity injuries. This study also found that first-time snowboarders sustained more injuries that required emergency care (e.g., concussion, fracture, dislocation, and dental injury).

In comparison to experts, beginning snowboarders have a higher rate of upper-extremity fractures, especially of the wrist,[3,9] more lacerations and contusions resulting from collisions,[4] and more head and spine injuries.[4] The higher rate of head and spine injuries is thought to reflect an increased risk of totally losing control of the board. Snowboard equipment type may affect injury patterns, but current data are inconclusive.[1,2,4,5,9,16]

Snowboarder's Ankle:
Fracture of the Lateral Process of the Talus

The injury that is most particular to snowboarding and until recently was largely unrecognized is fracture of the lateral process of the talus (LPT). Recent epidemiologic studies of snowboarding injuries have highlighted LPT fractures.[9,16] This is an unusual fracture, rarely seen in other clinical settings, with fewer than 65 cases reported in the English literature prior to the recognition of the fracture among snowboarders.[17] Mukherjee et al.[7] had estimated in 1974 that LPT fractures accounted for less than 1% of all ankle injuries.

Kirkpatrick et. al.,[16] however, recently published a prospective study documenting more than 3,000 snowboarding injuries, specifically looking at the pattern of foot and ankle injuries. Fifteen percent of all injuries affected the ankle, and 44% of these were fractures. Fractures of the lateral process of the talus accounted for 32% of ankle fractures and 15% of all ankle injuries.

Anatomy and mechanics: The talus is important in rotatory and hinge movements at the talocrural and subtalar joints. Fractures of the talus carry a risk of avascular necrosis and nonunion. The lateral process is a portion of the posterior talar facet. It is a large, wedge-shaped prominence spanning almost the entire lateral wall of the talus. The lateral process has two articular surfaces, one positioned inferomedial to the fibula and the other dorsolateral to the anterior portion of the posterior calcaneal facet. LPT fractures commonly involve the articular surface of the talus. In severe injuries, there may also be a chondral defect of the posterior calcaneal articular surface.

The mechanism of LPT fracture is controversial. Many authors believe sudden severe dorsiflexion with the hindfoot in inversion causes the fracture.[7,18] This motion produces a shearing force transmitted from the calcaneus to the LPT, resulting in fracture fragments of variable size.[2,11,19] This could occur when landing after an aerial maneuver, which is reportedly a common cause of injury in snowboarders[20] (Peter C. Janes, MD, personal communication, February 1999). This proposed injury mechanism, however, is not universally accepted.

Clinical features: Clinically, LPT fractures closely resemble inversion ankle sprains. Snowboarders report a dorsiflexion twisting injury, such as landing an aerial that included a twist. Often, but not always, they are unable to continue boarding. Symptoms include anterolateral ankle pain and swelling with painful weight bearing. Depending on the severity and the time interval since the injury, ecchymosis may be present.

Physical examination reveals swelling over and anterior to the lateral malleolus and pain with ankle dorsiflexion and plantar flexion and/or with subtalar inversion and eversion. The lateral process is tender on palpation just inferior to the tip of the lateral malleolus. Unfortunately, this potentially specific finding is often obscured by overlying swelling and soft-tissue tenderness. The location of pain from an LPT fracture contrasts with the site of pain in a lateral collateral ligament sprain, which typically is anteroinferior to the lateral malleolus.

In many regards, the history and physical exam findings parallel those of an inversion ankle sprain. Consequently, clinicians must have a high index of suspicion for LPT fractures in high-risk situations and seek a definitive diagnosis. LPT fractures should be considered in a "sprained ankle" that is persistently painful or unresponsive to treatment. Repeated clinical and radiologic examination are typically warranted.

Hawkins[8] and McCrory and Bladin[20] describe three different LPT fracture patterns (Figure 46.1): Type 1 is a chip fracture off the anterior and inferior portion of the articular process of the talus that does not extend to the talofibular articulation. Type 2 is a simple fracture of the lateral process that extends from the talofibular articular surface to the posterior talocalcaneal articular surface of the subtalar joint. The fracture fragment may or may not be displaced. Type 3 is a comminuted fracture involving both the fibular and posterior calcaneal articular surfaces of the talus and the entire lateral process.

Diagnostic imaging: LPT fractures are notoriously difficult to recognize on plain radiographs,[7,8,11,17,18] particularly if the clinician does not have a high level of suspicion. This fracture is best seen on a mortise view, just distal to the lateral malleolus, particularly with the foot in internal rotation.[7,11,20,21] Some fracture patterns, particularly small chip fractures, are best seen on a lateral projection through the overlapping malleoli.[8,11] McCrory and Bladin[20] recommend lateral radiographs be taken in 0° of dorsiflexion and 10° to 20° of inversion.

Computed tomography (CT) (Figure 46.2a.) is useful when an LPT fracture is clinically suspected but plain radiographs are normal, when the patient has persistent pain after what appears to be an inversion ankle sprain, and to determine the size of fragments and extent of comminution when plain radiographs reveal an LPT fracture. CT can guide treatment by delineating the fracture pattern more clearly.[19,22,23] Lateral tomography (Figure 46.2b.) is an alternative means of further evaluating LPT fractures, particularly if three-dimensional CT reconstruction is not readily available.[24]

Type 1   Type 2   Type 3

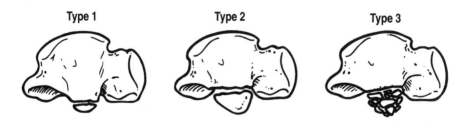

Figure 46.1. *Three types of fracture of the lateral process of the talus: Type 1, chip; Type 2, simple; and Type 3, comminuted. Type 2 fractures can be displaced, as shown, or non-displaced. Figure 46.1: Mary Albury-Noyes.*

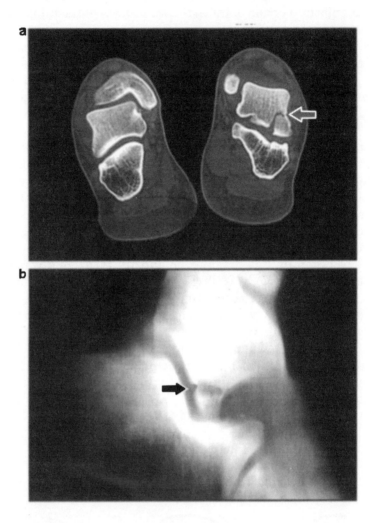

Figures 46.2. Two snowboarders were injured, each one when he fell forward with his ankle in acute dorisflexion. Each immediately felt pain. CT if one patient's ankles (a) and lateral tomography of the other's injured ankle (b) revealed fractures of the lateral process of the talus. Each patient was treated with immediate open reduction and internal fixation and had a good recovery, with some residual pain on six-month follow-up. Figures 46.2a. and 46.2b. courtesy of Peter C. Janes, MD.

A further finding that should not be overlooked is an inferior fibula avulsion fracture. These avulsion fractures are commonly associated with injuries of the lateral ankle ligaments and are typically managed the same as inversion ankle sprain. However, posterior fibular avulsion fractures (radiographically, the "flake sign") are diagnostic of peroneal tendon subluxation or dislocation and can be seen in association with LPT fractures[22] (Peter C. Janes, MD, personal communication, February 1999). It is helpful to note this preoperatively because surgery for peroneal tendon subluxation may involve deepening of the peroneal tendon groove on the fibula.

Management: Treatment of LPT fractures is evolving. The size of the LPT fracture and the degree of comminution and displacement are the primary determinants of treatment.

Type 1 and non-displaced Type 2 fractures may be treated with immobilization in a short non-weight-bearing cast for four weeks, followed by a walking cast for two weeks. When the non-weight-bearing cast is removed, the patient may bear weight as tolerated and should begin exercises for ankle flexibility, strength, stability, and proprioception.[25] Active assisted range of motion exercise may be required for stiff tibiotalar and subtalar joints.

For displaced Type 2 and for all Type 3 fractures, many authors recommend attempted closed reduction by an orthopedist with subsequent casting if reduction is successful.[8] If reduction cannot be achieved or maintained — or the fracture is comminuted — open reduction and internal fixation or excision is generally recommended.

Other authors suggest that prolonged casting is often unsuccessful in all LPT fractures.[7] These authors recommend early surgery to avoid prolonged subtalar stiffness. Kirkpatrick et al[16] recommend operative management for all but the smallest non-displaced LPT fractures. We favor early operative intervention for large displaced or any type of comminuted fractures.

Open reduction and internal fixation is used if possible. However, fracture comminution often prevents restoration of joint surface anatomy, necessitating debridement and possibly drilling of the chondral surface to salvage the joint.

Postoperatively, a short leg cast is applied for two to three weeks. During this time, active range of motion of the metatarsophalangeal joints is allowed. At three weeks, the cast is exchanged for a splint, and the patient begins ankle range-of-motion exercises. Weight bearing is typically allowed when osseous union is evident, at about six weeks.

Whether treatment is operative or non-operative, the patient can maintain conditioning through cross-training, including resistance training of the upper body and unaffected lower limb.

Prognosis: An unrecognized LPT fracture may result in nonunion, persistent pain, and long-term disability. Malalignment and osseous overgrowth are not uncommon in such cases. Despite the lack of epidemiologic data regarding the outcome of LPT fractures in snowboarders, it is well established that similar fractures among other populations have a poor prognosis, particularly if misdiagnosed or inappropriately managed non-operatively. Several studies[6,8,17-19,21,23] have evaluated outcomes when LPT fractures were managed with casting only. Unless anatomic alignment was maintained, there was significant residual disability. At this time there is a lack of formal outcome studies evaluating operative management of LPT fractures.

Recommendatons for Physicians and Patients

Physicians need to know the peculiar patterns of injury in snowboarders, such as more upper-extremity, ankle, and abdominal injuries and fewer serious knee injuries.[1,3-5,9,10] Clinicians must also raise awareness of the commonly misdiagnosed LPT fracture, which can masquerade as a simple ankle sprain. One must maintain a high index of suspicion, pursue an accurate diagnosis, and treat the injury promptly.

Novice snowboarders can reduce their injury risk by taking lessons, using protective equipment including helmets and knee and elbow pads, and wearing soft-shell or hybrid boots. The value of wrist guards would seem obvious because beginners have a significantly increased risk of wrist fracture. However, there is a legitimate concern that use of wrist guards may transmit forces proximally and lead to more shoulder injuries. More studies are needed to determine this.

References

1. Abu-Laban RB: Snowboarding injuries: an analysis and comparison with alpine skiing injuries. *Can Med Assoc J* 1991;145(9):1097-1103.

2. Bladin C, McCrory P: Snowboarding injuries: an overview. *Sports Med* 1995;19(5):358-364.

3. Chow TK, Corbett SW, Farstad DJ: Spectrum of injuries from snowboarding. *J Trauma* 1996;41(2):321-325.

4. Pigozzi F, Santori N, Di Salvo V, et al: Snowboard traumatology: an epidemiological study. *Orthopedics* 1997;20(6):505-509.

5. Pino EC, Colville MR: Snowboard injuries. *Am J Sports Med* 1989;17(6):778-781.

6. Sneppen O, Christensen SB, Krogsoe O, et al: Fracture of the body of the talus. *Acta Orthop Scand* 1977;48(3):317-324.

7. Mukherjee SK, Pringle RM, Baxter AD: Fracture of the lateral process of the talus: a report of thirteen cases. *J Bone Joint Surg* (Br) 1974;56(2):263-273.

8. Hawkins LG: Fracture of the lateral process of the talus: a review of thirteen cases. *J Bone Joint Surg* (Am) 1965;47(6): 1170-1175.

9. Bladin C, Giddings P, Robinson M: Australian snowboard injury data base study: a four-year prospective study. *Am J Sports Med* 1993;21(5):701-704.

10. Sacco DE, Sartorelli DH, Vane DW: Evaluation of alpine skiing and snowboarding injury in a northeastern state. *J Trauma* 1998;44(4):654-659.

11. Nicholas R, Hadley J, Paul C, et al: 'Snowboarder's fracture': fracture of the lateral process of the talus. *J Am Board Fam Pract* 1994;7(2):130-133.

12. Prall JA, Winston KR, Brennan R: Severe snowboarding injuries. *Injury* 1995;26(8):539-542.

13. Kocher MS, Dupre MM, Feagin JA Jr: Shoulder injuries from alpine skiing and snowboarding: aetiology, treatment and prevention. *Sports Med* 1998;25(3):201-211.

14. Ganong RB, Heneveld EH, Beranek SR, et al: Snowboarding injuries: a report on 415 patients. *Phys Sportsmed* 1992; 20(12):114-122.

15. O'Neill DF, McGlone MR: Injury risk in first-time snowboarders versus first-time skiers. *Am J Sports Med* 1999;27(1):94-97.

16. Kirkpatrick DP, Hunter RE, Janes PC, et al: The snowboarder's foot and ankle. *Am J Sports Med* 1998;26(2):271-277.

17. Mills HJ, Horne G: Fractures of the lateral process of the talus. *Aust N Z J Surg* 1987;57(9):643-646.

18. Heckman JD, McLean MR: Fractures of the lateral process of the talus. *Clin Orthop* 1985;199(Oct):108-113.

19. Paul CC, Janes PC: The snowboarder's talus fracture, in Mote CD, Johnson RJ, Hauser W (eds): *Skiing Trauma and Safety.* Philadelphia, ASTM, 1996, pp 388-393.

20. McCrory P, Bladin C: Fractures of the lateral process of the talus: a clinical review: 'snowboarder's ankle.' *Clin J Sport Med* 1996;6(2):124-128.

21. Dimon JH III: Isolated displaced fracture of the posterior facet of the talus. *J Bone Joint Surg (Am)* 1961;43(2):275-281.

22. Ebraheim NA, Skie MC, Podeszwa DA, et al: Evaluation of process fractures of the talus using computed tomography. *J Orthop Trauma* 1994;8(4):332-337.

23. Noble J, Royle SG: Fracture of the lateral process of the talus: computed tomographic scan diagnosis. *Br J Sports Med* 1992;26(4):245-246

24. Whitby EH, Barrington NA: Fractures of the lateral process of the talus: the value of lateral tomography. *Br J Radiol* 1995;68(810):583-586.

25. Laskowski ER, Newcomer-Aney K, Smith J: Refining rehabilitation with proprioception training: expediting return to play. *Phys Sportsmed* 1997;25(10):89-102.

— by Andrea J. Boon, MD; Jay Smith, MD;
and Edward R. Laskowski, MD

Dr. Boon is the chief resident, Dr. Smith a senior associate consultant, and Dr. Laskowski a consultant in the Department of Physical Medicine and Rehabilitation at the Mayo Clinic in Rochester, Minnesota. Dr. Smith also is an assistant professor at the Mayo Medical School and a staff physician at the Mayo Sports Medicine Center in Rochester. Dr. Laskowski also is an associate professor at the Mayo Medical School and a co-director of the Mayo Clinic Sports Medicine Center.

Chapter 47

Information for Amputees

David S. Barr of Bodfish, California, took an 80,000-mile motorcycle trip that spanned North and South America, Europe, Asia, and Africa.

"Only 70 people have ever done anything like it before," Barr said. "There've been more people in outer space than have made this trip."

What makes it more extraordinary is that Barr, 41, is a double amputee. Fighting in Angola in 1981, he lost one leg above the knee and the other below the knee. But that hasn't kept him from riding a two-wheel, 1972 Harley Davidson and writing a book about his around-the-world motorcycle trip.

And that is not all. Barr is one of only a handful of double-amputee parachutists who jump with special prosthetics. And he walks three or four miles a day and mows his own grass.

Advances in prosthetics, and the example set by amputees such as Barr, have shown more and more people that an amputation does not always mean confinement to a wheelchair. At private companies and key centers such as Northwestern University in Chicago and the University of Utah at Salt Lake City, research that sounds like something out of "The Six Million Dollar Man" could give amputees even more control over artificial limbs.

Physical therapist Marie A. Schroeder, chief of the Food and Drug Administration's restorative devices branch, explains that FDA regulates

"Big Steps Forward for Amputees," by Robert A. Hamilton, in *FDA Consumer*, March 1997, U.S. Food and Drug Administration (FDA).

prostheses, but manufacturers do not have to undergo a full review for each new device. Instead, they must register the products and keep a record of any complaints. "But if there's a significant change in the technology, we could get involved," Schroeder said.

For instance, she said, her branch has seen some interest in implantable electrodes for stimulating muscles in spinal cord injury cases. Such devices would require review by FDA. Some innovators are also exploring ways to use computers to design and manufacture custom prostheses, to attach muscles directly to a prosthesis, to develop powered fingers with microelectronics, and even to use brain waves to power prostheses.

For thousands of years, inventors have tried to replicate what nature cannot replace. Prostheses have been used since at least 300 B.C., when crude devices consisting of metal plates hammered over a wooden core, were attached to an amputated limb. Advances in the science of prosthetics burgeon during and immediately after wars, when large numbers of people need to be fitted with artificial limbs. The technology of modern prosthetics has changed little since shortly after World War II.

"There's a real need for revolution in design," said Giovani M. Ortega, research and development project manager at Sabolich Prosthetics & Research in Oklahoma City, Oklahoma, a division of NovaCare. "The systems that we have, have been around for a long time, and at best there have been only improvements. As far along as we've come, we're still far behind many other industries in terms of implementing new technologies."

Estimates of the amputee population in the United States vary widely, from fewer than 400,000 to more than 1 million. About nine out of 10 amputations involve the leg, from the foot to above the knee. Three-quarters of all amputations are the result of disease, often cancer or peripheral vascular disease. The latter is a narrowing of the arteries in the extremities that is often associated with diabetes. Most other amputations are the result of workplace or automobile accidents. And a small fraction, perhaps three percent, are due to birth defects that constrict bone growth.

Preventing Amputation

Because so many amputations result from disease, considerable attention has been paid to prevention. For example, the American Diabetes Association recommends people stop smoking, which can speed the progress of peripheral vascular disease. Patients with diabetes should monitor their blood glucose levels carefully, eat a healthy, balanced diet, see their doctors regularly, control their weight, and check their feet each day for small cuts or blisters.

Electric blankets and heating pads carry warning labels that say people with diabetes should not use them without talking to their doctors first. This is because people with diabetes may lose sensation in their limbs. Patients can be seriously burned by an electric blanket or heating pad because they cannot feel how hot it really is.

Patients are also advised to develop an exercise plan after consulting with their doctors. Regular exercise maintains strength, flexibility, and blood flow to damaged areas and can help control pain. However, it's important not to stress the legs, feet or joints. Some good exercises are bicycling or easy rowing on a rowing machine. Swimming and aqua aerobics are also good choices.

"We know of many things that can help people avoid amputation, but unfortunately, it's no fun to do daily foot care or wear only proper fitting, well-designed shoes," said Jennifer Mayfield, M.D., chairwoman of the association's Foot Care Council. "Everybody keeps waiting for a magic bullet, and that would be nice, but it's not coming anytime soon."

Richard J. Gusberg, M.D., chief of vascular surgery at Yale University, said one of the first signs of peripheral occlusive disease is claudication, an aching, tired feeling in the leg muscles when they are exercised.

"The vast majority of people with claudication remain stable, or nearly stable, for an indefinite period of time," Gusberg said. In most cases the progress of the disease can be slowed if people control the risk factors, which includes reducing blood pressure, controlling their diabetes through diet or insulin, and reducing cholesterol levels. Regular exercise has also proven effective because it can strengthen circulation, he said.

The drug Trental (pentoxifylline) is approved by the FDA for people with peripheral artery disease. Its use can decrease the thickness and stickiness of blood, and can reduce the deformities of red blood cells, so the blood can get through the narrowed arteries, but it is not effective in all patients, Gusberg said. The use of other drugs in treating occlusive disease has largely been abandoned, he said.

If the disease progresses, the patient might develop gangrene, or ulcers in the leg, as blood flow is reduced. "When people get to that stage, most of them need to be evaluated for a bypass operation," Gusberg said. Replacing the arteries in the lower leg is effective for five years or more in 70 to 80 percent of cases.

Sensory Loss

Another danger with diabetes is a deadening of the nerves in the extremities. John F. Glass, a biologist with FDA's pacing and neurological devices branch, said there are now a variety of devices that measure sensory loss in the affected limbs. In a patient with diabetes, loss of sensation because of nerve damage signals a need for diligence. Even minor injuries, undetected because the feeling is gone and thus left untreated, can become infected easily and lead to gangrene.

"If you're aware of sensory loss, you want to keep a close watch on it," Glass said. "There's a range of measurement devices, from those that detect general loss of sensation, to those that assess the specific degree of sensory loss, or that can quantify sensitivity to pressure or temperature."

Many of the devices are easy-to-use mechanical implements with no significant health risk to patients. One of the simplest is a hand-held device that looks like an old typewriter eraser with thin wires attached to it. The wires are placed on the toes or fingertips to see if there is tactile sensitivity.

Such simple devices are typically not reviewed by FDA before they are made available to the public. They are intended for use by the patient for monitoring only, not self-diagnosis. "Loss of sensation in an extremity could indicate a lot of other conditions or disorders, so we would encourage the patient to see a physician immediately for a complete physical examination," Glass said.

Unavoidable Limb Loss

Precautions such as Glass advocates can often delay the progression of the disease. Sometimes, though, the loss of a limb is unavoidable. In those cases, physical therapy starts a day or two after surgery. Since more than nine out of 10 amputations involve one or both legs, physical therapy usually involves the use of parallel bars, and later a walker or crutches. Part of the training involves how to fall and get up safely.

There are other adjustments as well. Barr said the loss of both legs, and covering the stumps with plastic, means his body has become much less effective at cooling itself, so he has to be on the lookout for hyperthermia. And he learned other tricks to cope, as well.

"I'm constantly on the move, never standing still, always readjusting my balance even when I'm staying in one place, because I don't want one particular area on the stump to get sore," Barr said.

Until recently, patients were not fitted with an artificial limb for four to eight weeks after surgery, but new techniques allow the use of a protective foam over a sterile bandage, and the prosthesis can be fit as soon as the day following surgery.

New Prosthetic Materials

For centuries, wood and leather were the only materials for prostheses, but today's physical therapist has a much wider range available, including advanced plastics and carbon fiber, which are much stronger and lighter and more durable. "The industry is really moving towards composite materials, because they're lighter in weight, easier to work with, and more durable," said Douglas McCormack, vice president of the Amputee Coalition of America.

Silicone-based compounds used to make prosthetic arms, for instance, give the appearance of real skin, unlike the rigid plastic or metal limbs of years ago, and they are more comfortable for the person wearing them. Women can get prosthetic feet with life-like toes for when they wear sandals; men can get legs with the appearance of hair. But even materials that work out in one application might not work in another.

"We tested a silicone foot at one point. On a machine it was subjected to 300 pounds of stress for a million cycles, and it didn't have any problems. But an amputee broke it within a few minutes. It really surprised us. Torque and other stresses can fatigue the material quickly," said Sabolich's Ortega. "You'd be amazed at the toll that a human body puts on even the strongest material."

New computer programs better determine where and what the forces are. But it's not just a question of choosing a material that will withstand those forces. "With some of the new materials being developed, we could make a foot to take any of the pressures that the human body will give it," Ortega said. "The problem is it might not have any springiness. You give up flexibility for strength. You have to balance all the considerations in a prosthetic."

Prostheses are typically sold as components, so that someone who has an above-the-knee amputation would be able to choose leg, knee and foot units, often from different manufacturers, depending on their individual needs.

Most of the units are adjustable. Shock absorbers in knees, for instance, can be made more flexible as a person gains controls over the artificial leg. Ankles can be adjusted to the weight and activity level of the patient.

Arm amputees today can choose between prostheses that are powered by a harness and cable attached to the residual limb, or externally powered devices. Powered arms can be controlled by switches mounted inside or outside the socket, that the patient can activate by flexing certain muscle groups.

Energy Requirements

Some prosthetics research is aimed at providing active devices, which do part of the work of the amputated limb, as opposed to passive devices that are controlled by the residual limb. An amputee with prostheses expends two to three times more energy than a non-disabled person to perform even the simplest activities, such as walking across a room or climbing stairs. "A semi-active system, in which the limb itself performs part of the function, could reduce that energy requirement significantly," said Sabolich's Ortega. "And there would also be a psychological benefit, because the prosthesis would no longer be just a dead limb, but something that is helping." Ortega said one area Sabolich is researching would provide sensory feedback from the prosthesis to the remaining limb. For instance, in an artificial leg, pressure sensors in the foot would send a mild electrical signal to the thigh muscles when there is pressure on the back, front or sides of the foot.

That kind of feedback would be similar to what they would get with the pressure of the ground against a natural foot, which would make their adjustment to the prostheses go more quickly, Ortega said.

Ortega said prosthetic designs are limited only by how large a power pack the amputee can carry. "The crucial issue when it comes to trying to introduce any new prosthesis is the energy requirements," said Ortega. "Our muscles are so efficient, in terms of the power that they produce versus the fuel that they use, that we have a difficult time matching it."

Scientists are also working to build a better socket—the part of the prosthesis that attaches to the residual limb. Dudley S. Childress, Ph.D., of Northwestern University's Rehabilitation Engineering Program, is working on applying the industrial practice known as rapid prototyping to socket production.

Sockets are now produced largely by hand. A cast is made of the residual limb, and plaster is poured into the cast to make a positive mold. The mold is then used to create a plastic or laminated polyester socket that fits over the residual limb.

Childress employs a computer-aided design program to measure the residual limb and design a socket. Then, using a modified "plastic deposition technology" called squirt shaping; a computer lays down small amounts of polypropylene to produce the desired shape, to very tight tolerances. In industry, the technology is used to quickly produce prototypes of everything from car parts to military weapons, to test them before starting mass production.

"Essentially, every socket is a prototype, and there are potentially some significant advantages to applying these techniques to prosthesis manufacture," Childress said. "We can make a socket in about 50 minutes, which isn't bad, but as people continue to work with the technology, it may be possible to get that down even faster."

The process would also allow manufacturers to make sockets out of different types of material than have been used in the past, or alter the thickness or characteristics of the material very quickly. Another innovation being explored at Northwestern is powered prosthetic fingers. That might be difficult if you were going to match real fingers, he acknowledged, but most of the time that's unnecessary. Picking up a spoon and holding a book don't require much power, just control. Small motor technology and power storage capability have both improved vastly in recent years.

"If you want to do something like squeeze orange juice, you need force," Childress said. "But even for people without a prosthesis, that's tiresome, so we have all kinds of devices to do those jobs for us. So the intent of the powered fingers would be to provide prehensile (wrap-around) force."

Childress said his laboratory is also looking at devices that would improve the "feel" of prostheses over current devices. It would be comparable, he said, to the way power steering reduces the muscle power needed to steer a car, but you can still "feel" the road through the wheel.

Cables in artificial fingers and hands would connect to the muscles of the forearm, either through holes in the muscle that are surgically lined with skin, or tendons could be taken outside the residual limb and covered with skin. Either option would give the muscle the sense of how hard it is working and how fast it is moving.

Mundane, But Important Needs

Joan E. Edelstein, Ph.D., director of Columbia University's physical therapy program, stresses the need for prosthetics research to focus not just on high-technology improvements, but to the more mundane but critical things such as fit, to make them as comfortable as possible, particularly among the elderly, whose needs may not be fully considered.

327

"Most patients are older people who have lost a limb because of diabetes, and the assumption is that they're going to be relatively undemanding of their prosthesis," Edelstein said.

Better prostheses for the elderly might prevent skin breakdown and infections, yet hardly any research dollars are being spent in that area, she said, explaining that, "It's not as glamorous as developing better prostheses for sport, or for children, and they are very difficult problems to overcome."

Research often proceeds along several courses at once, she noted, and you can never know which might yield the next major breakthrough.

—by Robert A. Hamilton

Robert A. Hamilton is a writer in Franklin, Connecticut.

Part Five

Additional Help and Information

Chapter 48

Glossary of Terms

A

Achilles tendinitis: Inflammation of the Achilles tendon.

Achilles tendon: The tendon located at the back of the ankle that is formed by the union of the gastrocnemius and the soleus muscles.

AIDS: Acquired immunodeficiency syndrome.

Amputation: Amputations are the loss of a body part. Amputations are divided into Traumatic Amputations (those involving loss of a body part caused by an injury) and Non-traumatic Amputations. The later often occurs secondary to diabetes, poor circulation, or infection.

Ankle joint: The joining of the talus, which is the largest bone in the foot, and the tibia and the fibula of the lower leg.

Apert's syndrome: A rare birth defect affecting approximately one child in every 160,00 live births, and characterized by a tower-shaped skull (craniosynostosis), an underdeveloped mid-face, eyes that are widely spaced and protruding, and webbed fingers and toes.

Arteries: The blood vessels that carry oxygenated blood from the lungs to the body.

Arthritis: "Artho" means joint and "itis" means inflammation. There are approximately 38 causes of arthritis and most of these conditions affect the human foot. The most common of these conditions is osteoarthritis. This is the simple wearing and tearing away of the cartilage of the joints. Age, excessive weight, ill-fitting shoes and trauma (injury) are the basic causes of osteoarthritis. Fortunately, this condition is very treatable.

The term "arthritis" is also used for more than 100 rheumatic diseases involving joint inflammation and pain, with loss of function. The diseases also may affect muscles, tendons, and ligaments, and organs.

Athlete's foot: A common, and uncomfortable fungal infection of the foot that may resist treatment and reoccur often.

B

Bone scan: A test using an injected radiation tracer to detect boney metastasis.

Brachymetatarsia: A congenital deformity in which one of the metatarsals is abnormally short resulting in an abnormally short toe.

Bunion: Also known as "hallux valgus," is characterized by a lump or bump that is red, swollen and/or painful on the big toe joint. The most common cause of bunions is tight-fitting shoes.

Bursa: Small sacs that contain fluid and serve to prevent friction and irritation.

Bursitis: A condition in which a bursal sac becomes inflamed due to irritation.

C

Calcaneus heel bone: The largest bone in the foot.

Calluses: Rough, thickened skin, usually on the bottom of the foot.

Cartilage: A tough, resilient connective tissue that covers and cushions the ends of the bones and absorbs shock.

Charcot foot: A condition associated with diabetes where the foot is usually injured but lack of feeling prevents the patient from recognizing the injury. The resulting damage can be very severe and includes arch collapse, fractures and deformity of the foot. Left untreated, the condition can result in amputation.

Charcot-Marie-Tooth disease: A progressive neuromuscular disease affecting the nerves in the arms, hands, legs and fee. Over time, the loss of nerve function causes degeneration of the associated muscles.

Clubfoot: The second most common birth defect in the United States, clubfoot is a congenital deformity resulting in the foot being twisted out of its normal position.

Corns: Thickened areas of skin resembling a kernel of corn that develop as the result of excessive pressure or friction on the area, usually on the top of the toes.

Corticosteroid: An anti-inflammatory hormone that is both produced by the body and produced synthetically as a medication.

D

Diabetes: A disease that occurs when the body lacks the ability to produce or use insulin, the hormone necessary to convert starches and sugars into energy.

E

Edema: Localized swelling of any part of the body cause by the build up of fluids.

Equinus: A deformity that cause the foot to point downward forcing the person to walk on the toes.

F

Flat feet: A condition characterized by the lack of arch in the foot.

Foot ulcers: Foot ulcers are painful sores on the bottom of the foot. They have many causes, but the most common are diabetes and poor circulation.

Fracture: A fracture is a break in a bone classified either as a "Traumatic Fracture" from an injury, or as a "Stress Fracture" from repeated trauma.

G

Gangrene: The death of body tissue due to loss of blood circulation, especially in the extremities.

Gout: A condition that causes severe painful attacks, usually in the big toe, but other joints can also be affected. The cause is the build-up of uric acid resulting in the formation of crystals in the joints.

H

Haglund's deformity: A painful condition on the back of the heel in the area of the Achilles tendon.

Hallux valgus: A condition where the big toe is forced over or under the second toe.

Hammertoes: The shortening of the tendons that control toe movement.

I

Inflammation: The reaction of body tissue to injury, resulting in swelling, redness, heat, and pain.

Ingrown toe nails: A painful condition caused when one or both sides of a toenail cut into the skin and continue to grow.

L

Ligament: Cord-like tissue that connect bone to bone or cartilage.

M

Morton's neuroma: A painful condition brought on by abnormal growth of the sheath covering the nerve of a toe.

N

Neuropathy: Damage to the peripheral nerves anywhere in the body resulting in a range of symptoms including pain, tingling, burning, loss of motor skills, and numbness.

Nonsteroidal anti-inflammatory drugs (NSAIDs): Aspirin and aspirin-like drugs commonly used to reduce inflammation, headaches and other minor pain.

O

Orthotics: Devices designed to correct or control an abnormal foot function. Orthotics are generally worn inside the shoe and help to relieve pain and discomfort by providing support to the bones and ligaments of the foot.

Osteoarthritis: A degenerative form of arthritis characterized by the break down of cartilage in the joints. It is most common after age 45 and affects about half of all Americans 65 or older.

Osteomeylitis: A serious bone infection that requires intense antibiotic treatment.

Overpronation: The result of the loss of arch (flat feet), and subsequent stress upon the foot resulting in inflammation and discomfort. Treatment may include the use orthotics and special footwear designed to provide necessary support.

P

Peripheral neuropathy: Injury to the nerves of the extremities causing loss of motion and sensation, as well as pain.

Plantar fasciitis: Also know as heel spurs, causes intense pain on the bottom of the heel and is caused by a bony overgrowth on the heel bone. Most often, an inflamed plantar fascia ligament on the bottom of the foot irritates the bone to the point that the bone creates the bony growth to protect itself.

Polydactyly: A birth defect caused by a genetic mutation and characterized by a tower-shaped skull (craniosynostosis), underdeveloped mid-face, prominent eyes, wide-set and/or crossed eyes, and broad fingers and toes.

R

Rheumatic diseases: A general term used to describe a variety of conditions affecting joints, muscles, bones, and connective tissues.

S

Shin splints: A common injury among untrained and out-of-shape athletes that results from the tearing away of the anterior tibial muscle from the bone. The injury can be avoided by building up muscle strength over time before beginning any strenuous physical activities.

Sprain: Damage to ligament fibers often resulting from a twist or repetitive strain.

Stress fractures: Stress fractures are usually the result of poor foot biomechanics or repetitive trauma and normally show no bone displacement, allowing for fast recovery.

Supination: Also known as "underpronation," it is the tendency of the foot to roll outward upon landing.

Syndactyly: A birth defect characterized by webbed hands or feet.

Synovial fluid: A lubricating liquid found around the joints.

T

Tarsal tunnel syndrome: A painful condition that affects the ankle when the posterior tibial nerve becomes inflamed.

Tendons: The fibrous tissues that connect a muscle to a bone.

Tinea pedis: See Athlete's foot.

U

Urea: A primary body waste that is flushed from the body in urine.

Uric acid: An organic substance that results from the breakdown of purines or waste products in the body. It is dissolved in the blood and passes through the kidneys into the urine, where it is eliminated. Persons with gout have high blood levels of uric acid resulting in the formation of crystals in the joints causing inflammation and pain.

V

Vein: A blood vessel that carries blood to the heart.

X

Xeorosis: The thickening and cracking of the bottom of the heels. In most cases, the problem is only cosmetic, however, diabetics and others with vascular diseases can be seriously affected.

Chapter 49

Medical Resources for Foot Care

Associations and Societies

American Association of Podiatric Sports Medicine
4414 Ives Street
Rockville MD 20853
Toll Free: 800-438-3355
Tel: 301-962-1540
Website: http://www.aapsm.org
E-Mail: info@aapsm.org

American College of Foot and Ankle Surgeons
515 Bussee Highway
Park Ridge IL 60068-3150
Toll Free: 888-843-3338
Tel: 847-292-2237
Fax: 897-292-2022
Website: http://www.acfas.org
E-Mail: mail@acfas.org

The American Orthopaedic Foot and Ankle Society
2517 East Lake Avenue, East
Suite 200
Seattle, WA 98102
Tel: 206-223-1120
Fax: 206-223-1178
Website: http://www.aofas.org
E-Mail: aofas@aofas.org

American Podiatric Medical Association
9312 Old Georgetown Road
Bethesda, MD 20814-1698
Telephone: 301-571-9200
Toll Free: 1-800-FOOTCARE
Fax: 301-530-2752
Website: http://www.apma.org
E-Mail: askapma@apma.org

Organizations listed in this chapter were compiled from many sources; inclusion does not constitute endorsement. Contact information was verified and updated as necessary in May 2001.

The Podiatry Institute
1459 Montreal Road, Suite 206
Tucker, GA 30084
Telephone: 770-939-0393
Toll Free: 888-833-5682
Fax: 770-493-7563
Website: http://
www.podiatryinstitute.com
E-Mail:
info@podiatryinstitute.com

Government and Public Service Organizations

Arthritis Foundation
1330 West Peachtree Street
Atlanta, GA 30309
Telephone: 404-872-7100
Toll Free: 800-283-7800
Fax: 404-872-0457
or call your local chapter (listed
in the telephone directory)
Website: http://
www.arthritis.org

**March of Dimes Birth
Defects Foundation**
National Office
1275 Mamaroneck Ave.
White Plains, NY 10605
Toll Free: 888-663-4637
Tel: 914-428-7100
Website: http://
www.modimes.org

**National Arthritis and
Musculoskeletal and Skin
Diseases Information
Clearinghouse (NAMSIC)**
National Institutes of Health
1 AMS Circle
Bethesda, MD 20892-3675
Toll Free: 877-22-NIAMS
Telephone: 301-495-4484
TTY: 301-565-2966
Fax: 301-718-6366
Website: http://www.nih.gov/
niams
E-Mail: niamsinfo@mail.nih.gov

**U.S. Food and Drug
Administration**
5600 Fishers Lane
Rockville, MD 20857-0001
Toll Free: 888-463-6332
Website: www.fda.gov

Medical Resources

Mayo Foundation for Medical Education and Research
200 First St. S.W.
Rochester, MN 55905
Tel: 507-284-2511
Fax: 507-284-0161
Website: http://www.mayohealth.org

New York Orthopaedics & Sports Medicine, PC
215 East 73rd Street
New York, NY 10021
Tel: 212-249-8200
Fax: 212-249-5727
Website: http://www.nyorthopaedics.com
E-Mail: nyortho@aol.com

Rice University
SportsMed Web
Website: http://www.rice.edu/~jenky

Seaford Foot Care Center
3650 Merrick Road
Seaford, NY 11783
Telephone: 516-221-5982
Fax: 516-221-0720
Website: http://www.seafordfootcare.com

Publications and Publishers

Advances in Wound Care: The Journal for Prevention and Healing
Springhouse Corp.
1111 Bethlehem Pike
P.O. Box 908
Springhouse PA 19477
Telephone: 215-646-8700
Fax: 215-646-4399
Website: http://www.springnet.com

Consultant
Cliggott Publishing Company
330 Boston Post Road
Darien, CT 06820
Telephone: 203-662-6400
Fax: 203-662-6776

FDA Consumer
U.S. Food and Drug Administration
5600 Fishers Lane
Rockville, MD 20857-0001
Toll Free: 888-463-6332
Website: http://www.fda.gov/fdac/fdacindex.html

Medical Multimedia Group
515 South Reserve, Suite 1
Missoula, MT 59804
Toll Free: 866-721-3072
Telephone: 406-721-3072
Fax: 406-721-3072
Website: www.medicalmultimediagroup.com
E-mail: info@medicalmultimediagroup.com

Occupational Hazards
Penton Media Inc.
1300 E. Ninth St.
Cleveland, OH 44114-1503
Telephone: 216-696-7000
Fax: 216-696-7658
Website: http://www.penton.com
Website: http://
www.occupationalhazards.com

Orthopaedic Nursing
National Association of Ortho-
paedic Nurses
East Holly Avenue/Box 56
Pitman, NJ 08071-0056
Telephone: 856-256-2310
Fax: 856-589-7463
Website: http://naon.inurse.com

Patient Care
Medical Economics
Five Paragon Drive
Montvale, NJ 07645-1742
Telephone: 201-358-7244
Fax: 201-722-2676
Website: http://pc.pdr.net

**The Physician and
Sportsmedicine**
McGraw-Hill
4530 W. 77th St.
Minneapolis, MN 55435
Telephone: 952-835-3222
Fax: 952-835-3460
Website: http://
www.physsportsmed.com

Podiatry Today
HMP Communications
950 West Valley Road, Suite
2800
Wayne, PA 19087
Telephone: 610-688-8220
Fax: 610-688-8050
Toll Free: 1-800-237-7285 (editor
at extension 214)
Website: http://
www.podiatrytoday.com

Orthotics

*The Prescription Foot
Orthotic Laboratory
Association*
36 South Last Chance Gulch,
Suite A
Helena, MT 59601
Toll Free: 800-347-6585
Fax: 406-443-4614
Website: http://www.pfola.org
E-Mail: info@pfola.org

Information for Diabetics

American Association of Diabetes Educators
100 West Monroe Street, Suite 400
Chicago, IL 60603
Toll Free: 800-338-3633
Telephone: 312-424-2426
Fax: 312-424-2427
Website: http://www.aadenet.org

American Diabetes Association
1701 N. Beauregard St.
Alexandria, VA 22311
Toll Free: 800-DIABETES (800-342-2383)
Toll Free: 800-232-3472 Professional Services
Website: http://www.diabetes.org
E-Mail: customerservice@diabetes.org

American Podiatric Medical Association
9312 Old Georgetown Road
Bethesda, MD 20814-1698
Telephone: 301-571-9200
Toll Free: 1-800-FOOTCARE
Fax: 301-530-2752
Website: http://www.apma.org
E-Mail: askapma@apma.org

Centers for Disease Control and Prevention
Division of Diabetes Translation
Program Development Branch
4770 Buford Highway, NE, Mailstop K-10
Atlanta, GA 30341-3724
Toll Free: 877-CDC-DIAB (877-232-3422)
Telephone: 770-488-5000
Fax: 770-488-5966
Website: http://www.cdc.gov/diabetes
E-Mail: diabetes@cdc.gov

Juvenile Diabetes Foundation International
120 Wall Street, 19th Floor
New York, NY 10005
Toll Free: 800-JDF-CURE (800-533-2873)
Website: http://www.jdfcure.org
E-Mail: info@jdrf.org

National Institute of Diabetes and Digestive and Kidney Diseases
National Diabetes Information Clearinghouse (NDIC)
1 Information Way
Bethesda, MD 20892-3560
Toll Free: 800-GET-LEVEL (800-438-5383)
Telephone: 301-654-3327
Fax: 301-907-8906
Website: http://www.niddk.nih.gov

Podiatry Information On-Line

Dancer.com
Gaynor Minden, Inc.
Website: www.dancer.com

Feet for Life
Website: www.feetforlife.org

Foot and Ankle Web Index
Website: www.footandankle.com

Foot Care Direct
Website:
www.footcaredirect.com
E-Mail:
footcaredirect@home.com

Foot Dr. Link
Website: www.footdrlink.com
E-Mail: footdrlink@home.com

Foot Health
Website: www.foothealth.com
E-Mail: fh@avonet.com

FootHealthNetwork.com, Inc.
Website:
www.foothealthnetwork.com

A Foot Talk Place on the Net
Website: www.foottalk.com

Podiatry Channel
Website:
www.podiatrychannel.com

PodiatryNetwork.com
Website:
www.podiatrynetwork.com
E-Mail:
info@podiatrynetwork.com

Chapter 50

Foot Safety Resources

American College of Occupational and Environmental Medicine
1114 N. Arlington Heights Road
Arlington Heights, IL 60004
Telephone: 847-818-1800
Fax: 847-818-9266
Website: http://www.acoem.org

American Podiatric Medical Association
9312 Old Georgetown Road
Bethesda, MD 20814-1698
Telephone: 301-571-9200
Toll Free: 1-800-FOOTCARE
Website: http://www.apma.org

Arnot Ogden Medical Center
300 Roe Ave.
Elmira, NY 14905
Toll Free: 800-952-2662
Website: http://www.aomc.org

Canadian Centre for Occupational Health and Safety
250 Main Street East
Hamilton, Ontario,
Canada L8N 1H6
Toll Free: 1-800-263-8466 (toll-free in Canada)
Telephone: 1-905-572-4400 (8:30 AM to 5:00 PM Eastern Time)
Fax: 1-905-572-4500
Website: http://www.canoshweb.org

Feet For Life
Website: http://www.feetforlife.org

*National Institute for Occu-
pational Safety and Health*
U.S. Department of Health and
Human Services
4676 Columbia Parkway
Cincinnati, OH 45226
Toll Free: 1-800-35-NIOSH (1-
800-356-4674)
Fax: 513-533-8573
Website: http://www.cdc.gov/
niosh

"Occupational Hazards"
Penton Media Inc.
1300 E. Ninth St.
Cleveland, OH 44114-1503
Telephone: 216-696-7000
Fax: 216-696-7658
Website: http://
www.occupationalhazards.com

U.S. Department of Labor
Occupational Safety and Health
Administration (OSHA)
200 Constitution Avenue, N.W.
Washington, D.C. 20210
Toll Free: 800-321-6742
Telephone: 202-693-1999
Website: http://www.osha.gov

Index

Index

Page numbers followed by 'n' indicate a footnote. Page numbers in *italics* indicate a table or illustration.

A

accessory navicular 45, 206–7
accommodative orthosis, described 84
Achilles tendinitis
  athletic shoes 66–67
  dancers 306
  defined 331
  described 302–3
  prevention 80
  treatment 56–57
Achilles tendon
  defined 331
  high-heeled shoes 40
Ackman, J.D. 175n
acquired immune deficiency syndrome (AIDS), foot disorders 237–39
Administration on Aging (AoA), publications 23n
adolescents, Sever's disease 247–49
"The Adult Foot" (AOFAS) 9n
Advances in Wound Care: The Journal for Prevention and Healing 341

age factor
  ingrown toenails 119
  onychomycosis 130
AIDS *see* acquired immune deficiency syndrome
"AIDS and Your Feet" (FootHealthNetwork.com, Inc.) 237n
alcohol use, gout 221
Alexander, M. 175n
allergic urticaria 130, 134
allopurinol 223
allylamines 146
aluminum chloride hexahydrate 151
Amendola, Ned 95–96
American Academy of Ambulatory Foot Surgeons, contact information 4
American Association of Diabetes Educators, contact information 32, 343
American Association of Podiatric Sports Medicine, contact information 339
American Board of Podiatric Surgery 4
American Board of Podiatry Orthopedics and Primary Podiatric Medicine 4

349

American College of Foot and Ankle
Surgeons, contact information 339
American College of Occupational
and Environmental Medicine, contact information 345
American Diabetes Association, contact information 343
American Orthopaedic Foot and
Ankle Society (AOFAS)
contact information 339
publications
adult feet 9n
arthritis 229n
Charcot joints 39n
children's shoes 35n
high heels 39n, 41
American Podiatric Medical Association (APMA), contact information 3,
25, 345
amorolfine 136
amputations
defined 331
diabetes mellitus 212–14
information 321–28
Syme's 126
Anaprox (naproxen) 223
ankle fractures 266–68, 313–18
ankle joint, defined 331
ankle sprains
described 60–61, 277
high-heeled shoes 40
treatment 277–79
"Ankle Sprains" (Rice University
SportsMed website) 277n
ankylosing spondylitis 231
antibacterial soap 149
antibiotics, foot odor 151–52
AoA *see* Administration on Aging
AOFAS *see* American Orthopaedic
Foot and Ankle Society
Apert's syndrome, defined 331
APMA *see* American Podiatric Medical Association
apophysitis, described 58
arch pain *see* plantar fasciitis
arch supports, athletic shoes 68
"Are You Picking the Right Foot Protection? (LaBar) 71n
Artane (trihexyphenidyl) 235, 236

arteries, defined 331
arthritis
defined 225, 332
described 54, 229–331
gout 219
treatment 231–33
see also osteoarthritis; rheumatoid
arthritis
Arthritis Foundation, contact information 224, 340
arthroplasty 104, 156
astemizole 135
athletes
foot disorders 53–69
shoes 64–69
socks 43–51
athlete's foot (tinea pedis)
causes 24
defined 332
described 115–17, 145–47, *146*
treatment 151–52
"Athlete's Foot--Skin Fungus Infection, Dermatophytosis, Tinea Pedis,
Ringworm" (White) 115n
athletic footwear 43–51
autonomic neuropathy, described
166
avulsion 123–24

B

baclofen 235–36
bacterial cellulitis 129, 130
bacterial infections
athlete's foot 116
ingrown toenails 119
socks 45
toenail surgery 125
see also foot odor; pitted keratolysis
Bahr, Roald 247n
BAPFOL *see* Board for Accreditation
of Prescription Foot Orthotic Laboratories
Benemid (probenecid) 223
benzoyl peroxide 151
"Big Steps Forward for Amputees"
(Hamilton) 321n
black heel *see* talon noir

children
  clubfeet 175–91
  flatfeet 205–6
  foot pain prevention 77
  genetic foot disorders 195–203
  intoeing 193–94
  Sever's disease 58, 247–49
  shoes 35–36
Childress, Dudley S. 326–27
chiriatry, described 5
chiropody, described 5
chondrocalcinosis *see* pseudogout
chondromalacia patellae (runner's
  knee) 62
chronic myotic infection 123
Churchill, R. Sean 281n, 296
Cincinnati incision 188
circulation, foot health 23, 30
cisapride 135
clawtoes
  described 153–56
  poorly fitting shoes 40
"Clawtoes and Hammertoes" (Orthopaedic Patient Education) 153n
clindamycin 151
clinodactyly 199
clonazepam 235–36
clotrimazole 146
clubfoot (talipes equinovarus) 175–
  91
  causes *178–81*
  defined 333
  described 175–86, *176, 200*
  genetic factors 202–3
  surgical procedure *188*
  treatment 186–88
colchicine
  defined 225
  gout 223
congenital, defined 196
connective tissue
  defined 225
connective tissue, defined 225
Consultant, contact information 341
contusions 300
corns
  causes 24
  defined 333
  described 12, 103, 141–43

corns, continued
  surgery 105
  treatment 29
corticosteroids
  defined 225, 333
  heel pain 245
cortisone 57, 169
Coughlin, Michael 119n
craniosynostosis, described 335
crystal deposition disease *see*
  pseudogout
crystal-induced arthritis, defined
  225
  see also gout; pseudogout
cyclobenzaprine 235–36
cyclosporine
  drug interactions 134
  gout 221

D

Dale, Stephen J. 205n, 301n
Dancer.com, website 344
dancers
  Achilles tendinitis 56–57
  foot injuries 305–9
  hallux valgus 282
David, Daniel J. 205n, 301n
Denis Browne splint 194
dermatophyte infections
  heredity 116
  socks 45
  see also athlete's foo
dermatophytid eruption 130
"Detecting and Treating Common
  Foot and Ankle Fractures"
  (Thordarson) 265n
diabetes mellitus
  athlete's foot 116
  defined 333
  foot amputations 212–14
  foot care 14–15, 27–33, 78–80
  foot ulcers 211–12
diabetic orthosis, described 85
"Diagnosing and Treating Onychomycosis" (Seraly; Fuerst) 129n
diazepam 134
didanosine 134

Health Reference Series
COMPLETE CATALOG

AIDS Sourcebook, 1st Edition

Basic Information about AIDS and HIV Infection, Featuring Historical and Statistical Data, Current Research, Prevention, and Other Special Topics of Interest for Persons Living with AIDS

Along with Source Listings for Further Assistance

Edited by Karen Bellenir and Peter D. Dresser. 831 pages. 1995. 0-7808-0031-1. $78.

"One strength of this book is its practical emphasis. The intended audience is the lay reader . . . useful as an educational tool for health care providers who work with AIDS patients. Recommended for public libraries as well as hospital or academic libraries that collect consumer materials."
—Bulletin of the Medical Library Association, Jan '96

"This is the most comprehensive volume of its kind on an important medical topic. Highly recommended for all libraries." — Reference Book Review, '96

"Very useful reference for all libraries."
— Choice, Association of College and Research Libraries, Oct '95

"There is a wealth of information here that can provide much educational assistance. It is a must book for all libraries and should be on the desk of each and every congressional leader. Highly recommended."
— AIDS Book Review Journal, Aug '95

"Recommended for most collections."
— Library Journal, Jul '95

AIDS Sourcebook, 2nd Edition

Basic Consumer Health Information about Acquired Immune Deficiency Syndrome (AIDS) and Human Immunodeficiency Virus (HIV) Infection, Featuring Updated Statistical Data, Reports on Recent Research and Prevention Initiatives, and Other Special Topics of Interest for Persons Living with AIDS, Including New Antiretroviral Treatment Options, Strategies for Combating Opportunistic Infections, Information about Clinical Trials, and More

Along with a Glossary of Important Terms and Resource Listings for Further Help and Information

Edited by Karen Bellenir. 751 pages. 1999. 0-7808-0225-X. $78.

"Highly recommended."
—American Reference Books Annual, 2000

"Excellent sourcebook. This continues to be a highly recommended book. There is no other book that provides as much information as this book provides."
— AIDS Book Review Journal, Dec-Jan 2000

"Recommended reference source."
—Booklist, American Library Association, Dec '99

"A solid text for college-level health libraries."
—The Bookwatch, Aug '99

Cited in Reference Sources for Small and Medium-Sized Libraries, American Library Association, 1999

Alcoholism Sourcebook

Basic Consumer Health Information about the Physical and Mental Consequences of Alcohol Abuse, Including Liver Disease, Pancreatitis, Wernicke-Korsakoff Syndrome (Alcoholic Dementia), Fetal Alcohol Syndrome, Heart Disease, Kidney Disorders, Gastrointestinal Problems, and Immune System Compromise and Featuring Facts about Addiction, Detoxification, Alcohol Withdrawal, Recovery, and the Maintenance of Sobriety

Along with a Glossary and Directories of Resources for Further Help and Information

Edited by Karen Bellenir. 613 pages. 2000. 0-7808-0325-6. $78.

"This title is one of the few reference works on alcoholism for general readers. For some readers this will be a welcome complement to the many self-help books on the market. Recommended for collections serving general readers and consumer health collections."
— E-Streams, Mar '01

"This book is an excellent choice for public and academic libraries."
— American Reference Books Annual, 2001

"Recommended reference source."
—Booklist, American Library Association, Dec '00

"Presents a wealth of information on alcohol use and abuse and its effects on the body and mind, treatment, and prevention." — SciTech Book News, Dec '00

"Important new health guide which packs in the latest consumer information about the problems of alcoholism." — Reviewer's Bookwatch, Nov '00

SEE ALSO Drug Abuse Sourcebook, Substance Abuse Sourcebook

Allergies Sourcebook, 1st Edition

Basic Information about Major Forms and Mechanisms of Common Allergic Reactions, Sensitivities, and Intolerances, Including Anaphylaxis, Asthma, Hives and Other Dermatologic Symptoms, Rhinitis, and Sinusitis

Along with Their Usual Triggers Like Animal Fur, Chemicals, Drugs, Dust, Foods, Insects, Latex, Pollen, and Poison Ivy, Oak, and Sumac; Plus Information on Prevention, Identification, and Treatment

Edited by Allan R. Cook. 611 pages. 1997. 0-7808-0036-2. $78.

Allergies Sourcebook, 2nd Edition

Basic Consumer Health Information about Allergic Disorders, Triggers, Reactions, and Related Symptoms, Including Anaphylaxis, Rhinitis, Sinusitis, Asthma, Dermatitis, Conjunctivitis, and Multiple Chemical Sensitivity

Along with Tips on Diagnosis, Prevention, and Treatment, Statistical Data, a Glossary, and a Directory of Sources for Further Help and Information

Edited by Annemarie S. Muth. 600 pages. 2001. 0-7808-0376-0. $78.

Alternative Medicine Sourcebook

Basic Consumer Health Information about Alternatives to Conventional Medicine, Including Acupressure, Acupuncture, Aromatherapy, Ayurveda, Bioelectromagnetics, Environmental Medicine, Essence Therapy, Food and Nutrition Therapy, Herbal Therapy, Homeopathy, Imaging, Massage, Naturopathy, Reflexology, Relaxation and Meditation, Sound Therapy, Vitamin and Mineral Therapy, and Yoga, and More

Edited by Allan R. Cook. 737 pages. 1999. 0-7808-0200-4. $78.

"Recommended reference source."
    —Booklist, American Library Association, Feb '00

"A great addition to the reference collection of every type of library." —American Reference Books Annual, 2000

Alzheimer's, Stroke & 29 Other Neurological Disorders Sourcebook, 1st Edition

Basic Information for the Layperson on 31 Diseases or Disorders Affecting the Brain and Nervous System, First Describing the Illness, Then Listing Symptoms, Diagnostic Methods, and Treatment Options, and Including Statistics on Incidences and Causes

Edited by Frank E. Bair. 579 pages. 1993. 1-55888-748-2. $78.

"Nontechnical reference book that provides reader-friendly information."
    —Family Caregiver Alliance Update, Winter '96

"Should be included in any library's patient education section." —American Reference Books Annual, 1994

"Written in an approachable and accessible style. Recommended for patient education and consumer health collections in health science center and public libraries." —Academic Library Book Review, Dec '93

"It is very handy to have information on more than thirty neurological disorders under one cover, and there is no recent source like it." —Reference Quarterly, American Library Association, Fall '93

SEE ALSO Brain Disorders Sourcebook

Alzheimer's Disease Sourcebook, 2nd Edition

Basic Consumer Health Information about Alzheimer's Disease, Related Disorders, and Other Dementias, Including Multi-Infarct Dementia, AIDS-Related Dementia, Alcoholic Dementia, Huntington's Disease, Delirium, and Confusional States

Along with Reports Detailing Current Research Efforts in Prevention and Treatment, Long-Term Care Issues, and Listings of Sources for Additional Help and Information

Edited by Karen Bellenir. 524 pages. 1999. 0-7808-0223-3. $78.

"Provides a wealth of useful information not otherwise available in one place. This resource is recommended for all types of libraries."
    —American Reference Books Annual, 2000

"Recommended reference source."
    —Booklist, American Library Association, Oct '99

Arthritis Sourcebook

Basic Consumer Health Information about Specific Forms of Arthritis and Related Disorders, Including Rheumatoid Arthritis, Osteoarthritis, Gout, Polymyalgia Rheumatica, Psoriatic Arthritis, Spondyloarthropathies, Juvenile Rheumatoid Arthritis, and Juvenile Ankylosing Spondylitis

Along with Information about Medical, Surgical, and Alternative Treatment Options, and Including Strategies for Coping with Pain, Fatigue, and Stress

Edited by Allan R. Cook. 550 pages. 1998. 0-7808-0201-2. $78.

"... accessible to the layperson."
    —Reference and Research Book News, Feb '99

Asthma Sourcebook

Basic Consumer Health Information about Asthma, Including Symptoms, Traditional and Nontraditional Remedies, Treatment Advances, Quality-of-Life Aids, Medical Research Updates, and the Role of Allergies, Exercise, Age, the Environment, and Genetics in the Development of Asthma

Along with Statistical Data, a Glossary, and Directories of Support Groups, and Other Resources for Further Information

Edited by Annemarie S. Muth. 628 pages. 2000. 0-7808-0381-7. $78.

"A worthwhile reference acquisition for public libraries and academic medical libraries whose readers desire a quick introduction to the wide range of asthma information." —Choice, Association of College and Research Libraries, Jun '01

"Recommended reference source."
    —Booklist, American Library Association, Feb '01

Back & Neck Disorders Sourcebook

Basic Information about Disorders and Injuries of the Spinal Cord and Vertebrae, Including Facts on Chiropractic Treatment, Surgical Interventions, Paralysis, and Rehabilitation

Along with Advice for Preventing Back Trouble

Edited by Karen Bellenir. 548 pages. 1997. 0-7808-0202-0. $78.

"The strength of this work is its basic, easy-to-read format. Recommended."
— Reference and User Services Quarterly, American Library Association, Winter '97

Blood & Circulatory Disorders Sourcebook

Basic Information about Blood and Its Components, Anemias, Leukemias, Bleeding Disorders, and Circulatory Disorders, Including Aplastic Anemia, Thalassemia, Sickle-Cell Disease, Hemochromatosis, Hemophilia, Von Willebrand Disease, and Vascular Diseases

Along with a Special Section on Blood Transfusions and Blood Supply Safety, a Glossary, and Source Listings for Further Help and Information

Edited by Karen Bellenir and Linda M. Shin. 554 pages. 1998. 0-7808-0203-9. $78.

"Recommended reference source."
— Booklist, American Library Association, Feb '99

"An important reference sourcebook written in simple language for everyday, non-technical users. "
— Reviewer's Bookwatch, Jan '99

Brain Disorders Sourcebook

Basic Consumer Health Information about Strokes, Epilepsy, Amyotrophic Lateral Sclerosis (ALS/Lou Gehrig's Disease), Parkinson's Disease, Brain Tumors, Cerebral Palsy, Headache, Tourette Syndrome, and More

Along with Statistical Data, Treatment and Rehabilitation Options, Coping Strategies, Reports on Current

Breast Cancer Sourcebook

Basic Consumer Health Information about Breast Cancer, Including Diagnostic Methods, Treatment Options, Alternative Therapies, Self-Help Information, Related Health Concerns, Statistical and Demographic Data, and Facts for Men with Breast Cancer

Along with Reports on Current Research Initiatives, a Glossary of Related Medical Terms, and a Directory of Sources for Further Help and Information

Edited by Edward J. Prucha and Karen Bellenir. 580 pages. 2001. 0-7808-0244-6. $78.

SEE ALSO Cancer Sourcebook for Women, 1st and 2nd Editions, Women's Health Concerns Sourcebook

Breastfeeding Sourcebook

Basic Consumer Health Information about the Benefits of Breastmilk, Preparing to Breastfeed, Breastfeeding as a Baby Grows, Nutrition, and More, Including Information on Special Situations and Concerns, Such as Mastitis, Illness, Medications, Allergies, Multiple Births, Prematurity, Special Needs, and Adoption

Along with a Glossary and Resources for Additional Help and Information

Edited by Jenni Lynn Colson. 350 pages. 2001. 0-7808-0332-9. $48.

SEE ALSO Pregnancy & Birth Sourcebook

Burns Sourcebook

Basic Consumer Health Information about Various Types of Burns and Scalds, Including Flame, Heat, Cold, Electrical, Chemical, and Sun Burns

Along with Information on Short-Term and Long-Term Treatments, Tissue Reconstruction, Plastic Surgery, Prevention Suggestions, and First Aid

Edited by Allan R. Cook. 604 pages. 1999. 0-7808-0204-7. $78.

"This key reference guide is an invaluable addition to all health care and public libraries in confronting this ongoing health issue."
— American Reference Books Annual, 2000

"This is an exceptional addition to the series and is highly recommended for all consumer health collections, hospital libraries, and academic medical centers." — *E-Streams, Mar '00*

"Recommended reference source."
—*Booklist, American Library Association, Dec '99*

SEE ALSO Skin Disorders Sourcebook

■

Cancer Sourcebook, 1st Edition

Basic Information on Cancer Types, Symptoms, Diagnostic Methods, and Treatments, Including Statistics on Cancer Occurrences Worldwide and the Risks Associated with Known Carcinogens and Activities

Edited by Frank E. Bair. 932 pages. 1990. 1-55888-888-8. $78.

Cited in *Reference Sources for Small and Medium-Sized Libraries*, American Library Association, 1999

"Written in nontechnical language. Useful for patients, their families, medical professionals, and librarians." — *Guide to Reference Books, 1996*

"Designed with the non-medical professional in mind. Libraries and medical facilities interested in patient education should certainly consider adding the *Cancer Sourcebook* to their holdings. This compact collection of reliable information . . . is an invaluable tool for helping patients and patients' families and friends to take the first steps in coping with the many difficulties of cancer." — *Medical Reference Services Quarterly, Winter '91*

"Specifically created for the nontechnical reader . . . an important resource for the general reader trying to understand the complexities of cancer." — *American Reference Books Annual, 1991*

"This publication's nontechnical nature and very comprehensive format make it useful for both the general public and undergraduate students." — *Choice, Association of College and Research Libraries, Oct '90*

■

New Cancer Sourcebook, 2nd Edition

Basic Information about Major Forms and Stages of Cancer, Featuring Facts about Primary and Secondary Tumors of the Respiratory, Nervous, Lymphatic, Circulatory, Skeletal, and Gastrointestinal Systems, and Specific Organs; Statistical and Demographic Data; Treatment Options; and Strategies for Coping

Edited by Allan R. Cook. 1,313 pages. 1996. 0-7808-0041-9. $78.

"An excellent resource for patients with newly diagnosed cancer and their families. The dialogue is simple, direct, and comprehensive. Highly recommended for patients and families to aid in their understanding of cancer and its treatment." — *Booklist Health Sciences Supplement, American Library Association, Oct '97*

"The amount of factual and useful information is extensive. The writing is very clear, geared to general readers. Recommended for all levels." — *Choice, Association of College and Research Libraries, Jan '97*

■

Cancer Sourcebook, 3rd Edition

Basic Consumer Health Information about Major Forms and Stages of Cancer, Featuring Facts about Primary and Secondary Tumors of the Respiratory, Nervous, Lymphatic, Circulatory, Skeletal, and Gastrointestinal Systems, and Specific Organs

Along with Statistical and Demographic Data, Treatment Options, Strategies for Coping, a Glossary, and a Directory of Sources for Additional Help and Information

Edited by Edward J. Prucha. 1,069 pages. 2000. 0-7808-0227-6. $78.

"This title is recommended for health sciences and public libraries with consumer health collections." — *E-Streams, Feb '01*

". . . can be effectively used by cancer patients and their families who are looking for answers in a language they can understand. Public and hospital libraries should have it on their shelves." — *American Reference Books Annual, 2001*

"Recommended reference source." — *Booklist, American Library Association, Dec '00*

■

Cancer Sourcebook for Women, 1st Edition

Basic Information about Specific Forms of Cancer That Affect Women, Featuring Facts about Breast Cancer, Cervical Cancer, Ovarian Cancer, Cancer of the Uterus and Uterine Sarcoma, Cancer of the Vagina, and Cancer of the Vulva; Statistical and Demographic Data; Treatments, Self-Help Management Suggestions, and Current Research Initiatives

Edited by Allan R. Cook and Peter D. Dresser. 524 pages. 1996. 0-7808-0076-1. $78.

". . . written in easily understandable, non-technical language. Recommended for public libraries or hospital and academic libraries that collect patient education or consumer health materials." — *Medical Reference Services Quarterly, Spring '97*

"Would be of value in a consumer health library. . . . written with the health care consumer in mind. Medical jargon is at a minimum, and medical terms are explained in clear, understandable sentences." — *Bulletin of the Medical Library Association, Oct '96*

"The availability under one cover of all these pertinent publications, grouped under cohesive headings, makes this certainly a most useful sourcebook." — *Choice, Association of College and Research Libraries, Jun '96*

366

SEE ALSO *Breast Cancer Sourcebook, Women's Health Concerns Sourcebook*

Cancer Sourcebook for Women, 2nd Edition

Basic Consumer Health Information about Specific Forms of Cancer That Affect Women, Including Cervical Cancer, Ovarian Cancer, Endometrial Cancer, Uterine Sarcoma, Vaginal Cancer, Vulvar Cancer, and Gestational Trophoblastic Tumor; and Featuring Statistical Information, Facts about Tests and Treatments, a Glossary of Cancer Terms, and an Extensive List of Additional Resources

Edited by Karen Bellenir. 600 pages. 2001. 0-7808-0226-8. $78.

SEE ALSO *Breast Cancer Sourcebook, Women's Health Concerns Sourcebook*

Cardiovascular Diseases & Disorders Sourcebook, 1st Edition

Basic Information about Cardiovascular Diseases and Disorders, Featuring Facts about the Cardiovascular System, Demographic and Statistical Data, Descriptions of Pharmacological and Surgical Interventions, Lifestyle Modifications, and a Special Section Focusing on Heart Disorders in Children

Edited by Karen Bellenir and Peter D. Dresser. 683 pages. 1995. 0-7808-0032-X. $78.

"... comprehensive format provides an extensive overview on this subject."
—*Choice, Association of College and Research Libraries, Jun '96*

"... an easily understood, complete, up-to-date resource. This well executed public health tool will make valuable information available to those that need it most, patients and their families. The typeface, sturdy non-reflective paper, and library binding add a feel of quality found wanting in other publications. Highly recommended for academic and general libraries. "
—*Academic Library Book Review, Summer '96*

SEE ALSO *Healthy Heart Sourcebook for Women, Heart Diseases & Disorders Sourcebook, 2nd Edition*

Caregiving Sourcebook

Basic Consumer Health Information for Caregivers, Including a Profile of Caregivers, Caregiving Responsibilities and Concerns, Tips for Specific Conditions, Care Environments, and the Effects of Caregiving

Along with Facts about Legal Issues, Financial Information, and Future Planning, a Glossary, and a Listing of Additional Resources

Edited by Joyce Brennfleck Shannon. 600 pages. 2001. 0-7808-0331-0. $78.

Colds, Flu & Other Common Ailments Sourcebook

Basic Consumer Health Information about Common Ailments and Injuries, Including Colds, Coughs, the Flu, Sinus Problems, Headaches, Fever, Nausea and Vomiting, Menstrual Cramps, Diarrhea, Constipation, Hemorrhoids, Back Pain, Dandruff, Dry and Itchy Skin, Cuts, Scrapes, Sprains, Bruises, and More

Along with Information about Prevention, Self-Care, Choosing a Doctor, Over-the-Counter Medications, Folk Remedies, and Alternative Therapies, and Including a Glossary of Important Terms and a Directory of Resources for Further Help and Information

Edited by Chad T. Kimball. 638 pages. 2001. 0-7808-0435-X. $78.

Communication Disorders Sourcebook

Basic Information about Deafness and Hearing Loss, Speech and Language Disorders, Voice Disorders, Balance and Vestibular Disorders, and Disorders of Smell, Taste, and Touch

Edited by Linda M. Ross. 533 pages. 1996. 0-7808-0077-X. $78.

"This is skillfully edited and is a welcome resource for the layperson. It should be found in every public and medical library." — *Booklist Health Sciences Supplement, American Library Association, Oct '97*

Congenital Disorders Sourcebook

Basic Information about Disorders Acquired during Gestation, Including Spina Bifida, Hydrocephalus, Cerebral Palsy, Heart Defects, Craniofacial Abnormalities, Fetal Alcohol Syndrome, and More

Along with Current Treatment Options and Statistical Data

Edited by Karen Bellenir. 607 pages. 1997. 0-7808-0205-5. $78.

"Recommended reference source."
— *Booklist, American Library Association, Oct '97*

SEE ALSO *Pregnancy & Birth Sourcebook*

Consumer Issues in Health Care Sourcebook

Basic Information about Health Care Fundamentals and Related Consumer Issues, Including Exams and Screening Tests, Physician Specialties, Choosing a Doctor, Using Prescription and Over-the-Counter Medications Safely, Avoiding Health Scams, Managing Common Health Risks in the Home, Care Options for Chronically or Terminally Ill Patients, and a List of Resources for Obtaining Help and Further Information

Edited by Karen Bellenir. 618 pages. 1998. 0-7808-0221-7. $78.

"Both public and academic libraries will want to have a copy in their collection for readers who are interested in self-education on health issues."
— American Reference Books Annual, 2000

"The editor has researched the literature from government agencies and others, saving readers the time and effort of having to do the research themselves. Recommended for public libraries."
— Reference and User Services Quarterly, American Library Association, Spring '99

"Recommended reference source."
— Booklist, American Library Association, Dec '98

∎

Contagious & Non-Contagious Infectious Diseases Sourcebook

Basic Information about Contagious Diseases like Measles, Polio, Hepatitis B, and Infectious Mononucleosis, and Non-Contagious Infectious Diseases like Tetanus and Toxic Shock Syndrome, and Diseases Occurring as Secondary Infections Such as Shingles and Reye Syndrome

Along with Vaccination, Prevention, and Treatment Information, and a Section Describing Emerging Infectious Disease Threats

Edited by Karen Bellenir and Peter D. Dresser. 566 pages. 1996. 0-7808-0075-3. $78.

∎

Death & Dying Sourcebook

Basic Consumer Health Information for the Layperson about End-of-Life Care and Related Ethical and Legal Issues, Including Chief Causes of Death, Autopsies, Pain Management for the Terminally Ill, Life Support Systems, Insurance, Euthanasia, Assisted Suicide, Hospice Programs, Living Wills, Funeral Planning, Counseling, Mourning, Organ Donation, and Physician Training

Along with Statistical Data, a Glossary, and Listings of Sources for Further Help and Information

Edited by Annemarie S. Muth. 641 pages. 1999. 0-7808-0230-6. $78.

"Public libraries, medical libraries, and academic libraries will all find this sourcebook a useful addition to their collections."
— American Reference Books Annual, 2001

"An extremely useful resource for those concerned with death and dying in the United States."
— Respiratory Care, Nov '00

"Recommended reference source."
— Booklist, American Library Association, Aug '00

"This book is a definite must for all those involved in end-of-life care." — Doody's Review Service, 2000

∎

Diabetes Sourcebook, 1st Edition

Basic Information about Insulin-Dependent and Non-insulin-Dependent Diabetes Mellitus, Gestational Diabetes, and Diabetic Complications, Symptoms, Treatment, and Research Results, Including Statistics on Prevalence, Morbidity, and Mortality

Along with Source Listings for Further Help and Information

Edited by Karen Bellenir and Peter D. Dresser. 827 pages. 1994. 1-55888-751-2. $78.

". . . very informative and understandable for the layperson without being simplistic. It provides a comprehensive overview for laypersons who want a general understanding of the disease or who want to focus on various aspects of the disease."
— Bulletin of the Medical Library Association, Jan '96

∎

Diabetes Sourcebook, 2nd Edition

Basic Consumer Health Information about Type 1 Diabetes (Insulin-Dependent or Juvenile-Onset Diabetes), Type 2 (Noninsulin-Dependent or Adult-Onset Diabetes), Gestational Diabetes, and Related Disorders, Including Diabetes Prevalence Data, Management Issues, the Role of Diet and Exercise in Controlling Diabetes, Insulin and Other Diabetes Medicines, and Complications of Diabetes Such as Eye Diseases, Periodontal Disease, Amputation, and End-Stage Renal Disease

Along with Reports on Current Research Initiatives, a Glossary, and Resource Listings for Further Help and Information

Edited by Karen Bellenir. 688 pages. 1998. 0-7808-0224-1. $78.

"This comprehensive book is an excellent addition for high school, academic, medical, and public libraries. This volume is highly recommended."
— American Reference Books Annual, 2000

"An invaluable reference." — Library Journal, May '00

Selected as one of the 250 "Best Health Sciences Books of 1999." — Doody's Rating Service, Mar-Apr 2000

"Recommended reference source."
— Booklist, American Library Association, Feb '99

". . . provides reliable mainstream medical information . . . belongs on the shelves of any library with a consumer health collection." — E-Streams, Sep '99

"Provides useful information for the general public."
— Healthlines, University of Michigan Health Management Research Center, Sep/Oct '99

Diet & Nutrition Sourcebook, 1st Edition

Basic Information about Nutrition, Including the Dietary Guidelines for Americans, the Food Guide Pyramid, and Their Applications in Daily Diet, Nutritional Advice for Specific Age Groups, Current Nutritional Issues and Controversies, the New Food Label and How to Use It to Promote Healthy Eating, and Recent Developments in Nutritional Research

Edited by Dan R. Harris. 662 pages. 1996. 0-7808-0084-2. $78.

"Useful reference as a food and nutrition sourcebook for the general consumer." —Booklist Health Sciences Supplement, American Library Association, Oct '97

"Recommended for public libraries and medical libraries that receive general information requests on nutrition. It is readable and will appeal to those interested in learning more about healthy dietary practices." —Medical Reference Services Quarterly, Fall '97

"An abundance of medical and social statistics is translated into readable information geared toward the general reader." —Bookwatch, Mar '97

"With dozens of questionable diet books on the market, it is so refreshing to find a reliable and factual reference book. Recommended to aspiring professionals, librarians, and others seeking and giving reliable dietary advice. An excellent compilation." —Choice, Association of College and Research Libraries, Feb '97

SEE ALSO Digestive Diseases & Disorders Sourcebook, Gastrointestinal Diseases & Disorders Sourcebook

Diet & Nutrition Sourcebook, 2nd Edition

Basic Consumer Health Information about Dietary Guidelines, Recommended Daily Intake Values, Vitamins, Minerals, Fiber, Fat, Weight Control, Dietary Supplements, and Food Additives

Along with Special Sections on Nutrition Needs throughout Life and Nutrition for People with Such Specific Medical Concerns as Allergies, High Blood Cholesterol, Hypertension, Diabetes, Celiac Disease, Seizure Disorders, Phenylketonuria (PKU), Cancer, and Eating Disorders, and Including Reports on Current Nutrition Research and Source Listings for Additional Help and Information

Edited by Karen Bellenir. 650 pages. 1999. 0-7808-0228-4. $78.

"This book is an excellent source of basic diet and nutrition information." —Booklist Health Sciences Supplement, American Library Association, Dec '00

"This reference document should be in any public library, but it would be a very good guide for beginning students in the health sciences. If the other books in this publisher's series are as good as this, they should all be in the health sciences collections." —American Reference Books Annual, 2000

"This book is an excellent general nutrition reference for consumers who desire to take an active role in their health care for prevention. Consumers of all ages who select this book can feel confident they are receiving current and accurate information." —Journal of Nutrition for the Elderly, Vol. 19, No. 4, '00

"Recommended reference source." —Booklist, American Library Association, Dec '99

SEE ALSO Digestive Diseases & Disorders Sourcebook, Gastrointestinal Diseases & Disorders Sourcebook

Digestive Diseases & Disorders Sourcebook

Basic Consumer Health Information about Diseases and Disorders that Impact the Upper and Lower Digestive System, Including Celiac Disease, Constipation, Crohn's Disease, Cyclic Vomiting Syndrome, Diarrhea, Diverticulosis and Diverticulitis, Gallstones, Heartburn, Hemorrhoids, Hernias, Indigestion (Dyspepsia), Irritable Bowel Syndrome, Lactose Intolerance, Ulcers, and More

Along with Information about Medications and Other Treatments, Tips for Maintaining a Healthy Digestive Tract, a Glossary, and Directory of Digestive Diseases Organizations

Edited by Karen Bellenir. 335 pages. 1999. 0-7808-0327-2. $48.

"This title would be an excellent addition to all public or patient-research libraries." —American Reference Books Annual, 2001

"This title is recommended for public, hospital, and health sciences libraries with consumer health collections." —E-Streams, Jul-Aug '00

"Recommended reference source." —Booklist, American Library Association, May '00

SEE ALSO Diet & Nutrition Sourcebook, 1st and 2nd Editions, Gastrointestinal Diseases & Disorders Sourcebook

Disabilities Sourcebook

Basic Consumer Health Information about Physical and Psychiatric Disabilities, Including Descriptions of Major Causes of Disability, Assistive and Adaptive Aids, Workplace Issues, and Accessibility Concerns

Along with Information about the Americans with Disabilities Act, a Glossary, and Resources for Additional Help and Information

Edited by Dawn D. Matthews. 616 pages. 2000. 0-7808-0389-2. $78.

"A much needed addition to the Omnigraphics Health Reference Series. A current reference work to provide people with disabilities, their families, caregivers or those who work with them, a broad range of information in one volume, has not been available until now. . . . It is recommended for all public and academic library reference collections." —E-Streams, May '01

Domestic Violence & Child Abuse Sourcebook

Basic Consumer Health Information about Spousal/ Partner, Child, Sibling, Parent, and Elder Abuse, Covering Physical, Emotional, and Sexual Abuse, Teen Dating Violence, and Stalking; Includes Information about Hotlines, Safe Houses, Safety Plans, and Other Resources for Support and Assistance, Community Initiatives, and Reports on Current Directions in Research and Treatment

Along with a Glossary, Sources for Further Reading, and Governmental and Non-Governmental Organizations Contact Information

Edited by Helene Henderson. 1,064 pages. 2000. 0-7808-0235-7. $78.

Drug Abuse Sourcebook

Basic Consumer Health Information about Illicit Substances of Abuse and the Diversion of Prescription Medications, Including Depressants, Hallucinogens, Inhalants, Marijuana, Narcotics, Stimulants, and Anabolic Steroids

Along with Facts about Related Health Risks, Treatment Issues, and Substance Abuse Prevention Programs, a Glossary of Terms, Statistical Data, and Directories of Hotline Services, Self-Help Groups, and Organizations Able to Provide Further Information

Edited by Karen Bellenir. 629 pages. 2000. 0-7808-0242-X. $78.

Ear, Nose & Throat Disorders Sourcebook

Basic Information about Disorders of the Ears, Nose, Sinus Cavities, Pharynx, and Larynx, Including Ear Infections, Tinnitus, Vestibular Disorders, Allergic and Non-Allergic Rhinitis, Sore Throats, Tonsillitis, and Cancers That Affect the Ears, Nose, Sinuses, and Throat

Along with Reports on Current Research Initiatives, a Glossary of Related Medical Terms, and a Directory of Sources for Further Help and Information

Edited by Karen Bellenir and Linda M. Shin. 576 pages. 1998. 0-7808-0206-3. $78.

Eating Disorders Sourcebook

Basic Consumer Health Information about Eating Disorders, Including Information about Anorexia Nervosa, Bulimia Nervosa, Binge Eating, Body Dysmorphic Disorder, Pica, Laxative Abuse, and Night Eating Syndrome

Along with Information about Causes, Adverse Effects, and Treatment and Prevention Issues, and Featuring a Section on Concerns Specific to Children and Adolescents, a Glossary, and Resources for Further Help and Information

Edited by Dawn D. Matthews. 322 pages. 2001. 0-7808-0335-3. $78.

Endocrine & Metabolic Disorders Sourcebook

Basic Information for the Layperson about Pancreatic and Insulin-Related Disorders Such as Pancreatitis, Diabetes, and Hypoglycemia; Adrenal Gland Disorders Such as Cushing's Syndrome, Addison's Disease, and Congenital Adrenal Hyperplasia; Pituitary Gland Disorders Such as Growth Hormone Deficiency, Acromegaly, and Pituitary Tumors; Thyroid Disorders Such as Hypothyroidism, Graves' Disease, Hashimoto's Disease, and Goiter; Hyperparathyroidism; and Other Diseases and Syndromes of Hormone Imbalance or Metabolic Dysfunction

Along with Reports on Current Research Initiatives

Edited by Linda M. Shin. 574 pages. 1998. 0-7808-0207-1. $78.

Environmentally Induced Disorders Sourcebook

Basic Information about Diseases and Syndromes Linked to Exposure to Pollutants and Other Substances in Outdoor and Indoor Environments Such as Lead, Asbestos, Formaldehyde, Mercury, Emissions, Noise, and More

Edited by Allan R. Cook. 620 pages. 1997. 0-7808-0083-4. $78.

Ethnic Diseases Sourcebook

Basic Consumer Health Information for Ethnic and Racial Minority Groups in the United States, Including General Health Indicators and Behaviors, Ethnic Diseases, Genetic Testing, the Impact of Chronic Diseases, Women's Health, Mental Health Issues, and Preventive Health Care Services

Along with a Glossary and a Listing of Additional Resources

Edited by Joyce Brennfleck Shannon. 664 pages. 2001. 0-7808-0336-1. $78.

Family Planning Sourcebook

Basic Consumer Health Information about Planning for Pregnancy and Contraception, Including Traditional Methods, Barrier Methods, Hormonal Methods, Permanent Methods, Future Methods, Emergency Contraception, and Birth Control Choices for Women at Each Stage of Life

Along with Statistics, a Glossary, and Sources of Additional Information

Edited by Amy Marcaccio Keyzer. 520 pages. 2001. 0-7808-0379-5. $78.

SEE ALSO Pregnancy & Birth Sourcebook

Fitness & Exercise Sourcebook, 1st Edition

Basic Information on Fitness and Exercise, Including Fitness Activities for Specific Age Groups, Exercise for People with Specific Medical Conditions, How to Begin a Fitness Program in Running, Walking, Swimming, Cycling, and Other Athletic Activities, and Recent Research in Fitness and Exercise

Edited by Dan R. Harris. 663 pages. 1996. 0-7808-0186-5. $78.

Fitness & Exercise Sourcebook, 2nd Edition

Basic Consumer Health Information about the Fundamentals of Fitness and Exercise, Including How to Begin and Maintain a Fitness Program, Fitness as a Lifestyle, the Link between Fitness and Diet, Advice for Specific Groups of People, Exercise as It Relates to Specific Medical Conditions, and Recent Research in Fitness and Exercise

Along with a Glossary of Important Terms and Resources for Additional Help and Information

Edited by Kristen M. Gledhill. 646 pages. 2001. 0-7808-0334-5. $78.

Food & Animal Borne Diseases Sourcebook

Basic Information about Diseases That Can Be Spread to Humans through the Ingestion of Contaminated Food or Water or by Contact with Infected Animals and Insects, Such as Botulism, E. Coli, Hepatitis A, Trichinosis, Lyme Disease, and Rabies

Along with Information Regarding Prevention and Treatment Methods, and Including a Special Section for International Travelers Describing Diseases Such as Cholera, Malaria, Travelers' Diarrhea, and Yellow Fever, and Offering Recommendations for Avoiding Illness

Edited by Karen Bellenir and Peter D. Dresser. 535 pages. 1995. 0-7808-0033-8. $78.

Food Safety Sourcebook

Basic Consumer Health Information about the Safe Handling of Meat, Poultry, Seafood, Eggs, Fruit Juices, and Other Food Items, and Facts about Pesticides, Drinking Water, Food Safety Overseas, and the Onset, Duration, and Symptoms of Foodborne Illnesses, Including Types of Pathogenic Bacteria, Parasitic Protozoa, Worms, Viruses, and Natural Toxins

Along with the Role of the Consumer, the Food Handler, and the Government in Food Safety; a Glossary, and Resources for Additional Help and Information

Edited by Dawn D. Matthews. 339 pages. 1999. 0-7808-0326-4. $48.

"This book is recommended for public libraries and universities with home economic and food science programs." — *E-Streams, Nov '00*

"This book takes the complex issues of food safety and foodborne pathogens and presents them in an easily understood manner. [It does] an excellent job of covering a large and often confusing topic."
— *American Reference Books Annual, 2000*

"Recommended reference source."
— *Booklist, American Library Association, May '00*

■

Forensic Medicine Sourcebook

Basic Consumer Information for the Layperson about Forensic Medicine, Including Crime Scene Investigation, Evidence Collection and Analysis, Expert Testimony, Computer-Aided Criminal Identification, Digital Imaging in the Courtroom, DNA Profiling, Accident Reconstruction, Autopsies, Ballistics, Drugs and Explosives Detection, Latent Fingerprints, Product Tampering, and Questioned Document Examination

Along with Statistical Data, a Glossary of Forensics Terminology, and Listings of Sources for Further Help and Information

Edited by Annemarie S. Muth. 574 pages. 1999. 0-7808-0232-2. $78.

"Given the expected widespread interest in its content and its easy to read style, this book is recommended for most public and all college and university libraries."
— *E-Streams, Feb '01*

"There are several items that make this book attractive to consumers who are seeking certain forensic data. . . . This is a useful current source for those seeking general forensic medical answers."
— *American Reference Books Annual, 2000*

"Recommended for public libraries."
— *Reference & User Services Quarterly, American Library Association, Spring 2000*

"Recommended reference source."
— *Booklist, American Library Association, Feb '00*

"A wealth of information, useful statistics, references are up-to-date and extremely complete. This wonderful collection of data will help students who are interested in a career in any type of forensic field. It is a great

resource for attorneys who need information about types of expert witnesses needed in a particular case. It also offers useful information for fiction and nonfiction writers whose work involves a crime. A fascinating compilation. All levels." — *Choice, Association of College and Research Libraries, Jan 2000*

■

Gastrointestinal Diseases & Disorders Sourcebook

Basic Information about Gastroesophageal Reflux Disease (Heartburn), Ulcers, Diverticulosis, Irritable Bowel Syndrome, Crohn's Disease, Ulcerative Colitis, Diarrhea, Constipation, Lactose Intolerance, Hemorrhoids, Hepatitis, Cirrhosis, and Other Digestive Problems, Featuring Statistics, Descriptions of Symptoms, and Current Treatment Methods of Interest for Persons Living with Upper and Lower Gastrointestinal Maladies

Edited by Linda M. Ross. 413 pages. 1996. 0-7808-0078-8. $78.

". . . very readable form. The successful editorial work that brought this material together into a useful and understandable reference makes accessible to all readers information that can help them more effectively understand and obtain help for digestive tract problems."
— *Choice, Association of College and Research Libraries, Feb '97*

SEE ALSO *Diet & Nutrition Sourcebook, 1st and 2nd Editions, Digestive Diseases & Disorders Sourcebook*

■

Genetic Disorders Sourcebook, 1st Edition

Basic Information about Heritable Diseases and Disorders Such as Down Syndrome, PKU, Hemophilia, Von Willebrand Disease, Gaucher Disease, Tay-Sachs Disease, and Sickle-Cell Disease, Along with Information about Genetic Screening, Gene Therapy, Home Care, and Including Source Listings for Further Help and Information on More Than 300 Disorders

Edited by Karen Bellenir. 642 pages. 1996. 0-7808-0034-6. $78.

"Recommended for undergraduate libraries or libraries that serve the public."
— *Science & Technology Libraries, Vol. 18, No. 1, '99*

"Provides essential medical information to both the general public and those diagnosed with a serious or fatal genetic disease or disorder."
— *Choice, Association of College and Research Libraries, Jan '97*

"Geared toward the lay public. It would be well placed in all public libraries and in those hospital and medical libraries in which access to genetic references is limited." — *Doody's Health Sciences Book Review, Oct '96*

Genetic Disorders Sourcebook, 2nd Edition

Basic Consumer Health Information about Hereditary Diseases and Disorders, Including Cystic Fibrosis, Down Syndrome, Hemophilia, Huntington's Disease, Sickle Cell Anemia, and More; Facts about Genes, Gene Research and Therapy, Genetic Screening, Ethics of Gene Testing, Genetic Counseling, and Advice on Coping and Caring

Along with a Glossary of Genetic Terminology and a Resource List for Help, Support, and Further Information

Edited by Kathy Massimini. 768 pages. 2001. 0-7808-0241-1. $78.

"Recommended for public libraries and medical and hospital libraries with consumer health collections."
— E-Streams, May '01

"Recommended reference source."
— Booklist, American Library Association, Apr '01

"Important pick for college-level health reference libraries." — The Bookwatch, Mar '01

Head Trauma Sourcebook

Basic Information for the Layperson about Open-Head and Closed-Head Injuries, Treatment Advances, Recovery, and Rehabilitation

Along with Reports on Current Research Initiatives

Edited by Karen Bellenir. 414 pages. 1997. 0-7808-0208-X. $78.

Health Insurance Sourcebook

Basic Information about Managed Care Organizations, Traditional Fee-for-Service Insurance, Insurance Portability and Pre-Existing Conditions Clauses, Medicare, Medicaid, Social Security, and Military Health Care

Along with Information about Insurance Fraud

Edited by Wendy Wilcox. 530 pages. 1997. 0-7808-0222-5. $78.

"Particularly useful because it brings much of this information together in one volume. This book will be a handy reference source in the health sciences library, hospital library, college and university library, and medium to large public library."
— Medical Reference Services Quarterly, Fall '98

Awarded "Books of the Year Award"
— American Journal of Nursing, 1997

"The layout of the book is particularly helpful as it provides easy access to reference material. A most useful addition to the vast amount of information about health insurance. The use of data from U.S. government agencies is most commendable. Useful in a library or learning center for healthcare professional students."
— Doody's Health Sciences Book Reviews, Nov '97

Health Reference Series Cumulative Index 1999

A Comprehensive Index to the Individual Volumes of the Health Reference Series, Including a Subject Index, Name Index, Organization Index, and Publication Index

Along with a Master List of Acronyms and Abbreviations

Edited by Edward J. Prucha, Anne Holmes, and Robert Rudnick. 990 pages. 2000. 0-7808-0382-5. $78.

"This volume will be most helpful in libraries that have a relatively complete collection of the Health Reference Series."
— American Reference Books Annual, 2001

"Essential for collections that hold any of the numerous Health Reference Series titles."
— Choice, Association of College and Research Libraries, Nov '00

Healthy Aging Sourcebook

Basic Consumer Health Information about Maintaining Health through the Aging Process, Including Advice on Nutrition, Exercise, and Sleep, Help in Making Decisions about Midlife Issues and Retirement, and Guidance Concerning Practical and Informed Choices in Health Consumerism

Along with Data Concerning the Theories of Aging, Different Experiences in Aging by Minority Groups, and Facts about Aging Now and Aging in the Future; and Featuring a Glossary, a Guide to Consumer Help, Additional Suggested Reading, and Practical Resource Directory

Edited by Jenifer Swanson. 536 pages. 1999. 0-7808-0390-6. $78.

"Recommended reference source."
— Booklist, American Library Association, Feb '00

SEE ALSO Physical & Mental Issues in Aging Sourcebook

Healthy Heart Sourcebook for Women

Basic Consumer Health Information about Cardiac Issues Specific to Women, Including Facts about Major Risk Factors and Prevention, Treatment and Control Strategies, and Important Dietary Issues

Along with a Special Section Regarding the Pros and Cons of Hormone Replacement Therapy and Its Impact on Heart Health, and Additional Help, Including Recipes, a Glossary, and a Directory of Resources

Edited by Dawn D. Matthews. 336 pages. 2000. 0-7808-0329-9. $48.

"A good reference source and recommended for all public, academic, medical, and hospital libraries."
— Medical Reference Services Quarterly, Summer '01

"Because of the lack of information specific to women on this topic, this book is recommended for public libraries and consumer libraries."
—*American Reference Books Annual, 2001*

"Contains very important information about coronary artery disease that all women should know. The information is current and presented in an easy-to-read format. The book will make a good addition to any library." —*American Medical Writers Association Journal, Summer '00*

"Important, basic reference."
—*Reviewer's Bookwatch, Jul '00*

SEE ALSO *Cardiovascular Diseases & Disorders Sourcebook, 1st Edition, Heart Diseases & Disorders Sourcebook, 2nd Edition, Women's Health Concerns Sourcebook*

■

Heart Diseases & Disorders Sourcebook, 2nd Edition

Basic Consumer Health Information about Heart Attacks, Angina, Rhythm Disorders, Heart Failure, Valve Disease, Congenital Heart Disorders, and More, Including Descriptions of Surgical Procedures and Other Interventions, Medications, Cardiac Rehabilitation, Risk Identification, and Prevention Tips

Along with Statistical Data, Reports on Current Research Initiatives, a Glossary of Cardiovascular Terms, and Resource Directory

Edited by Karen Bellenir. 612 pages. 2000. 0-7808-0238-1. $78.

"This work stands out as an imminently accessible resource for the general public. It is recommended for the reference and circulating shelves of school, public, and academic libraries."
—*American Reference Books Annual, 2001*

"Recommended reference source."
—*Booklist, American Library Association, Dec '00*

"Provides comprehensive coverage of matters related to the heart. This title is recommended for health sciences and public libraries with consumer health collections."
—*E-Streams, Oct '00*

SEE ALSO *Cardiovascular Diseases & Disorders Sourcebook, 1st Edition, Healthy Heart Sourcebook for Women*

■

Immune System Disorders Sourcebook

Basic Information about Lupus, Multiple Sclerosis, Guillain-Barré Syndrome, Chronic Granulomatous Disease, and More

Along with Statistical and Demographic Data and Reports on Current Research Initiatives

Edited by Allan R. Cook. 608 pages. 1997. 0-7808-0209-8. $78.

Infant & Toddler Health Sourcebook

Basic Consumer Health Information about the Physical and Mental Development of Newborns, Infants, and Toddlers, Including Neonatal Concerns, Nutrition Recommendations, Immunization Schedules, Common Pediatric Disorders, Assessments and Milestones, Safety Tips, and Advice for Parents and Other Caregivers

Along with a Glossary of Terms and Resource Listings for Additional Help

Edited by Jenifer Swanson. 585 pages. 2000. 0-7808-0246-2. $78.

"As a reference for the general public, this would be useful in any library." —*E-Streams, May '01*

"Recommended reference source."
—*Booklist, American Library Association, Feb '01*

"This is a good source for general use."
—*American Reference Books Annual, 2001*

■

Kidney & Urinary Tract Diseases & Disorders Sourcebook

Basic Information about Kidney Stones, Urinary Incontinence, Bladder Disease, End Stage Renal Disease, Dialysis, and More

Along with Statistical and Demographic Data and Reports on Current Research Initiatives

Edited by Linda M. Ross. 602 pages. 1997. 0-7808-0079-6. $78.

■

Learning Disabilities Sourcebook

Basic Information about Disorders Such as Dyslexia, Visual and Auditory Processing Deficits, Attention Deficit/Hyperactivity Disorder, and Autism

Along with Statistical and Demographic Data, Reports on Current Research Initiatives, an Explanation of the Assessment Process, and a Special Section for Adults with Learning Disabilities

Edited by Linda M. Shin. 579 pages. 1998. 0-7808-0210-1. $78.

Named "Outstanding Reference Book of 1999."
—*New York Public Library, Feb 2000*

"An excellent candidate for inclusion in a public library reference section. It's a great source of information. Teachers will also find the book useful. Definitely worth reading."
—*Journal of Adolescent & Adult Literacy, Feb 2000*

"Readable . . . provides a solid base of information regarding successful techniques used with individuals who have learning disabilities, as well as practical suggestions for educators and family members. Clear language, concise descriptions, and pertinent information for contacting multiple resources add to the strength of this book as a useful tool." — *Choice, Association of College and Research Libraries, Feb '99*

"Recommended reference source."
— *Booklist, American Library Association, Sep '98*

"This is a useful resource for libraries and for those who don't have the time to identify and locate the individual publications."
— *Disability Resources Monthly, Sep '98*

■

Liver Disorders Sourcebook

Basic Consumer Health Information about the Liver and How It Works; Liver Diseases, Including Cancer, Cirrhosis, Hepatitis, and Toxic and Drug Related Diseases; Tips for Maintaining a Healthy Liver; Laboratory Tests, Radiology Tests, and Facts about Liver Transplantation

Along with a Section on Support Groups, a Glossary, and Resource Listings

Edited by Joyce Brennfleck Shannon. 591 pages. 2000. 0-7808-0383-3. $78.

"A valuable resource."
— *American Reference Books Annual, 2001*

"This title is recommended for health sciences and public libraries with consumer health collections."
— *E-Streams, Oct '00*

"Recommended reference source."
— *Booklist, American Library Association, Jun '00*

■

Medical Tests Sourcebook

Basic Consumer Health Information about Medical Tests, Including Periodic Health Exams, General Screening Tests, Tests You Can Do at Home, Findings of the U.S. Preventive Services Task Force, X-ray and Radiology Tests, Electrical Tests, Tests of Blood and Other Body Fluids and Tissues, Scope Tests, Lung Tests, Genetic Tests, Pregnancy Tests, Newborn Screening Tests, Sexually Transmitted Disease Tests, and Computer Aided Diagnoses

Along with a Section on Paying for Medical Tests, a Glossary, and Resource Listings

Edited by Joyce Brennfleck Shannon. 691 pages. 1999. 0-7808-0243-8. $78.

"A valuable reference guide."
— *American Reference Books Annual, 2000*

"Recommended for hospital and health sciences libraries with consumer health collections."
— *E-Streams, Mar '00*

"This is an overall excellent reference with a wealth of general knowledge that may aid those who are reluctant to get vital tests performed."
— *Today's Librarian, Jan 2000*

Men's Health Concerns Sourcebook

Basic Information about Health Issues That Affect Men, Featuring Facts about the Top Causes of Death in Men, Including Heart Disease, Stroke, Cancers, Prostate Disorders, Chronic Obstructive Pulmonary Disease, Pneumonia and Influenza, Human Immunodeficiency Virus and Acquired Immune Deficiency Syndrome, Diabetes Mellitus, Stress, Suicide, Accidents and Homicides; and Facts about Common Concerns for Men, Including Impotence, Contraception, Circumcision, Sleep Disorders, Snoring, Hair Loss, Diet, Nutrition, Exercise, Kidney and Urological Disorders, and Backaches

Edited by Allan R. Cook. 738 pages. 1998. 0-7808-0212-8. $78.

"This comprehensive resource and the series are highly recommended."
— *American Reference Books Annual, 2000*

"Recommended reference source."
— *Booklist, American Library Association, Dec '98*

■

Mental Health Disorders Sourcebook, 1st Edition

Basic Information about Schizophrenia, Depression, Bipolar Disorder, Panic Disorder, Obsessive-Compulsive Disorder, Phobias and Other Anxiety Disorders, Paranoia and Other Personality Disorders, Eating Disorders, and Sleep Disorders

Along with Information about Treatment and Therapies

Edited by Karen Bellenir. 548 pages. 1995. 0-7808-0040-0. $78.

"This is an excellent new book . . . written in easy-to-understand language."
— *Booklist Health Sciences Supplement, American Library Association, Oct '97*

". . . useful for public and academic libraries and consumer health collections."
— *Medical Reference Services Quarterly, Spring '97*

"The great strengths of the book are its readability and its inclusion of places to find more information. Especially recommended." — *Reference Quarterly, American Library Association, Winter '96*

". . . a good resource for a consumer health library."
— *Bulletin of the Medical Library Association, Oct '96*

"The information is data-based and couched in brief, concise language that avoids jargon. . . . a useful reference source." — *Readings, Sep '96*

"The text is well organized and adequately written for its target audience." — *Choice, Association of College and Research Libraries, Jun '96*

". . . provides information on a wide range of mental disorders, presented in nontechnical language."
— *Exceptional Child Education Resources, Spring '96*

"Recommended for public and academic libraries."
— *Reference Book Review, 1996*

Mental Health Disorders Sourcebook, 2nd Edition

Basic Consumer Health Information about Anxiety Disorders, Depression and Other Mood Disorders, Eating Disorders, Personality Disorders, Schizophrenia, and More, Including Disease Descriptions, Treatment Options, and Reports on Current Research Initiatives

Along with Statistical Data, Tips for Maintaining Mental Health, a Glossary, and Directory of Sources for Additional Help and Information

Edited by Karen Bellenir. 605 pages. 2000. 0-7808-0240-3. $78.

"Well organized and well written."
—*American Reference Books Annual, 2001*

"Recommended reference source."
—*Booklist, American Library Association, Jun '00*

■

Mental Retardation Sourcebook

Basic Consumer Health Information about Mental Retardation and Its Causes, Including Down Syndrome, Fetal Alcohol Syndrome, Fragile X Syndrome, Genetic Conditions, Injury, and Environmental Sources

Along with Preventive Strategies, Parenting Issues, Educational Implications, Health Care Needs, Employment and Economic Matters, Legal Issues, a Glossary, and a Resource Listing for Additional Help and Information

Edited by Joyce Brennfleck Shannon. 642 pages. 2000. 0-7808-0377-9. $78.

"Public libraries will find the book useful for reference and as a beginning research point for students, parents, and caregivers."
—*American Reference Books Annual, 2001*

"The strength of this work is that it compiles many basic fact sheets and addresses for further information in one volume. It is intended and suitable for the general public. The sourcebook is relevant to any collection providing health information to the general public."
—*E-Streams, Nov '00*

"From preventing retardation to parenting and family challenges, this covers health, social and legal issues and will prove an invaluable overview."
—*Reviewer's Bookwatch, Jul '00*

■

Obesity Sourcebook

Basic Consumer Health Information about Diseases and Other Problems Associated with Obesity, and Including Facts about Risk Factors, Prevention Issues, and Management Approaches

Along with Statistical and Demographic Data, Information about Special Populations, Research Updates, a Glossary, and Source Listings for Further Help and Information

Edited by Wilma Caldwell and Chad T. Kimball. 376 pages. 2001. 0-7808-0333-7. $48.

"Recommended pick both for specialty health library collections and any general consumer health reference collection." — *The Bookwatch, Apr '01*

"Recommended reference source."
—*Booklist, American Library Association, Apr '01*

■

Ophthalmic Disorders Sourcebook

Basic Information about Glaucoma, Cataracts, Macular Degeneration, Strabismus, Refractive Disorders, and More

Along with Statistical and Demographic Data and Reports on Current Research Initiatives

Edited by Linda M. Ross. 631 pages. 1996. 0-7808-0081-8. $78.

■

Oral Health Sourcebook

Basic Information about Diseases and Conditions Affecting Oral Health, Including Cavities, Gum Disease, Dry Mouth, Oral Cancers, Fever Blisters, Canker Sores, Oral Thrush, Bad Breath, Temporomandibular Disorders, and other Craniofacial Syndromes

Along with Statistical Data on the Oral Health of Americans, Oral Hygiene, Emergency First Aid, Information on Treatment Procedures and Methods of Replacing Lost Teeth

Edited by Allan R. Cook. 558 pages. 1997. 0-7808-0082-6. $78.

"Unique source which will fill a gap in dental sources for patients and the lay public. A valuable reference tool even in a library with thousands of books on dentistry. Comprehensive, clear, inexpensive, and easy to read and use. It fills an enormous gap in the health care literature." — *Reference and User Services Quarterly, American Library Association, Summer '98*

"Recommended reference source."
— *Booklist, American Library Association, Dec '97*

■

Osteoporosis Sourcebook

Basic Consumer Health Information about Primary and Secondary Osteoporosis and Juvenile Osteoporosis and Related Conditions, Including Fibrous Dysplasia, Gaucher Disease, Hyperthyroidism, Hypophosphatasia, Myeloma, Osteopetrosis, Osteogenesis Imperfecta, and Paget's Disease

Along with Information about Risk Factors, Treatments, Traditional and Non-Traditional Pain Management, a Glossary of Related Terms, and a Directory of Resources

Edited by Allan R. Cook. 584 pages. 2001. 0-7808-0239-X. $78.

SEE ALSO *Women's Health Concerns Sourcebook*

Pain Sourcebook

Basic Information about Specific Forms of Acute and Chronic Pain, Including Headaches, Back Pain, Muscular Pain, Neuralgia, Surgical Pain, and Cancer Pain

Along with Pain Relief Options Such as Analgesics, Narcotics, Nerve Blocks, Transcutaneous Nerve Stimulation, and Alternative Forms of Pain Control, Including Biofeedback, Imaging, Behavior Modification, and Relaxation Techniques

Edited by Allan R. Cook. 667 pages. 1997. 0-7808-0213-6. $78.

"The text is readable, easily understood, and well indexed. This excellent volume belongs in all patient education libraries, consumer health sections of public libraries, and many personal collections."
— *American Reference Books Annual, 1999*

"A beneficial reference." — *Booklist Health Sciences Supplement, American Library Association, Oct '98*

"The information is basic in terms of scholarship and is appropriate for general readers. Written in journalistic style ... intended for non-professionals. Quite thorough in its coverage of different pain conditions and summarizes the latest clinical information regarding pain treatment." — *Choice, Association of College and Research Libraries, Jun '98*

"Recommended reference source."
— *Booklist, American Library Association, Mar '98*

Pediatric Cancer Sourcebook

Basic Consumer Health Information about Leukemias, Brain Tumors, Sarcomas, Lymphomas, and Other Cancers in Infants, Children, and Adolescents, Including Descriptions of Cancers, Treatments, and Coping Strategies

Along with Suggestions for Parents, Caregivers, and Concerned Relatives, a Glossary of Cancer Terms, and Resource Listings

Edited by Edward J. Prucha. 587 pages. 1999. 0-7808-0245-4. $78.

"A valuable addition to all libraries specializing in health services and many public libraries."
— *American Reference Books Annual, 2000*

"Recommended reference source."
— *Booklist, American Library Association, Feb '00*

"An excellent source of information. Recommended for public, hospital, and health science libraries with consumer health collections." — *E-Streams, Jun '00*

Physical & Mental Issues in Aging Sourcebook

Basic Consumer Health Information on Physical and Mental Disorders Associated with the Aging Process, Including Concerns about Cardiovascular Disease, Pulmonary Disease, Oral Health, Digestive Disorders,

Musculoskeletal and Skin Disorders, Metabolic Changes, Sexual and Reproductive Issues, and Changes in Vision, Hearing, and Other Senses

Along with Data about Longevity and Causes of Death, Information on Acute and Chronic Pain, Descriptions of Mental Concerns, a Glossary of Terms, and Resource Listings for Additional Help

Edited by Jenifer Swanson. 660 pages. 1999. 0-7808-0233-0. $78.

"Recommended for public libraries."
— *American Reference Books Annual, 2000*

"This is a treasure of health information for the layperson." — *Choice Health Sciences Supplement, Association of College & Research Libraries, May 2000*

"Recommended reference source."
— *Booklist, American Library Association, Oct '99*

SEE ALSO *Healthy Aging Sourcebook*

Podiatry Sourcebook

Basic Consumer Health Information about Foot Conditions, Diseases, and Injuries, Including Bunions, Corns, Calluses, Athlete's Foot, Plantar Warts, Hammertoes and Clawtoes, Clubfoot, Heel Pain, Gout, and More

Along with Facts about Foot Care, Disease Prevention, Foot Safety, Choosing a Foot Care Specialist, a Glossary of Terms, and Resource Listings for Additional Information

Edited by M. Lisa Weatherford. 380 pages. 2001. 0-7808-0215-2. $78.

Pregnancy & Birth Sourcebook

Basic Information about Planning for Pregnancy, Maternal Health, Fetal Growth and Development, Labor and Delivery, Postpartum and Perinatal Care, Pregnancy in Mothers with Special Concerns, and Disorders of Pregnancy, Including Genetic Counseling, Nutrition and Exercise, Obstetrical Tests, Pregnancy Discomfort, Multiple Births, Cesarean Sections, Medical Testing of Newborns, Breastfeeding, Gestational Diabetes, and Ectopic Pregnancy

Edited by Heather E. Aldred. 737 pages. 1997. 0-7808-0216-0. $78.

"A well-organized handbook. Recommended."
— *Choice, Association of College and Research Libraries, Apr '98*

"Recommended reference source."
— *Booklist, American Library Association, Mar '98*

"Recommended for public libraries."
— *American Reference Books Annual, 1998*

SEE ALSO *Congenital Disorders Sourcebook, Family Planning Sourcebook*

Prostate Cancer Sourcebook

Basic Consumer Health Information about Prostate Cancer, Including Information about the Associated Risk Factors, Detection, Diagnosis, and Treatment of Prostate Cancer

Along with Information on Non-Malignant Prostate Conditions, and Featuring a Section Listing Support and Treatment Centers and a Glossary of Related Terms

Edited by Dawn D. Matthews. 358 pages. 2001. 0-7808-0324-8. $78.

■

Public Health Sourcebook

Basic Information about Government Health Agencies, Including National Health Statistics and Trends, Healthy People 2000 Program Goals and Objectives, the Centers for Disease Control and Prevention, the Food and Drug Administration, and the National Institutes of Health

Along with Full Contact Information for Each Agency

Edited by Wendy Wilcox. 698 pages. 1998. 0-7808-0220-9. $78.

"Recommended reference source."
— Booklist, American Library Association, Sep '98

"This consumer guide provides welcome assistance in navigating the maze of federal health agencies and their data on public health concerns."
— SciTech Book News, Sep '98

■

Reconstructive & Cosmetic Surgery Sourcebook

Basic Consumer Health Information on Cosmetic and Reconstructive Plastic Surgery, Including Statistical Information about Different Surgical Procedures, Things to Consider Prior to Surgery, Plastic Surgery Techniques and Tools, Emotional and Psychological Considerations, and Procedure-Specific Information

Along with a Glossary of Terms and a Listing of Resources for Additional Help and Information

Edited by M. Lisa Weatherford. 374 pages. 2001. 0-7808-0214-4. $48.

■

Rehabilitation Sourcebook

Basic Consumer Health Information about Rehabilitation for People Recovering from Heart Surgery, Spinal Cord Injury, Stroke, Orthopedic Impairments, Amputation, Pulmonary Impairments, Traumatic Injury, and More, Including Physical Therapy, Occupational Therapy, Speech/ Language Therapy, Massage Therapy, Dance Therapy, Art Therapy, and Recreational Therapy

Along with Information on Assistive and Adaptive Devices, a Glossary, and Resources for Additional Help and Information

Edited by Dawn D. Matthews. 531 pages. 1999. 0-7808-0236-5. $78.

"This is an excellent resource for public library reference and health collections."
— American Reference Books Annual, 2001

"Recommended reference source."
— Booklist, American Library Association, May '00

■

Respiratory Diseases & Disorders Sourcebook

Basic Information about Respiratory Diseases and Disorders, Including Asthma, Cystic Fibrosis, Pneumonia, the Common Cold, Influenza, and Others, Featuring Facts about the Respiratory System, Statistical and Demographic Data, Treatments, Self-Help Management Suggestions, and Current Research Initiatives

Edited by Allan R. Cook and Peter D. Dresser. 771 pages. 1995. 0-7808-0037-0. $78.

"Designed for the layperson and for patients and their families coping with respiratory illness. . . . an extensive array of information on diagnosis, treatment, management, and prevention of respiratory illnesses for the general reader." — Choice, Association of College and Research Libraries, Jun '96

"A highly recommended text for all collections. It is a comforting reminder of the power of knowledge that good books carry between their covers."
— Academic Library Book Review, Spring '96

"A comprehensive collection of authoritative information presented in a nontechnical, humanitarian style for patients, families, and caregivers."
— Association of Operating Room Nurses, Sep/Oct '95

■

Sexually Transmitted Diseases Sourcebook, 1st Edition

Basic Information about Herpes, Chlamydia, Gonorrhea, Hepatitis, Nongonoccocal Urethritis, Pelvic Inflammatory Disease, Syphilis, AIDS, and More

Along with Current Data on Treatments and Preventions

Edited by Linda M. Ross. 550 pages. 1997. 0-7808-0217-9. $78.

Sexually Transmitted Diseases Sourcebook, 2nd Edition

Basic Consumer Health Information about Sexually Transmitted Diseases, Including Information on the Diagnosis and Treatment of Chlamydia, Gonorrhea, Hepatitis, Herpes, HIV, Mononucleosis, Syphilis, and Others

Along with Information on Prevention, Such as Condom Use, Vaccines, and STD Education; And Featuring a Section on Issues Related to Youth and Adolescents, a Glossary, and Resources for Additional Help and Information

Edited by Dawn D. Matthews. 538 pages. 2001. 0-7808-0249-7. $78.

"Recommended pick both for specialty health library collections and any general consumer health reference collection." — *The Bookwatch, Apr '01*

"Recommended reference source."
— *Booklist, American Library Association, Apr '01*

■

Skin Disorders Sourcebook

Basic Information about Common Skin and Scalp Conditions Caused by Aging, Allergies, Immune Reactions, Sun Exposure, Infectious Organisms, Parasites, Cosmetics, and Skin Traumas, Including Abrasions, Cuts, and Pressure Sores

Along with Information on Prevention and Treatment

Edited by Allan R. Cook. 647 pages. 1997. 0-7808-0080-X. $78.

". . . comprehensive, easily read reference book."
— *Doody's Health Sciences Book Reviews, Oct '97*

SEE ALSO Burns Sourcebook

■

Sleep Disorders Sourcebook

Basic Consumer Health Information about Sleep and Its Disorders, Including Insomnia, Sleepwalking, Sleep Apnea, Restless Leg Syndrome, and Narcolepsy

Along with Data about Shiftwork and Its Effects, Information on the Societal Costs of Sleep Deprivation, Descriptions of Treatment Options, a Glossary of Terms, and Resource Listings for Additional Help

Edited by Jenifer Swanson. 439 pages. 1998. 0-7808-0234-9. $78.

"This text will complement any home or medical library. It is user-friendly and ideal for the adult reader."
— *American Reference Books Annual, 2000*

"Recommended reference source."
— *Booklist, American Library Association, Feb '99*

"A useful resource that provides accurate, relevant, and accessible information on sleep to the general public. Health care providers who deal with sleep disorders patients may also find it helpful in being prepared to answer some of the questions patients ask."
— *Respiratory Care, Jul '99*

Sports Injuries Sourcebook

Basic Consumer Health Information about Common Sports Injuries, Prevention of Injury in Specific Sports, Tips for Training, and Rehabilitation from Injury

Along with Information about Special Concerns for Children, Young Girls in Athletic Training Programs, Senior Athletes, and Women Athletes, and a Directory of Resources for Further Help and Information

Edited by Heather E. Aldred. 624 pages. 1999. 0-7808-0218-7. $78.

"Public libraries and undergraduate academic libraries will find this book useful for its nontechnical language." — *American Reference Books Annual, 2000*

"While this easy-to-read book is recommended for all libraries, it should prove to be especially useful for public, high school, and academic libraries; certainly it should be on the bookshelf of every school gymnasium." — *E-Streams, Mar '00*

■

Substance Abuse Sourcebook

Basic Health-Related Information about the Abuse of Legal and Illegal Substances Such as Alcohol, Tobacco, Prescription Drugs, Marijuana, Cocaine, and Heroin; and Including Facts about Substance Abuse Prevention Strategies, Intervention Methods, Treatment and Recovery Programs, and a Section Addressing the Special Problems Related to Substance Abuse during Pregnancy

Edited by Karen Bellenir. 573 pages. 1996. 0-7808-0038-9. $78.

"A valuable addition to any health reference section. Highly recommended."
— *The Book Report, Mar/Apr '97*

". . . a comprehensive collection of substance abuse information that's both highly readable and compact. Families and caregivers of substance abusers will find the information enlightening and helpful, while teachers, social workers and journalists should benefit from the concise format. Recommended."
— *Drug Abuse Update, Winter '96/'97*

SEE ALSO Alcoholism Sourcebook, Drug Abuse Sourcebook

■

Transplantation Sourcebook

Basic Consumer Health Information about Organ and Tissue Transplantation, Including Physical and Financial Preparations, Procedures and Issues Relating to Specific Solid Organ and Tissue Transplants, Rehabilitation, Pediatric Transplant Information, the Future of Transplantation, and Organ and Tissue Donation

Along with a Glossary and Listings of Additional Resources

Edited by Joyce Brennfleck Shannon. 600 pages. 2001. 0-7808-0322-1. $78.

Traveler's Health Sourcebook

Basic Consumer Health Information for Travelers, Including Physical and Medical Preparations, Transportation Health and Safety, Essential Information about Food and Water, Sun Exposure, Insect and Snake Bites, Camping and Wilderness Medicine, and Travel with Physical or Medical Disabilities

Along with International Travel Tips, Vaccination Recommendations, Geographical Health Issues, Disease Risks, a Glossary, and a Listing of Additional Resources

Edited by Joyce Brennfleck Shannon. 613 pages. 2000. 0-7808-0384-1. $78.

"Recommended reference source."
— *Booklist, American Library Association, Feb '01*

"This book is recommended for any public library, any travel collection, and especially any collection for the physically disabled."
— *American Reference Books Annual, 2001*

■

Women's Health Concerns Sourcebook

Basic Information about Health Issues That Affect Women, Featuring Facts about Menstruation and Other Gynecological Concerns, Including Endometriosis, Fibroids, Menopause, and Vaginitis; Reproductive Concerns, Including Birth Control, Infertility, and Abortion; and Facts about Additional Physical, Emotional, and Mental Health Concerns Prevalent among Women Such as Osteoporosis, Urinary Tract Disorders, Eating Disorders, and Depression

Along with Tips for Maintaining a Healthy Lifestyle

Edited by Heather E. Aldred. 567 pages. 1997. 0-7808-0219-5. $78.

"Handy compilation. There is an impressive range of diseases, devices, disorders, procedures, and other physical and emotional issues covered . . . well organized, illustrated, and indexed." — *Choice, Association of College and Research Libraries, Jan '98*

SEE ALSO *Breast Cancer Sourcebook, Cancer Sourcebook for Women, 1st and 2nd Editions, Healthy Heart Sourcebook for Women, Osteoporosis Sourcebook*

Workplace Health & Safety Sourcebook

Basic Consumer Health Information about Workplace Health and Safety, Including the Effect of Workplace Hazards on the Lungs, Skin, Heart, Ears, Eyes, Brain, Reproductive Organs, Musculoskeletal System, and Other Organs and Body Parts

Along with Information about Occupational Cancer, Personal Protective Equipment, Toxic and Hazardous Chemicals, Child Labor, Stress, and Workplace Violence

Edited by Chad T. Kimball. 626 pages. 2000. 0-7808-0231-4. $78.

"Provides helpful information for primary care physicians and other caregivers interested in occupational medicine. . . . General readers; professionals."
— *Choice, Association of College and Research Libraries, May '01*

"Recommended reference source."
— *Booklist, American Library Association, Feb '01*

"Highly recommended." — *The Bookwatch, Jan '01*

■

Worldwide Health Sourcebook

Basic Information about Global Health Issues, Including Malnutrition, Reproductive Health, Disease Dispersion and Prevention, Emerging Diseases, Risky Health Behaviors, and the Leading Causes of Death

Along with Global Health Concerns for Children, Women, and the Elderly, Mental Health Issues, Research and Technology Advancements, and Economic, Environmental, and Political Health Implications, a Glossary, and a Resource Listing for Additional Help and Information

Edited by Joyce Brennfleck Shannon. 614 pages. 2001. 0-7808-0330-2. $78.

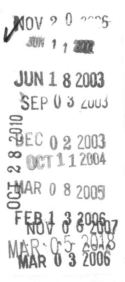

380